A. VOGEL · SWISS NATURE DOCTOR

D0925525

A. VOGEL

SWISS NATURE DOCTOR

AN ENCYCLOPEDIC COLLECTION OF HELPFUL HINTS GATHERED FROM THE SWISS FOLKLORE OF HEALING

1980 · Edition A. Vogel · CH-9053 Teufen/Switzerland

44th Edition
Third Revised and Enlarged English Edition

Over 1.000.000 Books
in eleven languages

Copyright 1952, 1960, 1980
by Edition A. Vogel, Teufen AR (Switzerland)
Color photograph on front cover: Ruth Vogel

Printed by Druckerei und Verlagsanstalt Konstanz GmbH
D-7750 Konstanz (Germany)

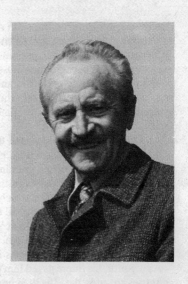

Dr. h.c. Vogel, almost eighty years old, is a living monument to good health. In addition to enjoying, to the full, physical and mental activities, he is always busy about the work he loves so much. Rising early in the morning, before dawn he spends his first few hours answering his mail. Besides writing a monthly health magazine he finds time to supervise the six large herb and fruit gardens that are dotted around Switzerland, in the lush valleys and high in the Engadine mountains. He is in great demand as a speaker and is well known on the lecture circuit where he speaks before clinics, medical groups, and many organizations dedicated to better health all over the world. In addition to his native land he appears before various groups in Germany, France, Great Britain, the Low Countries, Sweden and Norway, Australia, South Africa and many parts of the United States as well as in Central and South America. He is particularly known as a champion of "good health through good nourishment". His treatment of the ill and ailing through naturopathy, a system of treatment of disease emphasizing assistance to nature and including the use of natural plant extracts and tinctures, has established him as an expert nature doctor.

His extensive background and training sets him apart as a peer among his contemporaries and Dr. Vogel commands the respect and confidence of all who know him for his mature grasp and analysis of human ailments and how to cope with them.

At a very early age he learned to be on familiar terms with plants and animals. He is a third generation herbalist, following in the footsteps of his grandmother and his father, who themselves, were well known in the field of naturopathy. His close association with them helped him immeasurably in becoming well acquainted with all the middle European plants and herbs. Further knowledge acquired in school helped him lay a solid foundation for his eminent career, but he has always maintained that Nature itself was his favorite university.

As a youth, his interests led him to many strange and foreign countries to study the effects of nutrition, mode of life and the health of primitive people. His experiences in Africa, Asia, the Americas (North, Central and South), the Orient and the Middle East proved to him that greater success can be achieved by Nature with skillful assistance and direction than by all the physical and chemical arts of man.

For many years Dr. Vogel operated a clinic in Switzerland serving patients from many different countries and he has, by reason of his wide experience, become convinced of the superiority and success of combatting ailments through natural, biological methods in conjunction with carefully chosen diets. Although in his twilight years, his stamina and vigor command attention wherever he goes. You will enjoy meeting him through these pages.

PREFACE

During my travels in Great Britain, Africa, Canada and the U.S.A. friends have constantly asked me to publish a revised and enlarged English edition similar to the latest German edition of "Der Kleine Doktor". Since the second edition in English has been out of print for some time now, they have expressed a need and desire for a newer book with additional information. Letters, too, from all over the world where more than 50,000 of the later German edition have been distributed, have encouraged me to bring out a new and greatly enlarged edition in the English language.

Thus, "Der Kleine Doktor" is once again available to English speaking people all over the world. Those who became acquainted with the earlier editions as well as those who have never had the opportunity, will, I believe, value the well-proven natural healing methods suggested in this latest book and, I am sure, will make good use of it.

"The Nature Doctor" does not contain any revolutionary scientific theories. It is based upon practical knowledge gained through a period of 55 years and combined with age-old healing methods that have stood the test of time and are still widely used by the peasant folk of the Swiss mountains and valleys.

It does not, nor indeed could it, attempt to replace your family doctor. It will, however, very often help you to help yourself should an emergency arise and no professional or outside help is available. It will also teach you how to insure your general well-being by directing you through channels that lead to a healthy approach to good health in conformity with the laws of nature. This book may well be of interest to the scientist and doctor, too, for it shows how very little known remedies and curative measures have aided and alleviated various ailments and health problems, serious and minor, in the towns, country and mountain districts of Switzerland.

It is hoped that "The Nature Doctor" will be a friend indeed wherever it goes; that it will help you to return to nature's ways! And may it be a guide to the natural way of life, bringing with it physical health, mental stability and spiritual awareness! Both a French and Dutch translation have been published to satisfy the needs of the friends in those countries and shortly a new Spanish translation may be made available for the Spanish friends who love good health.

Teufen (Switzerland), July 1980

The Author

Dr. h.c. A. Vogel with Family

A DOCTOR IN YOUR HOUSE

Two things are certain. One is that I do not know where you live, whether on the side of a mountain or in a valley; in a pretty little village or an average size town; in one of the many large cities of the earth, contaminated by air pollution, or in one of the many suburbs where fumes from automobile traffic and factories choke out the real joy of country life; perhaps you live closer to nature on a large or small farm far from the cramped quarters of noisy urban life or perhaps you may spend many months out of the year on a ship earning your living as a fisherman. Or by chance you may live in the Arctic or the tropics in either a mansion or a plain grass hut. It is highly improbable that I could guess correctly where you really live.

Nevertheless, the second thing that is certain is, that whoever you may be, "butcher, baker or candlestick maker" and no matter where you live, you can be sure "The Nature Doctor" will be constantly at your side and will be a source of ready assistance in your hour of need, at least, until you can call your other doctor who may be able to give you further aid. Often, however, in an emergency the immediate help offered by this book may be sufficient to overcome your problem because proper remedies given in time, more often than not, result in successful treatments.

Thus, the purpose of "The Nature Doctor" is to awaken and kindle your interest in the many natural healing resources that are readily available in your immediate locality. This book is dedicated to the important task of demonstrating how simple and harmless remedies found in nature are often more effective than artificially created chemical drugs found in your local pharmacy that are manufactured to "cure" you but, additionally, may bring with the "cure" unpleasant and harmful side effects. Simply stated, self-administered first aid may prove to be the only aid you require, because many times a permanent improvement will be achieved if the correct remedy is used early enough to avoid complications.

You may feel that you and your family are assured of good health because "it runs in the family" and because illness is foreign to your way of life. That may be so. Certainly it often happens that day after day one goes about one's business and varied tasks without giving a second thought to the interruption of the even rhythm of life when, suddenly something happens, an unaccountable rash, a sudden fever, an ache, a pain, acute indigestion or some other inexplicable feeling occurs and the question of what to do immediately arises. At such a time you will be glad you have appropriate help from "The Nature Doctor" at hand.

What have you in your house or its surroundings that give you swift, sure and reliable help? Although you may have a large medicine chest, if the remedies in it are inadequate, to where will you turn? In an emergency you will find many little friends among the plants, those staunch helpers in times of distress, that will provide remedies and even preventative measures. If you live in the city it may be more difficult to find these plants but if you live in the country, the fields and forests offer abundant help. Plant aids found hidden in the woods, sprouting in fields and meadows, growing along the banks of rivers are an inexhaustible supply and "The Nature Doctor" could easily become a "real" doctor if it aspired to offer all the treasures which can be found in nature.

Welcome "The Nature Doctor" into your home. Read it carefully. By studying it you will become acquainted with many hitherto secret, yet easily accessible remedies which are only waiting to be discovered and put to good use by you. At first glance, the colorful collection of helpful hints from the Swiss folklore of healing may have a kaleidoscopic effect upon you and the multitude of suggestions may appear confusing but, a careful examination of the index at the back of the book will help you to find quickly the information you are seeking.

Welcome to our large family numbering hundreds of thousands of persons all over the earth who through "The Nature Doctor" have unlocked the secrets of nature and have benefited greatly by the use of natural remedies.

CONTENTS

PART I

SOME DOMESTIC EXPERIMENTS

A SELECTION FROM THE PLANT KINGDOM

WILD FRUITS

A SELECTION OF HOMEOPATHIC REMEDIES

SOME EXAMPLES FROM BIOCHEMISTRY

SEASONINGS

VARIOUS REMEDIES AND TREATMENTS

NUTRITIONAL QUESTIONS

MISCELLANEOUS

PART I

SOME DOMESTIC EXPERIMENTS

Although you may be skeptical of these simple home remedies, it will be to your advantage to give them a fair trial when the opportunity presents itself. The more successful you find these domestic experiments the more your confidence will increase and you will be encouraged to seek further advice from this book.

BURNS AND SCALDS

Burns from flame or fire and *scalds* from boiling water or hot oil need quick action. First immerse the affected part in cold water. If the burn is on a part of the body that cannot be readily immersed, wet a towel in cold water and continuously apply to the burn. Keep cooling until the pain abates. Then cover the burned part with any of the following items. Easiest of all to find in your grocery cabinet would be flour. Make a paste with flour and water and apply. If you happen to be out of flour, use olive oil, salad oil, honey, icing sugar (confectionary sugar). Sprinkle on generously over the burned part. A poultice made with Slippery Elm powder and water has been found to be effective as well as St. John's wort oil. Newer remedies have appeared in recent years, the use of which, many claim effective in the treatment of burns and scalds. Two most prominently mentioned are *Vitamin E* and *Wheat Germ oil.*

21

SUNBURN

A century-old remedy if the *sunburn* isn't too severe is the application of cider vinegar to the affected parts. It will sting but usually brings relief in a very short time. Wheat Germ oil also has a soothing effect and when liberally applied will soothe sufficiently to permit you to sleep. Much of the burning sensation will have disappeared upon awakening. Re-apply oil liberally if burn is still uncomfortable. Stay out of the sun for a day or two.

WOUNDS

Superficial scratches and small wounds which refuse to heal quickly can be simply dealt with by using *whey*. Whey is obtained by letting buttermilk clabber at room temperature in a cloth gauze suspended over a bowl. The liquid that drips from the buttermilk is called *whey*. Also the liquid left over after making butter from sweet cream is whey. This is a first class *antiseptic,* especially in concentrated form. Rinse the wound with whey and afterwards dust it with calcium powder and cover with soft curd which is simply fresh cottage cheese. Should whey be unavailable soak wheat kernels or bran until a paste is formed, using raw milk or water. Before wetting the wheat kernels mince or mash with mortar and pestle. Apply liberally, as this will cleanse the wound, and after two days of treatment dry the wound and apply calcium powder. Instead of curd, pulped cabbage leaves may be used. A variety of cabbage known as Savoy is best. They are wonderfully curative and have been known to miraculously heal when everything else has failed. If the wound is stubborn it is important to continue treatment with cabbage leaves poultice for weeks or even months. Alleviation will be experienced even in apparently hopeless cases and complete cure will be achieved if perseverance is pursued. The lowly cabbage is convincing evidence of nature's power.

EYE INFLAMMATION

If your eyes have become inflamed through continuous exposure to the reflection of the sun on water or snow, take the white of an egg, beat it lightly, spread it on a cloth and bandage this poultice over the eyes. The burning will subside and you will be able to sleep. When you awaken in the morning, it is very likely that the inflammation will have disappeared. If no egg is available, cottage cheese will once again come in very handy, producing the same effect. Even a piece of raw veal will produce good results. Also, you can turn to these well-proven remedies in case of sun-blindness which frequently occurs if your eyes are exposed to large expanses of snow and ice.

COLDS

A "streaming" cold, the symptoms of which are a bland lachrymation (tearing) and an excoriating (raw) nasal discharge always will be helped by *onions*; the Latin name is *Allium cepa* and this name is known by every Homeopath. To rid yourself of this type of cold is simple enough; just slice a fresh raw onion and immerse it in a glass of hot water. Do not let it remain for more than a second or two. Cool the water and sip it throughout the day. If the symptoms mentioned above correspond with your own, your cold will have soon left you. Many people have found it effective to cut an onion in half, place it on the night table beside the bed and breathe in the smell while sleeping. Another remedy is to place an onion poultice around the neck. The practice of sniffing up the nostrils either salt water, lemon juice or calcium powder has been found to have a beneficial effect in helping to terminate a cold and to dry up a constantly running nose.

CATARRH

The discomfort of an inflamed condition of the nose or throat which causes a discharge of mucus can be promptly reduced by using the buds of a fir, larch or any other conifer tree. In all seasons there are always plenty of buds on them, either open, sprouting or closed. Gather the buds and chew them thoroughly throughout the day, changing to fresh buds from time to time. You will be agreeably surprised to see the catarrh resulting from mucus and phlegm disappear within a few days. Before retiring at night sip a cup of hot tea made from camomile, coltsfoot or lemon balm. Dampen a cloth with camphor oil and wrap it around the neck. Cover with a woolen scarf and this will help to clear up any irritating cough.

HOARSENESS

Nearly everyone is familiar with the *Mountain Ash* also known as the *Rowanberry (Fructus sorbi)* tree belonging to the rose family with pinnate leaves, white flowers and red berries. There must be one in your neighborhood. The bright-red berries, either fresh or dried, will help you find your lost voice again. Chew them well so the juice can run down your throat and do its work. Failing Mountain Ash, you can always look for the *Pimpernell (Pimpinella saxifraga) plant,* a small scarlet, purple or white flower that closes at night, also called *Burnet.* It is a herbaceous perennial that grows in meadows and fields in a wild state. Steep the crushed root in a small amount of boiling water, strain and cool. Drink slowly a half a cup three or four times a day. Either of the two treatments will be found to be very effective. *Pimpernel plant* water is an excellent antidote for sour stomach.

CHILBLAINS AND COLD FEET

It is unlikely that you will be troubled with these unless your circulatory system needs attention. It is especially venous congestions that encourage the formation of *chilblains.* Hot, followed by cold foot baths will improve the circulation in the lower extremities and thus reduce the risk of continuing chilblains. Always begin by putting the foot in hot water first and then change over to the cold. Repeat this change from six to eight times. Time measurement is important. Keep your feet in the hot water for 2 to 3 minutes but in the cold water for only 2 to 3 seconds. Remember, it's 2–3 minutes in hot and 2–3 seconds in cold. Finish off with the cold then dry your feet thoroughly, rubbing with a towel vigorously. Rub into the skin St. Johns wort oil to which a little lemon or lanolin cream has been added. Persevere with this treatment and the circulation will soon be restored to normal again.

In the winter, an older but no less efficient method for the treatment of *chilblains*, is snow-walking, really running barefoot in the snow. If you live in a snow zone, try it and you will be surprised how much good it will do you. For a start, practice it for 10 seconds, gradually increasing to 2–3 minutes or even a little longer. It is important to be warmly dressed before going outside. After this exercise return to the house without drying your feet. Repeat several days in a row. If you are fortunate enough to have a garden, go out warmly clothed, take off your house slippers and start stamping your feet in the snow, then rub them well with snow and go back inside. After several treatments the chilblains will have disappeared. To avoid a relapse the next winter you will do well to go barefoot once in a while during the summer and fall months and take regularly Wild Thyme baths soaking your feet for about half an hour.

If you live in a southern climate use lemon juice rubbed well into the skin and let dry naturally without a towel. Rub with St. Johns wort oil or olive oil.

If you live anywhere near a cheese-making district or a dairy, you may be able to obtain either sweet or sour *whey*. This can be added to bath water. It is helpful not only in cases of chilblains but also when you suffer from moist skin eruption like ringworm infections, etc. Sour whey is always to be preferred to sweet because it acts more powerfully. These baths can be taken in winter as an alternative to hot and cold foot baths and snow stamping. The temperature of the bath should be kept at blood heat (98.6° F. – 37° C) and bathe for at least half an hour. Afterwards, rub feet with fresh cut lemon and apply pulped cabbage leaves as a poultice. This will benefit your circulation and dissipate the chilblains.

TIRED FEET AND LEGS

Should you be troubled with this you will find potato or vegetable water a great help. Bathe the feet in the water and then wrap them in a cloth on which you have sprinkled hot *salt* that has been heated in a pan. Repeat this procedure a few times and you will find that the tiredness will disappear. Wild Thyme or Hayflower can be added together with salt to the foot bath and this will help, too. Hot, burning feet also will be relieved by using the same procedure. Swollen feet, especially ankles, can be a sign of heart trouble but we shall consider this later.

HAEMORRHAGES AND "BLEEDERS"

If, amongst your friends or acquaintances, there is someone who constantly suffers from *nose bleeding* or one who is a *"bleeder"* apply ice or very cold water on the lower forehead just above the nose and also on the nape or back of the neck while the person is seated with the head tilted back. Do not try to stem the flow of blood by applying pressure on back of neck as this will stanch or stop the flow of blood to the head. Surprisingly, a piece of fresh raw chicken inserted in the nose will control the bleeding. If it is only a temporary disturbance it can be effectively dealt with by means of the little herb *Tormentil* or *Bloodwort*, applying a poultice made from the leaves and applied to the affected area.

CALCIUM DEFICIENCY

Sometime you will have occasion to advise a mother whose children have bad teeth and weak bones, children who suffer from calcium deficiency which prevents them from developing properly and makes them more likely to "catch" *colds* frequently. If the mother cannot afford to buy a good natural calcium preparation, you can tell her to make one up herself. Nettle can be found almost everywhere and egg or oyster shells can be obtained easily. Dry the nettles, then crush the shells, mix them both together and pulverise the mixture with pestle and mortar. A light green powder will result and the child should take one teaspoon three times daily. After a few months the teeth will become noticeably stronger, the bones will benefit also and colds and catarrhs will diminish in frequency and intensity.

PHLEBITIS (Inflammation of the veins)

For alleviation of acute inflammation of the veins you can do no better than to apply an alcohol compress. Be sure to add a few drops of tincture of *Arnica (Arnica montana), Yarrow (Achillea millefolium)* or *St. Johns wort oil (Hypericum perforatum).* As soon as inflammation has subsided a little, apply a poultice made from *potter's clay* and water followed in an hour or so by a poultice of cabbage leaves pulped. Eat sparingly, adhering to a vegetarian diet, drink plenty of fruit and vegetable juices, all of which will help to reduce the inflammation very quickly.

ABDOMINAL DISORDERS

Girls and women frequently suffer from venous congestions in the abdomen. Water treatment is excellent for this and if it is decided upon, a hip bath should be taken once or twice a week. For married women, this kind of treatment will not only make confinement easier, but benefit the baby as well and in addition prevent difficulties during menopause. The body will respond to such regular care and reward you by giving you far less trouble at these critical times than it would otherwise give.

RETENTION OF URINE (Difficulty in passing water)

Elderly men who find themselves unable to pass water during the night will likewise benefit from the water treatment. In their case, however, a herbal *steam bath* will be more effective. Camomile can be infused by pouring boiling water over the leaves and letting it steep. Pour into a large container while still hot and place a narrow board across the container so you can sit above the hot, rising steam which can be retained by covering yourself with a blanket. Your body will be heated up, urinary spasms will be released and the water once more will begin to flow. In this way you will relieve yourself and earn your doctor's appreciation who would, no doubt, dislike the idea of having to perform a catheterization in the middle of the night.

HIGH BLOOD PRESSURE AND ARTERIOSCLEROSIS

Although grandparents suffer from this combined malady, younger people also have been known to be affected by it. A change of diet is invariably necessary and instead of eggs, cheese, peas, beans and meat, *blood pressure* reducing buckwheat and unpolished rice should appear on the table. Buckwheat can be prepared in the same way as rice and a little enterprising imagination will enable you to serve them in such a variety of ways that monotony will be avoided. These dishes should be salt-free, but a vegetable extract which contains salt in biochemically balanced form can be used. Kitchen herbs will provide added piquancy and if these dishes are served in conjunction with artistically prepared raw salads, seasoned with oil and lemon or sour whey, even grandparents can be pursuaded to submit to new health ideas. Sharp seasonings should be avoided. Lightly steamed vegetables are permissible as long as they do not cause stomach gas. During the spring, *wild leek (Allium ursinum)* provides a beneficial raw salad or steamed vegetable. *Garlic* is one of its close relatives and used in the same way provides the same therapeutic benefits.

Mistletoe (Viscum Album), Hawthorn (Crataegus Oxy-acantha) and *Arnica (Arnica montana)* are further valuable helps, but they should be prescribed by a competent herbalist. Wild leek wine, however, is quite safe and can be easily prepared at home. Gather this herb on your walks through the country in the spring and extract the juice. To one pint of fresh juice add 5 fluid ounces of brandy. This will preserve the leek juice for a long time. Sip a small glass occasionally. If you follow all this advice you will most certainly achieve good results.

HEART TROUBLE

Carry dried *currants* and *raisins* with you and chew them slowly as you work. Your heart muscles will be grateful to you for this, and especially if you chew the tops of *rosemary* first thing in the morning before breakfast.

Relief from continuous heart pains can be obtained from the woody interior dividing walls of *walnuts*. Boil these for a few minutes and steep for about ten minutes with a lid covering. Drink this infusion to calm the heart and if you continue drinking it, the pains will gradually disappear.

More serious heart diseases cannot be cured by these simple, soothing remedies, although there are other natural medicines and therapeutic measures that will. These demand more understanding and will be dealt with later in greater detail.

HEARTBURN

This is a result of hyperacidity of the stomach and at times becomes so bad that the acid rises into the mouth. The lowly potato is recommended as a reliable help. All you need to do is to grate finely a medium size *potato*, fold the resulting pulp into a cheesecloth and press out the juice. Dilute with 2–3 times the amount of warm water and drink first thing in the morning, before lunch and at night before retiring. For best results, prepare fresh each time. Since one remedy may not work equally well for everyone, you might want to consider using other remedies. Some have found that a teaspoon of woodash in a cup of warm water is effective, or an infusion with the *woodash* in the same way you make a cup of tea, straining the solution through a fine sieve or cheesecloth. Another remedy is to crush *charcoal* (preferably from lime trees), but be careful not to use the commercial kind, mix the resulting powder with *oatflakes* and water and in this form it can be easily swallowed. Potter's clay dissolved in water also will neutralize *gastric acidity*. Raw milk will give temporary relief. Uncooked oatflakes, well masticated, are known to alleviate heartburn. The above remedies are much to be preferred to bicarbonate of soda or any of the over-the-counter chemical lozenges from the drug store. To regulate the secretion of gastric juice and cure acidity permanently, you will have to abstain from excessively flavored and spiced dishes. Also, cross off your list of foods white sugar and white flour products. If these applications fail to produce the desired effect, the heartburn may be caused from gall-bladder disfunction or even intestinal worms. In this case a different remedy will be required.

GASTRIC ULCERS

Raw potato and cabbage juice taken, if necessary, for several months will do more good than many of the expensive patent medicines. Take the juice of a small raw potato three times daily before meals and three tablespoons of raw cabbage juice after each meal. The cabbage juice can be added to soup after it has been taken from the stove; it must not be added while soup is boiling. Also, if you take woodash or charcoal (as directed under "heartburn") you may even expect a cure. Since gastric ulcers are usually triggered by anger and worries, one should exercise the art of positive thinking.

LIVER TROUBLE

If sweet and fatty dishes do not agree with you, you may assume that it is possible that your liver is malfunctioning. *Radishes* are excellent for the *liver* but must be taken in small quantities. A teaspoon of raw radish juice a day is the largest dose permissible. Raw *carrot* juice is almost a specific for the liver and obtained in the same way as the juice of *potatoes* will work wonders if taken for a few days to the exclusion of everything else. If you find it too time consuming to extract the juice from the carrots you can take them finely grated. You can add to the favorable effect of the carrots by adding to your diet bitter salads consisting of *dandelion* leaves, chicory and other bitter herbs. Sugar, or any sweet foods as well as all fatty foods, should be eliminated from your diet while undergoing this treatment and before long the liver will function in a normal manner again.

LIVER DIET

Follow these suggestions to avoid mistakes while you are dieting to overcome a liver problem:

Mornings: 1 glass of carrot juice, a slice of melba toast or crisp bread with very little butter, a tablespoon of wheat germ.

Midday: Vegetable soup, brown rice, or potatoes steamed in their jackets, chicory and raw carrot salad (or any other salad such as bitter endive). Other steamed vegetables may be added to the luncheon. All fried and sweet dishes as well as desserts must be avoided.

Vary the lunch menu as follows:

1st day: Brown rice, fennel root, mixed salad.

2nd day: Potatoes steamed in their skins with a little butter, cottage cheese, and mixed salad of your choice.

3rd day: Vegetable soup, rye or whole wheat bread sandwiches prepared with butter, yeast extract, garlic, onion and sliced tomatoes, salad of your choice. A cereal coffee with a little milk but no sugar can be served after the meal.

Evening: Oat, barley, or unpolished rice soup with a few added vegetables, lettuce, endive salad seasoned with lemon juice, sour whey or sour milk (never with vinegar). For the sake of variety, sandwiches and different salads may be served followed by cereal coffee. Just remember that FRUIT is taboo while the liver is out of order.

INFLAMMATION OF THE GALL BLADDER

A cold milk compress will eliminate the worst pain until you can get to a doctor. If the inflammation is severe, the milk compress should be renewed because it loses its soothing effect as soon as it reaches body temperature. Less severe inflammations will usually respond to this simple measure within a few hours.

DIGESTIVE UPSETS

Overeating or taking the wrong kind of foods can cause the pancreas to go on strike and the result will be intestinal cramps. A hot shower will help dispel the cramps, if you remain under it for 10–15 minutes until the skin is flushed. Follow up with a raw *onion* poultice, placed on stomach. If no shower is available, use a hot water bottle or an electric heating pad. A *cabbage* poultice can be used in place of the onion, whichever you have in the house. If you follow this procedure the fermentation intestinally will cease and the cramps will gradually vanish. To avoid attacks, take care not to overeat, to masticate your food well and to avoid those foods that disagree with you. If these simple applications do not help, see your doctor, since there is a possibility of a perforation of the stomach, a gall stone or an inflammation of the appendix.

DIABETES

If sugar is found in your blood it is because the cells in the pancreas known as islets of Langerhans do not produce sufficient insulin. Once more you can resort to hot showers as mentioned in "Digestive Upsets". Showers taken two or three times daily for sustained periods of time will stimulate the secretion of insulin. It would aid considerably if you can procure from a dairy sour *whey*. Drink at least two pints a day until your thirst abates and then gradually reduce the quantity to be taken. Plenty of *raw vegetables* should be eaten and be sure to eat generous amounts of onions with your salads and sandwiches. Bitter salads like *chicory, dandelion* and *endive* as well as tea made from the leaves of *walnut* trees, *bilberries* (similar to blueberries), french bean pods and *alfalfa* clover *(Medicago sativa)* are all curatives and will greatly help you. *Alfalfa sprouts* can be added to your salads. Regular open air exercise, walking, hiking, bicycling and deep breathing are absolutely essential, for without them, a complete regeneration is unlikely to take place. A word should also be said about the "technique of *eating*"; hurried eating is definitely harmful. If you are all "keyed up", excited, or tense or angered before a meal, sit down and relax until you have recovered your peace of mind. Then, and then only, sit down and eat your meal slowly, masticate your food thoroughly and be cautious about eating until you feel full. If you eat too much you will experience indigestion and it will prevent your utilizing your food properly. The more moderately you eat the more easily will your digestion work. Therefore, leave the table feeling like you could still eat more. Remember, in all cases where the pancreas does not function properly, the problem is the quantity you must digest rather than the quantity you eat. If you follow this program you will give your doctor a pleasant surprise when he tests your blood and your urine for sugar next time.

CONSTIPATION

Soaked *prunes*, taken the first thing in the morning and the last thing at night, will frequently remedy the problem of *constipation*. Young spring nettles boiled in milk have helped others. These should be taken upon rising in the morning. This simple measure also stops *migraine headaches* which are associated with bilious vomiting. The *nettles* are wonderful purifiers of the blood. The simplest remedy for constipation is the drinking of a glass of hot water first thing in the morning. Another successful remedy is fig paste which you can make yourself in the following manner: Take 3 ozs. of figs, 3 ozs. of *raisins*, ⅓ oz. powdered *senna* pods, 1–2 ozs. ground *flaxseed*. Mix all ingredients together, put through a mincer, shape into rolls and store in a cool place. Eat three times a day.

There also is a special soup for *intestinal sluggishness*. It consists of freshly ground whole-wheat, a small chopped onion, a crushed clove of garlic boiled in water. The soup should be eaten with crisp bread or bran. You can also add to the soup some chopped parsley and a spoonful of olive oil. This simple breakfast has cured many of their constipation, but for more stubborn cases, psyllium seeds or linseeds should be added. Alternatively, a special herb soup, the recipe of which will be given later, can be taken. Sometimes a change in diet alone will accomplish more regular bowel action. It is quite possible that constipation has its origin in some psychological state, a nervous weakness, fatigue or certain mental disturbances. Primarily, the nerves must be calmed to ensure sufficient sleep and relaxation. Exercise must be taken, especially by those who engage in sedentary occupations.

DIARRHEA

Grated apples are without a doubt one of the most palatable remedies for this problem. Infants are easily persuaded to take this treatment. Follow up by making an *oatmeal* gruel which helps stop diarrhea too. Older children can take the *oatflakes* raw. They should chew them thoroughly and should not be given anything else to eat for a few hours. However, there is a little plant that will put an end to this unpleasant trouble almost without exception. It is called *Tormentilla (Potentilla Tormentilla)*. The presence of tannic acid and other substances gives this plant antidiuretic properties. It is the same plant previously recommended for haemorrhages.

Other treatments for bad cases of diarrhea are herbal teas. For a child, start the treatment by giving nothing but herbal teas for 6, 12, or 24 hours depending upon the age of the child. The following herbs are effective: *Bilberry (Vaccinium myrtillus)* leaves, sage, *Iceland moss (Cetraria islandica), Silverweed (Potentilla anserine)*. White potters clay can be used also. Mix 1 teaspoon of clay in a wine glass of water. Poisons can find entrance into the intestinal tract, not only from the outside, but can actually have their origin inside through putrefaction or excessive fermentation of the wrong kind. Coffee charcoal will be found useful for combating this fermentation.

REDUCING (SLIMMING)

Have you lost your slim figure? If so, beware of the majority of advertised reducing cures. Some of them can cause irreparable damage to the body, as well as the mind. For example, do not eat 5 or 6 lemons a day for the sake of a shapely waist because your liver is sure to dislike this program and rebel. No matter what any faddist says, calories do count and you can never ignore the counting of them. A sensible reducing diet will serve you better. Leave all starchy foods alone and if you must have meat, choose a little veal. For effective reducing, the bulk of your meals should consist of a wide variety of salads. And don't forget steamed vegetables such as *leek, fennel, chicory, celery, asparagus* and *carrots*. Top off your diet with an abundance of *fruit* for breakfast and supper. You will find it very beneficial to set aside a "juice-day" on which you drink nothing but fruit and vegetable juices such as *carrot, apple,* and *grape juice,* not canned, but from the garden, freshly ripened. Never attempt to follow a drastic reducing diet like those that advertise that you will lose 10 pounds in three days. They are loaded with all kind of dangers and especially so if you lack nutritional knowledge. Above all, avoid fats and highly seasoned foods and rich desserts such as cake and ice cream. They should be on the prohibited list. Along with your sensible diet try a *hip-bath* with sea salt and herbs. Baths are quite harmless to the health and are very good for obesity because they stimulate the circulation. Use only sea salt for seasoning in the kitchen as it will stimulate the internal metabolism and, at the same time, will help to dispose of many ounces of superfluous fat. Don't forget that a successful diet must be accompanied by regular exercise, push-ups, walking, riding a bicycle, jogging, etc.

HEADACHES

Headaches of any sort that come again and again can be relieved by applying *onion* or *horseradish poultices* to the nape of the neck, the calves and soles of the feet. This has the effect of drawing the blood pressure from the head. Many an inflammation such as sinusitis, can be relieved in this manner and terminated.

In reality, most headaches are merely symptomatic of deeper-lying disturbances and for this reason it is futile or useless to take any kind of drugs, for they are unrelated to the cause of the trouble. Instead, try to analyze your problem; try to find out what factors or circumstances bring on these headaches. Could it be indigestion, constipation, eyestrain, worry, nervousness? If you can pinpoint the cause of frequently recurring headaches and try to avoid them, then you are on the way to solving your problem. This is the sensible approach to eliminate the cause and it is definitely more sensible than to resort to "pain-killing" pills which have no permanent curative effect and merely induce a false sense of security which tends to make one dependent upon them. Continued use of aspirins, barbiturates and quick-relieving medication can be very dangerous to your physical health and well-being and some of them will leave you depressed.

FACIAL NEURALGIA

Unbearable, cramp-like pains in the face have their origin in the facial nerves. The best and most effective remedy for them is a hot shower directed against the face or, failing that, a hot water compress; severe cases will need a hot, moist herbal pack. This can be made from *Bitterroot (Apocynum androsaemifolium), celery, Peppermint, Nettle (Urtica),* etc. steeped in water that has been boiled and poured over the herbs or put the herbs into a small bag (cloth) on which boiling water has been poured. Wring out the excess water and apply to the affected part as hot as you can stand it. Reheat and apply repeatedly. It may require a half hour before alleviation takes place. In the case of a festering tooth (granulome), resulting in an inflammation of the sinuses, this simple application will not remedy the problem and it is suggested that you immediately consult your dentist.

CARE OF THE KIDNEYS

Chopped *parsley* used raw in soups, stews and salads stimulates and strengthens the kidneys. It can be also mixed with any spread prepared for a sandwich. Additional stimulation can be provided by using a poultice of finely chopped *onions* and applying it to the kidney region. Avoid as much as possible, salt and meat, as well as white flour and highly spiced condiments. Hot herbal poultices or compresses, herbal hip-baths and hot showers are excellent, too. One reminder you must observe with any kind of water treatment: make sure you never feel cool or chilly before applying it. Exercise well to increase your circulation beforehand.

You may find it hard to believe, but a piece of *fur* wrapped around the body and covering the kidney area will help relieve pain. Why does it work? It seems that with the movement of the body the rubbing of the fur against it creates static which penetrates into the kidney area and thus provides relief. For herbal poultices over kidney area try infusions of *Goldenrod (Solidago virgaurea)*, *Horsetail (Equisetum arvense)*, *Rosehip kernels* and *Juniper berries (Fructus juniper)*, especially if you can collect them fresh when they are in season.

PRURITIS (ITCHING OF THE SKIN)

This condition is always exceedingly troublesome and embarrassing. Externally, you can rub the affected part with a slice of raw potato or grate the potato finely and apply the pulp as a poultice. While this treatment may be used on the face, by itself it is not sufficient. Often the kidneys are to blame, therefore, use the treatment prescribed as outlined above. By this means much of the offending substances in the blood will be eliminated by properly functioning kidneys. It is possible that the liver needs attention, in which case you should follow the suggestions in the paragraphs dealing with the Liver diet.

ECZEMA AND OTHER SKIN INFECTIONS

Chronic skin infection marked by *pimples* and ugly *rashes* commonly called eczema have long plagued teenagers especially in their early years of puberty. It cannot be said with certainty that one remedy will work for all and it may be necessary to try different herbal treatments to find the one that works best. In the end, consultation with a dermatologist may be indicated. First, though, try bathing the affected area with warm sour *whey*, the watery part of the milk that separates from the curd when milk sours and becomes coagulated. You can make your own whey by leaving a bottle of milk at room temperature until it sours. Admittedly, the cure of skin diseases is frequently very difficult and may require much patience, time and trials. Many times the cause can be traced to malfunction of the kidneys, liver or intestines. So, the first thing one should do is make sure that these basic organs are working properly. On the other hand, skin infections can often be traced to a number of different things, i.e. plants, foods, fabrics, floor polishes, paints and even medicines. An analysis of what you eat may lead to the discovery of a culprit in the fruit family that can have a marked allergic effect on you. Instances of fruit *allergies* are quite common in warm climates and in the tropics. One fruit that comes to mind, which has caused skin rashes and swellings among a number of people, is the mango. It's skin has a resinous substance related to turpentine. As a result, those who have a bad allergic reaction to paints, varnishes and products that contain turpentine will immediately react to mangos. Plants such as poison ivy and poison oak afflict many whose skin is sensitive to these type of plants. For example, the otherwise harmless camomile plant as well as the Primula (Cowslip) and the less innocent Poison Ivy *(Rhus toxicodendron)* are known as urticaria-provoking plants. The effects of the latter plant can be treated successfully with *Grindelia (Grindelia robusta)* that can be cultivated in small gardens.

Children contract *nettle rash* and noticeably when they overindulge in too many *strawberries*. Some suffer badly, others less so, but however mild or severe, it is distressing to the little patients.

Skin troubles can have their origin in a deficiency of vitamins, especially B and E. Also dried fruits which have been sulphured and fresh fruits that have been sprayed chemically as well as sprayed vegetables. Chronic *skin ailments* will respond to various herbs individually as well as collectively. Some of the outstanding herbs that can be used are *Comfrey (Symphytum off.), Goldenseal, Arctium lappa (Burdock), Vinca major (Periwinkle) Walnut leaves,* to name a few. A decoction of one or more can be made by boiling the water and steeping the herbs in it and then straining through cheese cloth the cooled solution. Apply as you would use an astringent to the face or body or a moist poultice can be used cool. Liquid from steeping the common *dandelion* as well as the *plantain* which is abundant in almost every back yard, has produced beneficial results in many reported cases.

THE FIGHT AGAINST URIC ACID

When we speak of *uric acid* we automatically think of rheumatic ailments, painful joints, etc. and this would indicate it is time to form another partnership, in particular, with *parsley tea* and hot baths. These will go a long way towards eliminating this crippling unwanted host from your blood and tissues. If you add infusions of herbs, i.e. Common or *European Ash, Burdock* to the bath, all the better. Even steeped lawn-mowings, which have not been treated with insecticides, when added to the bath will have a salutary effect but make sure the bath water has a temperature approximating blood heat. Remain in it completely submerged letting only your nose emerge and if you can stand it, have someone turn on the faucet so that the bath temperature can rise to 100 degrees F. (38 C.) While submerged have someone brush you vigorously with a stiff brush. If you take this soaking bath regularly you will almost certainly rid yourself of your aching joints. For additional treatment to insure improvement, place a *poultice* of pulped *cabbage* on the aching joints and drink plenty of raw vegetable juices.

THE CURE OF RHEUMATIC AND ARTHRITIC AILMENTS WITHOUT MEDICINE

Begin your treatment the first thing in the morning before breakfast by drinking a half glass of raw *potato* juice diluted with warm water. All meals should consist of natural, organically grown foods. Detailed information concerning this diet will be found in another section of this book under "natural foods."

An hour before lunch eat 2–3 *juniper berries*, chewing them well. After lunch swallow 2–4 mustard seeds and during the day drink only the water in which *potatoes* have been boiled. Painful or arthritically affected parts should be covered with a *poultice* consisting alternately of pulped cabbage leaves, of potter's clay and of sour milk curd.

Anyone suffering from sciatic or *rheumatic pains* has the old but excellent formic acid therapy to fall back on. All that is necessary is to bury the painful limb in an ant-heap about once every two weeks. After the ants have done their work, brush them off and tender your thanks for the free formic acid injection they have given you. It is probably more effective than injections received in hospitals. Anyone who will follow these recommendations conscientiously not only will alleviate the problem, but cure it, even though the doctors have pronounced this ailment incurable.

BOILS

Whenever you suspect the formation of matter under a red and hot swelling in the skin, or when the swelling has already come to a "head", boil ground linseeds, add water to make a paste and apply to the affected part. Another alternative is pulverized Fenugreek seeds. You can mix it with *charcoal* powder and then make a paste; apply to the boil. If you have difficulty finding a source from which to obtain the seeds, you can resort to a well-known old fashion remedy: Peel and boil a *potato*, mash it, and apply it to the skin affect as hot as you can stand it. This will draw the pus to the surface enabling you to discharge it from the wound. The wound should be cleansed with boiled water to which a few drops of tincture of *Marigold* (Calendula off.) has been added. Next, sprinkle icing sugar (*Confectionary sugar*) or *milk sugar* (*lactose*) on the wound. An alternative is biological calcium powder. As added precaution, cover the treated part with *cabbage leaves* that have been crushed to a pulp. Internally, an extract of yeast or even dehydrated yeast may be taken twice a day. You will be surprised at the good results that this treatment offers. When treating boils, remember, cleanliness is of utmost importance to avoid the possibility of infection.

WHITLOWS (ABSCESSES)

A *whitlow* is an abscess on a finger or toe, usually near the nail. This throbbing, painful swelling is sometimes known as a "gathering." It is something that suddenly and unexpectedly appears and by its discomfort, impels you to take immediate steps to get rid of it. What to do! The simple remedy is to soak the finger or toe affected in warm water (100° F. – 38° C) three times a day for an hour each time. Keep the digit warm and in cold weather, wear a wollen glove or sock. Within the day improvement will be noted.

INSECT STINGS

What a shock to be stung by a bee or a wasp! Instinctively we try to pull out the stinger and forcefully suck out the poison that has been injected. What should we do next? If there is an ivy vine on your garden wall or in a nearby forest, pulp a leaf between your fingers and rub the pulp into the sting. A remedy of *Tincture of Ivy* can be prepared easily. Gather young ivy leaves and bark and mince. Pour alcohol over it and let stand for a week or so to permit the alcohol to extract substances from the ivy. Press off the liquid through a clean blotting paper and bottle. The tincture will be a handy addition to your medicine chest for future emergencies. A drop of the tincture rubbed into the sting will immediately relieve the pain. Some folks add a little salt water to the tincture as a precautionary antiseptic. If ivy is not at hand use plantain leaves crushed and rub into sting. These treatments will prevent extensive swelling and neutralize the poison. *Bracken* (fern) is one of the best antidotes for *gnat* and *insect stings*.

Rub the juice from the plant into the bite for quick and permanent relief. If you are bit by a mosquito and the above remedies are unavailable, quickly rub lemon juice or *Hamamelis* (*Witchhazel*) on the sting.

Stuff bracken generously into pillows and mattresses for relief from rheumatic problems and at the same time, repel insects and bugs.

INSECT STINGS IN THE THROAT

It has happened many times. A speaker, addressing an audience, was gesticulating and propounding when all of a sudden a gnat flew right into his open mouth. His voice suddenly squeaked and words refused to come out. In this particular case, a glass of water washed down the gnat and he was able to proceed with his talk. However, to be stung in the throat by a bee or a wasp is quite another thing. It can be a painful and dangerous experience. "Not possible," you will say! Oh yes it is. It is quite possible to swallow a bee or a wasp while eating fruit or honey and the insect, feeling the presence of the palate, will react in a most natural manner. It requires quick action to combat this danger. The quickest solution is to take 2 teaspoons of salt mixed with a little water. This will prevent the imminent danger of choking and reduce swelling. Use the solution as a gargle several times repeatedly. The salt water will draw out the poison from the palate or throat and by dispersion, render it harmless. *Calcium* tablets taken orally are also recommended. If you have Tincture of Ivy in your medicine chest, add it to the salt water.

SWELLING AND BRUISES

Swelling and *bruises* respond well to cabbage leaf poultices. If this appears too strong change to a clay pack. Mix an infusion of *Horsetail* (*Equisetum arvense*) with it for a better therapeutic effect. Or change alternatively from *cabbage poultice* to

43

clay because the cabbage cleanses and heals and the clay reduces the swelling. This double action ensures a rapid cure.

CONVULSIONS

Convulsions are quite frequent among children and parents will want to know about a treatment that is readily available, one that answers the need so well. There is a little-known remedy for convulsions which you can find almost anywhere throughout the year, and more than likely, you'll find it in your own backyard. It is *Stellaria media*, more popularly known as *Chickweed*. Prepare an infusion from either the fresh or dried plant and administer it frequently orally. Do not be afraid of an overdose because this herb is not only a curative but also a nutritious food that can be eaten as a salad as well. It is specifically indicated when the condition is worse in the morning and when pain shifts from one place to another. Because its use is quite limited, Chickweed is seldom mentioned as an herbal treatment for other ailments. Nevertheless, you will greatly prize *Chickweed* as a sure remedy for convulsions if you ever need it.

SEXUAL OVERSTIMULATION

The problem can be rather disturbing and unpleasant but it can be mitigated by drinking an infusion of *Wormwood* (*Artemisia absinthium*) and *Hops* (*Humulus lupulus*) alternating them for several weeks. Add to this treatment vegetables boiled with soda.

Although this method is used in prisons to keep inmates calm, it is most definitely harmful if resorted to for long periods and, therefore, not recommended as a regular treatment. Depending on the sensitivity of the individual, the general health will sooner or later suffer from this practice.

Non-stimulating foods and plenty of lemon juice are much to be preferred. Certainly they are less harmful and no less effective. Abstain from eggs, shellfish, i.e. oysters, clams, etc. Take cold showers and douse the genitals with cold water for a calming effect.

Having come to the end of our domestic experiments, "The Nature Doctor" has provided simple remedies for many ailments. It is hoped that, by giving them a fair trial, the simplicity and effectiveness of the suggestions thus far will persuade you to consult the book on other matters of health as well.

The following pages are written with the object of acquainting you with a natural health philosophy as well as with the best of natural treatments for various diseases and ailments. This should enable you to avoid costly medical bills with respect to the majority of afflictions that may come your way. At least it is worth trying and in the end, if you have to, you can always seek medical advice.

*

In the second part of this volume we present new sources of information that will be of positive help to those who suffer from many different afflictions. The physical problems of life will give rise to many more questions. The answers, some of which the earlier volume could not provide, now are available to you in this new edition. A careful reading of it by those who appreciate nature's counsel and aid will result in a profitable experience and a wealth of practical, healthful information that will be of lasting benefit. Unlike Ponce de Leon who searched diligently to find the "fountain of youth" and ultimately failed, we cannot guarantee that our revelation of the "secrets of nature" will "turn back the clock" for you, but, we can guarantee that it will enable you to maintain your body in a healthy condition and thus give more meaning and enjoyment to your life – and isn't that what we are searching for? All of us value health for without it life would be valueless. Thus, if only one "key" to nature's treasure house has been unlocked for you, we will consider that this new volume has accomplished its mission.

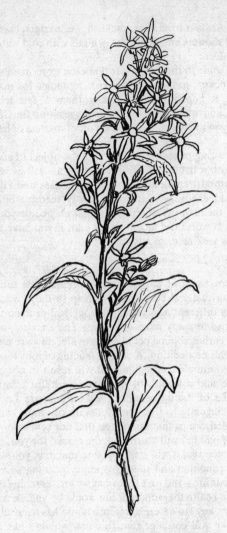

European goldenrod (Solidago virgaurea)

PART II

THE FEVER AS AN ALARM SIGNAL

Fever in itself is not a disease at all. It actually is a defense measure of the body against the invasion of a disease and, as such, provides a positive curative reaction. If this reaction is checked or altogether suppressed, the disease unopposed by the fever will, like an advancing army, completely invade and subjugate the body. In our mistaken fear and ignorance all too often we rush to take aspirin or quinine to reduce a temperature which by its very nature is our ally rather than our foe. It is a natural process, designed to aid us in our struggle for survival. We cannot hope to be wiser than nature. She is always working within us for our own good and if we ourselves do not sufficiently understand her ways, we should at least listen to those who have searched and have come to understand them. A wise prophet once said: " . . . show your concern for the earth, and it will instruct you."

Even in ancient times, the curative power of a *fever* was recognized and the statement of a famous physician of that era: "Give me the power to induce a fever and I will cure all disease," no doubt may be somewhat exaggerated but nevertheless, contains a fundamental truth.

It is well known that a sub-normal temperature indicates a dangerous condition and if complications set in, the art of the physician may be in vain unless he is able to induce fever. It is therefore the better part of wisdom to listen to the teachings of the ages and give fever its due respect as a curative agency. It is an important ally in the fight against disease and we

47

should be aware of this truth at all times. What happens though, if you are faced with an untimely demise with a temperature rising out of control? Did we not learn that we are in mortal danger with a temperature of 105 F? This is only true if we neglect to deal with the *fever* in a proper manner. Let us illustrate: We all know that for a stove to work well it must be properly ventilated. If it is clogged up and the current of air is insufficient, the fuel will not be consumed and leave a minimum of ashes. It will smolder, produce smoke and only partially consume the coals, eventually dying because of lack of air.

We can apply the same principle to *fever:* The body also needs ventilation, oxygen, to keep the flame of life alive or burning. As in the case of a fire, we also must keep removing the ashes (metabolic waste products) which might cause the flame to go out. The main channels of elimination in the body are the kidneys, the bowels, the skin and the lungs. These we might compare with the grate in the stove, for through them these "ashes" will leave the body. If they cannot do so and one or more channels are blocked up, they will accumulate inside the body. Since they consist of toxic substances which the blood is trying to throw off, auto-intoxication (self-poisoning) can kill the fire of life and cause death to the patient.

Therefore, as soon as a high fever becomes noticeable, the bowels should be thoroughly cleansed. An enema can be made from an infusion of herbs, i.e. *Chickweed, Bayberry bark* and particularly *Purple Cone flower (Echinacea)* which is very effective. Or, in place of an enema a natural laxative can be taken by mouth, such as unprocessed wheat bran.

A diuretic will help to stimulate the *kidneys.* One of the best is *Golden Rod (Solidago virgaurea)* or if not readily available use Horsetail (Equisetum arv.) Household vegetables such as parsley, onion or juniper berries are quite effective. Finally, an infusion of *Roseship kernels,* although not very strong in its effect, is still better than nothing.

Attention to the skin must now be given. The application of hot compresses will dilate the pores, bringing the blood to the surface where it can cool and throw off waste matter. If you are uncertain as to the correct procedure, ask for a practical demonstration at a home-nursing class or ask for written instructions. To go about it the wrong way can do more harm than good. However, a simple chest or buttock compress should not be too difficult to handle; just be careful there are not hollow spaces between the skin and the compress. If the patient is well wrapped, the desired perspiration will result. If he complains of being too hot, you can always apply cold compresses to his calves or put socks on his feet that have been soaked in vinegar. He will soon feel comfortable and probably doze off to sleep.

How simple the natural solution is. There is really no need to give way to fear and make use of harmful pills and potions of the apothecary. Nature's ways are always simple but man tends to seek a far more complicated solution to his troubles. A Latin prescription gives him more confidence perhaps because his inability to read the prescription lends an aura of mystery to it making nature's remedies seem too simple a solution. The sometimes dire consequences of such actions are, of course, never attributed to the drugs because they are considered scientific and almost infallible while natural remedies are relegated to a backward and unorthodox treatment.

Another factor that is very important in controlling a fever is nutrition. Normally a *fever* patient is not hungry. Nature thus indicates that feeding would not only be useless but actual y harmful, because the fever is trying to dispose of what is already in the body. The digestive system is at such times almost inactive, for the fever process demands most of the patient's vitality. Encouraging him to eat is kindness in reverse, so stifle that desire to prepare appetizing dishes for him. Avoid above everything else those foods that are rich in protein, i.e. eggs, cheese, fish, meat as well as heard to digest foods. He is much more likely to digest a little milk and honey, fruit juices, herbal teas, alcohol-free wine or just plain water sweetened with honey. The best liquids of course are fruit juices of the sub-acid kind and the fever patient will welcome them more than anything else. *Grapes* and freshly squeezed *oranges* will refresh him at the same time as it is seldom that patients cannot tolerate fruit juices.

NATURAL CONSEQUENCES

If the *fever* process is assisted rather than suppressed, the temperature will not rise to dangerous proportions but slowly decrease. It must not be reduced quickly for everything done in haste is unnatural. It should be allowed to remain reasonably high as long as there is any toxic waste matter to be eliminated and then it will come down of its own accord. It is a delusion and deceit to believe that medicinal drugs which force the *fever* down will, at the same time, remove the cause – the underlying disease, the accumulated systemic refuse. At best, a sort of armistice will be achieved, but that is all. Everything not eliminated through perspiration, the urine and the stool will be left in the body and will cause the trouble to flare up again, although not necessarily in the same way. Instead of having a fever resulting from one cause, complications such as pericarditis, articular rheumatism or pneumonia can plague you. We are all too familiar with the story of how a new drug discovery can cure a disease with amazing speed, but we are also familiar with the evil side effects it brings with it. Gradually, even orthodox medicine must conclude from experience that wonder drugs do not penetrate to the root of the disease and that nature can neither be circumvented or overpowered with impunity. In this 20th century we are living in an age of speed where "quick" cures are an accepted part of daily life and therein lies a fallacy. Unlike animals who are motivated by instinct when trying to overcome illness, man's instincts have become blunted and he depends upon his intellect to solve his problems. It therefore is not surprising that many of his theories fail. We should obey nature's laws as far as we are aware of them. If we ignore them, we are the ones who suffer. Let us regard a fever as nature's warning that all is not well within us and then assist her instead of resist her, to our mutual benefit.

PAIN AS AN ALARM SIGNAL

What has been said about fever equally applies to *pain*. Whenever it manifests itself, we must realize that by ignoring it or trying to deaden it, we give the condition responsible for it a greater chance to spread and increase its destructive power. It is true that pain, at times, can be very annoying but this is no excuse for tossing its warning to the winds. *Pain* is symptomatic of a heart attack if it occurs in the chest and particularly if it is accompanied by hot flashes, sweating and upset stomach. Sharp pains in the abdomen are symptoms of ulcers, ruptured appendix, gall stones, and it is not unusual that women feel pain in the abdomen at the beginning of pregnancy. *Pains* in the shoulder, back or legs are sometimes symptoms of rheumatism and neuralgia. Since *pain* is nature's most valuable clue to our bodily ills, it is important to diagnose correctly the cause. By taking drugs to numb the *pain* we are ignoring the cause and delaying improvement. The cost of freedom from *pain* by means of this method is too high a price to pay for relief and we must realize, that it is only by remedying the underlying condition to which the pain leads us, that we can finally get rid of both the symptom and the cause.

CORRECT ACTION: From the foregoing it will be seen that the conscientious doctor will try to track the *pain* to its source. For example, if you have reason to complain about *pain* over the liver, he will not consider his duty done by merely giving you a pain-relieving pill, but will check the color of your stool, check to find out what fats disagree with you and will take every precaution to diagnose the problem and get at the root of the trouble. Naturally, a correct diagnosis is half the battle and prescribing the proper medicine will bring prompt relief.

If the kidneys are suspect he will try to establish the nature of the *pain,* finding out if the skin covering that area feels tight, and he will check color of the urine and if he is suspicious that it is a case of kidney disease, he will go one step further and analyze the urine. He may find any one or several things in the *urine* which supplies the clue, i.e. albumen, bacteria, red and white blood corpuscles or cylindrical or epithelial cells from the bladder or kidneys. Even if he finds only traces of foreign bodies in the urine, he will take precautions and advise a saltless diet, warm clothing to protect from chills and any other measures he may deem necessary. An Herbalist would prescribe infusions of horsetail, birch leaves or parsley as well as warm compresses over the affected area to dissipate any congestions that may exist.

Pain manifests itself in so many different ways but always as a danger signal that something is wrong with the body. It signals a migraine or a bilious or nervous or sick headache and warns of many other malfunctions of the body. But mere palliation is harmful and does not get at the root cause. Millions of people, year in and year out, swallow pills to stop headaches without it occuring to them that the pills may lead to stubborn *constipation* which produce intestinal poisons which reach the brain through the bloodstream and thus lead to more troubles. Would it not be wiser to establish proper bowel function in the first place? This would avoid a "merry-go-round" that results from continued pill taking. Today it's a pill for the headache, tomorrow, for constipation and the next day, a reverse procedure. If this continues over a long enough period, intestinal cancer can result even though there has been no history of cancer in the family.

NATURAL CONSEQUENCES

Even the medical profession frequently ignores *constipation* and it is mere routine for some doctors to prescribe a laxative for it instead of waging a tireless war to get rid of the cause.

52

Similarly, abdominal pains in women, *leucorrhoea* (a whitish discharge from female genital organs), and *menstrual cramps* are often neglected and the cause, congestions in the venous system, remain untouched and untreated.

The proper course to take would suggest *hip-baths* to which have been added infusions of either *hayflowers*, *camomile* or *juniper* needles. The temperature of the bath should be maintained at blood heat because a bath too hot will send the blood rushing to the head. Since the bath should be taken for a minimum of a half hour, continue adding hot water from time to time to maintain the required temperature. These hip-baths will do much good and definitely relieve the cramps and if you continue the baths for a period of time even the leucorrhoea may be made to disappear. It is important, when first signs of discomfort are noticed, to attend to it at once because, if neglected, major complications may result.

The female abdomen should have the best of care possible for it contains vital organs, the functions of which are easily endangered by congestions, irritations and inflammations. It is simple enough to deal with the small beginnings of trouble, but if they are repeatedly neglected, in the end there will be no other way out than an operation or other drastic measures. A forester does not wait until a tree is badly diseased before taking action to cure it; at the first sign of a diseased shoot he pinches it off and thereby avoids having to take drastic measures later on. In this way he takes measures to eliminate the problem when it is small and easy to handle.

DANGEROUS INFLUENCES DURING PREGNANCY

Nothing gives greater happiness to a woman than to give birth to a healthy baby. No young person can fully understand the meaning of parental bliss until parenthood is realized. But how great is the distress when a sick child is born, or worse, a malformed child with limbs twisted or hands or feet missing, or with any other of those terrible malformations which occurred

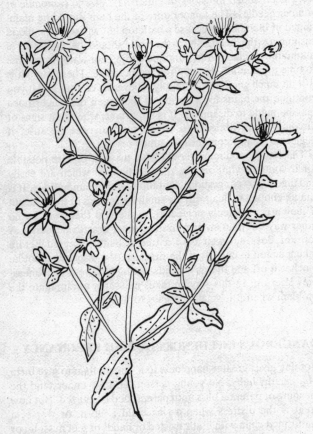

St. John's wort (Hypericum perforatum)

a few years ago in Europe and especially in Germany. How terrible is the guilt of a mother when she silently has to admit to herself that she bears most of the blame for this calamity. Scientific research has shown the first four to eight weeks, that is the first three months of pregnancy, are of greatest importance as far as harmful influences on the new germinating life are concerned. Following are some suggestions on how one may try during this time, in the best possible way, to prevent malformation in the developing baby.

NUTRITION AND EXERCISE

Anyone who appreciates the importance of *nutrition* will readily understand that the food of the mother-to-be should be as natural as possible, free of contaminating additives, preservatives and chemicals. A normal diet should be maintained as it is not necessary to eat greater amounts of food than one used to eat before *pregnancy*.

A pregnant woman should definitely inhale sufficient oxygen to ensure the best conditions for the proper development of the child. This benefit is gained by activities outdoors in the fresh air and by walks through green country areas, through woods and fields. Highways and streets with a lot of traffic polluting the air should be avoided.

THE DANGERS OF ALCOHOL, NICOTINE AND RADIATION

It should be sufficiently well known today that the intake of *alcohol* at the time of conception and during pregnancy may have frightful consequences. It is therefore utterly irresponsible to bear a child while drinking *alcohol* liberally. If you find it difficult to resist drinking at parties and celebrations, better not to attend during pregnancy because heavy drinking can lead to regret and possible lifelong tragedy. Every mother-to-be should know the disadvantages of alcohol and should resolve firmly to abstain from alcohol during her *pregnancy*.

It is equally irresponsible of women to smoke during pregnancy and particularly during the times of breast feeding. Research has shown that only a few hours after smoking, nicotine is already present in the mother's milk. Who can guarantee that during pregnancy the poison from *nicotine* will not reach the placenta and do irreparable damage to the unborn child? Precaution should be taken to avoid X-rays, *radium* therapy and any other type of rays that are used all too frequently nowadays. Unfortunately, it is impossible to avoid radio-active *radiation* that is contaminating the air as a result of atomic explosion drifts.

CHEMICAL MEDICINES

Of great significance is the use of headache remedies, *sedatives* or *soporifics* (sleep-inducing drugs), which should be avoided by every pregnant woman. The alarming articles about the thalidomide tragedy, which is said to have led to thousands of malformed babies, should alert any pregnant woman of the utter danger of taking chemical medicines. Today it is thalidomide, tomorrow, it will perhaps be a sulfanilamide, and soon it may be another product that will cause the damage. Thus, it is better to use chemistry to clean your clothes, floors and windows and put it to other technical uses than to ingest its preparations. *Pregnant* women should take notice and value their maternal duties much more than the desire to use strong chemical agents to quickly combat headaches, indispositions or insomnia. There are plenty of harmless remedies made from plants that will alleviate such temporary problems. So why expose yourself to the dangers resulting from hasty action. Every day we receive more confirmation of how nature in its harmless form can truly aid a person without harmful after-effects. Because of the unnatural conditions and unhealthy pollutions to which we are exposed to in this day and age, many people seem to find it expedient to take recourse to palliatives rather than curing their ailment through nature's process. The results of this deceptive thinking are disappointing but if one takes the detour via the natural way of healing the rewards are well worth while.

ADVANTAGES AND DISADVANTAGES OF HORMONE TREATMENTS

Women, who would love to have children but are unable to, often summon up all their energy to find fulfillment of their natural desire. This can easily be understood, for an unfilled longing in this respect may lead to severe mental suffering. There are, of course, women who have little or no desire for a child. Although they do not suffer from childlessness, they do forfeit a happy motherhood and miss the many natural pleasures which children bring to the home. But for those who wish to have children and are unable to conceive there may be a solution.

TWO SOLUTIONS TO CONSIDER:

The suspicion that has been confirmed is that the inability to have children may be connected with a *hormone deficiency*. In such cases two courses are open. First, there is the possibility of stimulating the body in such a way as to improve its ability to produce hormones. On the one hand this can be achieved through physical applications such as *hip-baths*, alternating baths, Kehne-baths and similar methods of treatment. On the other hand, stimulation of the circulatory system will increase the supply of blood to the abdomen. This in turn will stimulate the production of hormones and may eventually lead to pregnancy. Agents such as *Urtica* and *Aesculus hippocastannum (Horse chestnuts)* are extremely useful in aiding circulation. Of additional advantage would be the taking of wheat germ or wheat germ oil. Although outdoor exercises and deep breathing in the open air are part of the natural recovery for the body, sport activities should not be overdone. The whole way of life should be directed into normal channels. This is the natural and harmless course that should be first taken.

Yet, others, without second thought take the alternative course to overcome their infertility since it may possibly assure greater success. This is the hormonal treatment, especially the application of gonadotropins to the organ in which reproductive cells develop. But, to be sure, it involves risks. The degree of sensitiveness of the female body varies greatly from individual to individual and therefore it is not easy for a doctor to find the right dose. In an article which appeared in the "Weltwoche" magazine, Dr. Jurg Baer explained that an overdose of *hormones* can have strange results, because it is possible that a number of eggs are ready to be fertilized. The result could be twins, triplets or even a greater number of children. This would certainly be too much of a good thing, even for the woman who may have suffered previously due to her childlessness. It would be preferable, in any case, to try the first way out and to stimulate the *hormone* producing glands in a natural way. Only if these efforts fail should one contemplate hormonal treatment as a last resort.

OTHER IMPORTANT OBSERVATIONS

In this context it is important to take a closer look at the opposite method, the curbing of normal hormone production in the female body. Gynecologists have observed that the curbing effect lasts only as long as the appropriate agent, for example, the anti-pregnancy pill is taken. If a woman stops taking the "pill" her body may react in such a way that the end result will lead to multiple births. Considering the risks involved of the possibility of having triplets or quintuplets may prompt some women to have second thoughts about the advantages of taking the "pill". In addition to this, some doctors believe that the taking of hormonal preparations like anti-pregnancy pills may cause varicose veins and increase the danger of thrombosis. This underlines the warning to women not to commit gross abuse against nature because of the suffering and detrimental side effects that may result from this indiscretion.

THE CARE OF BABIES

It would be quite impossible for anyone who can appreciate modern hygiene to go back to the ways and customs of her parents although some of their ways may have had some value due to their experience. However, the superstitious fear of water, among other things, which led them to believe that bathing would actually be harmful is rightly laughed at today, although there are still many elderly people who have never sat in a bath tub. Our enlightened age can no longer uphold the conviction that children should not be brought into intimate contact with light, air, water and sun, although these things were actually frowned upon and feared even in the time of our grandparents. They also held the belief that children would develop crooked limbs if they were not tightly wrapped and rendered practically immobile. Even today we find evidence of bandaging up babies in the Orient and even in Italy. It is, therefore, not surprising that infant mortality was once much greater than it is today.

Today it is taken for granted that frequent baths are most beneficial for an infant, not only for hygienic reasons but also, because they encourage skin-activity, remove congestions and stimulate the functions of internal organs and of the ductless glands. We must not forget that the infant came from the warm, even temperature of the mother's womb, protected from outside discomforts of the outside world and it takes time to adjust to a cooler atmosphere. For this reason, the infant's first baths should be kept at blood heat, close to 98° F. The lively splashing and joyful shouts bear witness to the pleasure babies derive from their baths.

Any medicinal additions to a baby's bath should be chosen with the greatest care. It is impossible to stop little fingers wet

59

with bath water from going into little mouths. Therefore, avoid additions like commercial pine needle cubes which contain Natrium fluorescentum; it gives the water a nice green coloring but it can be harmful to the baby. The same applies to acrid herbs like Cranesbill (Geranium pratense) and Greater Celandine (Chelidonium majus) which, although of unquestioned benefit in eczematous skin troubles and scabies, if used at all, should be used in only the smallest quantities. Infant's skin is very sensitive and such seemingly harmless measures as herbal additions to baby's bath can cause unexpected reactions. The following *bath herbs* can, however, be confidently recommended, singly or in combination.

Horsetail (Equisetum arvense) contains organic silica and exerts a beneficial influence upon the skin.

Lemon Balm (Melissa officinalis) is indicated for nervous babies and is very soothing.

Common Lady's Mantle (Alchemilla vulg.) will give elasticity and firmness to the tissues when they are spongy and flabby. If there is a tendency to hernia (rupture), this herb will assist in rendering the affected tissues stronger but, for a complete cure, other measures will have to be resorted to as well.

Camomile (Anthemis nobilis) the infusion of which is good for digestive and metabolic disturbances as well as for stomach aches, gastric pains of the child.

Marigold (Calendula off.) is useful when the skin is sensitive and affected with rashes, etc. Use the flowers as well as the leaves.

Wild Thyme (Thymus serpyllum), also called "Mother of Thyme", has proved its worth as a bath herb and is especially valuable for infants who catch colds easily or suffer from hereditary pulmonary weakness. Therefore, remember this little herb for your baby if you have reason to suspect weak lungs in either yourself or your husband.

Plantain (Plantago lanceolata) is of great help in bladder weakness which, however, does not become apparent in infants until they are toilet trained. This herb is not to be

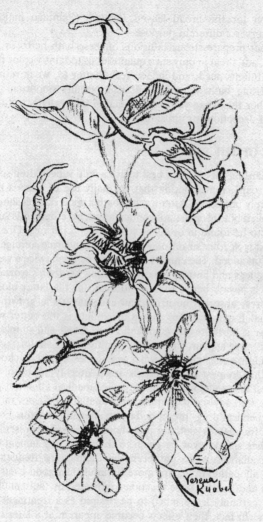

Nasturtium (Tropaeolum majus)

mistaken for the broad leaved *Plantain* (Plantago major) which serves a different purpose.

Do not prepare strong infusions of these bath herbs or, if you do, add them in only such quantities as to faintly color the water. Infants need, and indeed react better to, weak rather than strong bath stimulants. It is especially important to remember this when you prepare herbal teas, whether in the form of decoctions or infusions.

CARE OF THE SKIN

For cleansing the skin it is best to use a mild super-fatted soap (baby soap), remembering that the daily use of soap is not absolutely necessary. After a warm bath a good skin oil should be applied but this must not contain any acrid etheric oils such as are to be found in ordinary commercial toilet oils. One of the best is *St John's wort oil* with a little mandarine, orange or lemon oil added. The entire body should be oiled twice a week and the legs and buttocks every day using *St. John's wort oil.* Oiling is always better than powdering, for the latter blocks the pores, absorbs the urine und encourages the growth of bacteria. Experience has shown that oiling is the better way because it lubricates the skin and keeps it soft and supple. If redness does appear, rub the skin lightly with Lanolin.

Children's remedies and toilet accessories should be chosen with the greatest care. Infants react quickly to even the smallest doses and whenever they need medical attention you will be well advised to employ homeopathic medicines rather than chemical drugs prescribed by an allopathic doctor. Especially for babies nothing but homeopathically prescribed remedies should ever be given to them and it is lamentable that pediatricians do not prescribe them more frequently. Many allopathic drugs are more harmful than good even for adults and their adverse reactions, indicated by the manufacturer, certainly leave much to be desired as a treatment for infants. In fact, their effects become apparent at a later date when even the doctor fails to realize that the new condition he is called upon to treat is the direct result of the drug he prescribed a long time ago. Homeopathy works gently, safely and surely. The results achieved by skillful prescribing have nothing to do with "imaginary" and "psychological" effects which can hardly be expected with infants.

It should be re-emphasized that infusions (teas) for small children should be exceedingly weak, indeed, barely colored. You will find the following teas very useful and effective if given as indicated:

Fennel, Anise, Caraway, and *Dill* belong to the so-called "warming teas." Whenever there is anything wrong with the digestion of your baby, do try a weak Fennel infusion. Many times this will be sufficient to bridge any temporary difficulties you may experience with your child.

Yarrow is very good for diarrhea and loss of appetite but, again, it must be given very weak. If it does not produce sufficient improvement add a small pinch of Bloodwort (Tormentil) and give three or four teaspoonsful of this infusion throughout the day and into the evening.

Goldenrod (Solidago virgaurea) is a reliable remedy when the *kidneys* are out of order. The fresh plant extract from this herb is one of the best and most effective medicines for the kidneys and the bladder and should always be resorted to when something appears to be wrong with urination. If Goldenrod is not handy or available, a weak *Rose-hip* or *Horsetail tea* can be used.

For purposes of disinfection you will find a *whey*-concentrate, available in powder form, and mixed with water, very effective and it is certainly more harmless than iodine, the place of which it can take. *Hypericum* 1x can be also used as an antiseptic and *St. John's wort oil* has been recommended by such a well known child specialist as Dr. Joseph Schier for the prevention of tetanus.

Calcium deficiency shows itself in various ways and can be still found among small children. If, in addition, there is a deficiency of Vitamin D as well, then you have the fundamental cause of rickets. This disease is easily recognized by skeletal deficiencies evidenced by bowed legs and hunched backs and its victims have extremely soft teeth and a tendency to break bones in minor accidents. Preventative measures require taking *olive oil,* as well as *Vitamin D, calcium* and *phosphorus.* Symptoms of *rickets* in its mild form can be readily observed in children. They are very lively and react to everything quickly and their facial expression is almost too intelligent for their years. It reminds one of an apple grown ripe too soon and which, on closer examination, proves to be worm-eaten. These children can be helped. Homeopathic or biochemical *Calcium Phosphate* 6x, *Calcium Fluoride* 12x (to harden tooth enamel) and *Silica* 12x should be given. A Calcium-complex fortified with *Urtica (Nettles)* as a *Vitamin D* carrier is eminently suitable for such cases too. *Orange juice* and *codliver oil* are rich in *Vitamin D* and can be highly recommended. Raw *carrot juice* is another natural and efficacious remedy for calcium deficiency.

INFANT NUTRITION

Mothers often complain that their babies become constipated when they are fed *brown rice cereal.* It may very well be that rice is more constipating than barley gruel but because of its wonderful nutritional value it should not, on any account, be left out of the child's diet. The constipation can always be counteracted by natural means, such as giving *linseed* mucilage, which can be added to the rice gruel. The amount to be added depends upon the child's reaction, but a teaspoonful will usually be adequate. In this way the child will not be deprived of the good effects of the rice gruel.

Another valuable food, especially during teething time, is *whole rye.* It contains not only calcium but also calcium fluoride which is so necessary for the enamel of the teeth. Best of all diets is to feed the baby alternatively rice, barley, oat, millet and buckwheat gruels which can be used as a base for either carrot or any of the fruit juices. Care must be taken not to mix vegetable juices with fruit juices and it would be just as well to avoid using more than one kind of fruit juice per meal. If the baby's digestion is weak, mixing several fruit juices might lead to flatulence and similar digestive upsets. If this happens, despite the fact that the baby received only one vegetable or fruit juice at a time, you will be well advised to mix the fruit or vegetable juice with an already prepared *Almond cream*. It is readily available from health food stores. Mix with an electric blender or electric mixer and the resulting food will not only be the best you can give to your baby but it is equally valuable for older children and even adults.

Babies who suffer from *milk scabs (Crusta lactaea)* should have animal milk entirely removed from their diet. Put them on almond milk instead and give them in addition a weak infusion of Heartsease plant *(Viola tricolor)* which is also known as *Wild Pansy*. Calcium in the form mentioned before will also be needed and this will without doubt clear up this troublesome complaint.

SUCCESSFUL TREATMENT OF CRUSTA LACTAEA

This problem is not due to external factors like infections and the like. It is simply an abnormal over-sensitivity of the child's constitution with which it may have been born while the underlying cause may be found in some sort of deficiency. If one deals with the causes, then the rash will disappear without giving further trouble. In the first place, good digestion should be encouraged and if anything should be wrong in this respect, the bowels should be regulated with buttermilk, brown rice gruel or similar foods, using other gruels made from natural cereals.

In the case of breast-fed children, *Crusta lactaea* may be due to substances in the mother's milk. Few mothers pay much attention to the fact that what they take medicinally or as laxatives may be responsible for infant disorders. The mother's bloodstream absorbs whatever she takes and, as her milk is a product affected by the medicine, the baby will be affected also. For example, a mother suffering from constipation thoughtlessly takes a laxative. As a result the baby develops diarrhia which is unsuccessfully treated with all manner of things, until at last artificial feeding has to be resorted to in order to stop the problem. Thus the infant is deprived of the best food it could possibly have in a natural way, the mother's milk. With a little knowledge and forethought such a situation would never have arisen. If *constipation* is to be successfully dealt with, only harmless *laxatives* such as *linseed* preparations or *psyllium seed* should be used. These will regulate the bowels effectively during the period of *lactation*. Other medicines are known to enter into the composition of the milk when the mother has taken them. Luminal and many other barbiturates which go to make up various sedatives and sleeping pills, Morphia preparations, Mercury, Quinine and numerous rheumatic remedies containing salicylic acid directly affect the milk. Iodide of Potassium is another medication to watch out for, but it does not do as much damage as alcohol and nicotine in poisoning the baby's milk.

If a child is given such drastic medicines and drugs in its most tender years – the fact that it receives them indirectly via the mother's milk does not render them less harmful – we must not be surprised if its health is seriously affected. Consider these things if your baby develops *Crusta lactaea:* If you *smoke* you should certainly give it up while you are breast feeding. You wouldn't want to deliberately injure your baby's health, would you? Even in pregnancy it has been proved that smoking has an adverse effect on the unborn child. You can prove this yourself by a simple experiment. Place a stethoscope on the mother's abdomen under natural conditions and count the child's heartbeat. Let the mother *smoke* a cigarette and then count them again. You will note that the beats increase by eight per minute. This gives you an idea of how the baby's heart is overstimulated by smoking just one cigarette.

Articles of diet can affect the mother's milk just as well. It has been observed that a child's *Crusta lactaea* disappears within a few days if the mother avoids eating certain foods like eggs or those containing animal protein. Since she eats for both the child and herself she must pay particular attention to her diet while she is breast feeding. You will find health diets set out in other parts of this book.

A mother should also try to breast feed her baby as long as possible. If, in spite of changing diet, the child's condition remains unaltered, she should occasionally forego the usual meals and take almond or *buttermilk* instead for a day or two. To enhance the curative effects of these foods – and they are foods, not merely drinks – a little fresh plant extract of *Wild Pansy (Viola tricolor)* can be added to the buttermilk. If the general diet is kept free from fat, it seems to influence the child's condition favorably.

If the ailing child is already weaned, the following suggestions will prove very beneficial: Instead of cow's milk give the child *almond milk* only. This, however, necessitates accurate weight control. Some babies cannot assimilate vegetable protein and will lose weight or not gain enough. In this case soya milk should be tried and if this does not appear to improve matters, animal milk will have to be resorted to once more. Frequently *goat's or sheep milk* is better tolerated than cow's milk. Older children suffering from very stubborn cases of milk scabs should be given *wheat germ*. In all cases, natural measures and remedies should be employed only, even if the cure demands more perseverance than usual. Each child is different, some respond more rapidly while others take a little more time. As an example, a worried mother wrote and asked for advice on how to cure her little daughter's *Crusta lactaea*. She also sent a sample of the child's urine. An analysis revealed a liver problem existed. First *almond milk* and diluted *carrot juice* was suggested. Then a biological *calcium* preparation was recommended to rectify a mineral deficiency and *Goldenrod* tea was advised to give needed stimulation to the kidneys. Other remedies, chief of which is *Wild Pansy,* was also prescribed and as an external measure *St. John's wort oil* and *Urtica* powder was recommended.

Later, the mother wrote: "Your recommendation for treating our little one worked beautifully. The *Crust lactaea* disappeared within a very short time. Many thanks!" Another letter from a nurse reads: "At present I am alone with two children in a chalet. The boy, now 15 months old, had *Crusta lactaea* last year. You sent me a *Calcium* complex, *Viola tricolor* and *Whey* concentrate. Thanks to your excellent remedies the rash disappeared within fourteen days." In this case, diluted *Whey* concentrate was used externally. A fresh plant preparation from *Echinacea* would have worked equally well. Never use soap and water on *Crusta lactaea*. It is better to use *St. John's wort oil* to cleanse the skin.

It is exceedingly useful to know how nature furnishes it's wonderful provisions for treating this problem sparing children permanent harm.

INFLAMMATION OF THE BREAST
(MASTITIS)

An inflammation which has been improperly treated, or not treated at all, frequently leaves a hardening of the breasts. This can possibly be the cause of breat cancer later on. Not long ago, a well known gynecologist mentioned that she felt somewhat inhibited, having to examine the breasts of women, since breast cancer is very often detected. Because the breast is a very sensitive organ, it should be given more than the usual care.

Inflammation of the breast can develop from a simple bruise. Quite often, however, the inflammation appears after delivery or during the period of lactation or at the time of weaning. It is important to treat an inflammation immediately, since lumps may form that lead to abscesses. In case an *abscess* forms it is best to permit it to ripen (come to a head) in order that it may break open by itself. Or it is possible to open it surgically. In either case scars will remain, due to the fact that the scar tissue has lost its elasticity.

TREATMENT AND PRECAUTIONS

An inflammation of the breast is treated externally as well as internally by medication. In order to exert an internal influence an infusion of the *Echinacea* plant has proved to be extremely valuable. For external use Arnica and Echinacea ointments are excellent. Rub them over the affected surface gently, alternating between the two, and gradual improvement will be seen. If the area is sensitive, apply regularly a warm compress of Mallow tea to which has been added five to ten drops of Arnica and Echinacea plant extract. Women who are breast feeding and would like to stop the production of milk, may do so by rubbing the breasts with an ointment. In case of miscarriage or spontaneous abortion the milk has to be removed with a breast pump until the flow is decreased and then use the ointment. By doing this milk fever and inflammation of the breasts may be prevented. St. John's wort oil or Carob oil are excellent for this purpose. Rubbing the nipples und surrounding area with the oil will help to prevent chapping.

CHILDREN'S DISEASES

Admittedly children's diseases can be beneficial insofar as the fever disposes of pathological material within the system that would otherwise cause more serious conditions later on. This, however, does not mean we should take uncalculated risks and expose children to a disease because it purifies. When a child's disease strikes all we need to do is give the best care possible to encourage a strong and healthy body, because healthy children's bodies will easily overcome these diseases and will acquire new strength in doing so. To make this possible it is necessary to treat the disease properly. The *fever* not only destroys the poisons accumulated but it also eliminates many of the toxins which have been accumulating from the embryonic stage of development. Doctors concur that those who have never had any of the children's diseases, succumb to all sorts of diseases, even malignant ones, later on in life. There is sufficient proof that fevers are wonderfully curative, that they protect us from, rather than expose us to diseases. The majority of children readily recover from *feverish* conditions due to childhood diseases and if the child doesn't, it is not the fever but the treatment that is to blame. The medicinal suppression of "normal" disease symptoms such as fevers and rashes (Exanthems) is the worst form of "treatment" a child can receive. The purifying processes are halted and the toxins, instead of being eliminated, remain in the system and can severely damage the heart, the nervous system or the lungs. Indeed, no organ is really safe from damage.

The most "effective" and at the same time most harmful medicines used for the suppression of *fever* and diseases in general are the so-called family of Chemotherapeutics. It is hoped that enough has been said to discourage you from using them, no matter what the opinion of the medical profession may be. On the other hand, biochemical and homeopathic remedies are safe because they assist rather than suppress the natural curative processes. To assist in the oxidation of toxins *Ferrum Phosphoricum* 12x should always be given to *feverish* children, while *Aconitum* 4x helps to eliminate the toxins through the skin. If you do not know what course an infectious disease will take, try alternating *Aconitum* 4x with *Belladonna* 3x. It is important that the bowels should be clean and work properly. If not it may be necessary to give a small enema.

Do not use soap, just lukewarm water. Drinking of *Horsetail tea* every few hours will aid the kidneys discharge their functions effectively. The third organ to receive attention is the skin. You can hardly go wrong with warm water compresses. Cold ones demand knowledge and skill, and they should not be used when the patient is chilly and feverish. Cold packs reduce the internal body heat by drawing it to the surface of the skin where it is dissipated. In the case of a high *fever* no undue fear should be entertained about applying cold packs because a thoroughly heated body is not likely to chill easily.

Vitamin deficiencies as well as lack of proper nutrition open the door to all kinds of infectious diseases that affect adults as well as children. *Immunizations* are generally recommended in some form or other, but as the effects are uncertain and usually do not confer immunity for a sufficiently long period, they hardly deserve so much attention as they receive. Apart from that, the natural immunity and ability of the body to defend itself is greatly reduced through their indiscriminate use. As has been already pointed out, "infections" with their accompanying *fevers* serve a good purpose and if they cannot be prevented by natural means such as nutritionally sensible living, it would be just as well to encourage their normal course once they have established themselves. If the correct treatment is given, nothing need be feared. Complications are unlikely and as far as the heart is concerned, in the case of a high fever, remember that a child's heart can endure much more than that of an adult, at least in proportion to its size.

INFANTILE ECZEMA

The eczema infantum or children's *dermatitis* is a sad story, since it is not only a strain on the child, but also on the mother, due to the constant care and attention the child has to receive.

In 1964 at the Convention of the German Society for Child Therapy held in Munich, Dr. Holt, the American Pediatrician of New York University, presented the viewpoint that the *"Tar Therapy"* is still the best method for the treatment of infantile eczema. A tar extract of 5% is also more economical than a treatment with the expensive steroid ointments. Of considerable interest was Dr. Holt's concession that children's dermatitis is rather easy to suppress but very difficult to cure.

With the help of the *tar therapy*, it is relatively easy to decrease the severity of the case from degree IV to degree I, but for a complete cure the *tar therapy* is not sufficient, he stated. If, however, the tar therapy treatment is discontinued the little patient will quickly experience a worsening of the condition. This fact, however, was not mentioned at the convention; neither was mentioned that tar with its 11 hydrocarbons, including Naphthalin and Benzopyrene, has been recognized as a treatment that could lead to cancer.

RECOMMENDED TREATMENT

Unfortunately, no other pediatrician present could offer a better therapy. But there are several treatments available that are highly successful. Following are a few: First, a milk and protein free diet; treatment with milk enzymes, such as *Whey* concentrate. Not one of those present at the convention could explain why treating infantile eczema with Whey-concentrate results in such unexpected success. It is unfortunate that this treatment is not better known among the professionals considering it has been in use for a long time. Centuries ago it had already been noticed that eczemas began to heal when bathing in fresh or even better yet, sour *whey*. With a simultaneous application of *Viola tricolor*, which is known as a fresh botanical wild pansy preparation, the success is even more striking. In children, who suffer from a calcium deficiency, the taking of a calcium complex will also prove helpful. A calcium preparation in powder form is helpful if used externally since it prevents harmful bacteria from entering through the pores of the skin. Instead of steroid ointments, Lanolin should be used. Every pediatrician will be enthusiastic about the success achieved. Obviously the diet is very important too. Since milk proteins must be eliminated from the diet completely, the substitution of vegetable protein takes on added importance. Soy protein or almond protein, if available, have been proven excellent substitutes. Special attention should be given to a salt-free diet, although this was not even considered at the pediatric convention in Munich. The nutritional question brought out an interesting discovery. A pediatric report revealed that among the more affluent families of Nigeria, who live according to European standards, infantile eczema was much more frequent than it was among the natives among whom, it was hardly known at all. On the basis of this finding it can be concluded that the nutritional habits of the natives were superior to those families with higher incomes, and that living habits of an indulgent civilization makes its contribution to the incidence of dermatitis in children. The claim that dermatitis is an allergy does not have much support. The search for a harmless antigen or a specific antibody probably will not be successful. So why not look to a natural therapy that proves to be simple and harmless in treating infantile eczema, and which in the end, does not offer temporary relief but in most cases results in a complete cure.

MEASLES

This is probably the most harmless infectious disease of childhood. The causative virus was not discovered until recently, for it can be observed and studied only through the aid of an electronic microscope. The course it takes and the fact that children "catch" it easily from one another marks it as a highly infectious disease. Most mothers are familiar with the large spotted rashes that are accompanied by a high temperature. If you are uncertain of the nature of the child's illness in its early stages, take a look at the mucous membranes of the cheeks in the region of the molars. If it is a case of measles, you will discover a day or two before the rash breaks out, bright red spots with small white dots approximately one-eighth of an inch in diameter. This is what is called the "Koplik's Sign" which is an unmistakable indication of measles.

The disease has an incubation period of 14 days and it is therefore not surprising, that within another ten or twelve days, the next case will beak out either in your house or your neighbors and if it is not isolated or confined, the whole neighborhood will contract it.

The first symptoms are never exactly the same. Frequently a sneezing cold, nose bleeding, bronchial catarrh or conjunctivitis with lachrymation and burning of the eyes herald the onset. Soon a fever appears and rises to perhaps 100° F. It will decline and on the fourth day it may go as high as 103° F. It usually falls again as soon as the rash appears but if it remains high for more than three or four days after its first appearance, complications are likely to set in and energetic treatment must begin. Give the child Lachesis 10x to combat the septic development and apply flannels wrung out in a hot infusion of Wild Thyme repeatedly to the affected area. This will draw out internal toxins through the skin. Even when the disease takes its normal course, apply these hot packs to bring the rash out properly.

During the fever, give the child fruit juices, orange or grape, and carrot juice if the liver needs a tonic. If you have ready access to Yarrow, Marigold or Elderflowers, make an infusion of one of them and sweeten with honey.

Infectious diseases demand oral hygiene. For tiny children, wrap a clean cloth around your finger tip, dip it in diluted *Whey* concentrate and disinfect the gums with it as well as the mucous membranes and the tongue which in such cases is furred. For bigger children use a soft tooth brush. The following *homeopathic* remedies should be given as follows: Aconitum 3x or 4x, 5 drops every half hour. When perspiration has been induced and the temperature lowered, give less frequently.

Ferr. phos. 6x (for babies use 12x), 1 tablet every 1–2 hours.

Belladonna 4x: Use when the blood flushes to the head or with croup, conjunctivitis and ear complications. 5 drops every 2–3 hours.

Antimonium sulph. 2x or 3x, to be given when the fever subsides and no complications occur. It is to be given by itself, without additional medication, and it will suffice for completing the cure. In the beginning, give 1 tablet every 2 hours and reduce after 3 days to 2 tablets, three times daily.

Calcium complex preparation: Add 5 drops to fruit juice which should be the only liquid given while the fever lasts. This helps rid the kidneys of toxins.

Cuprum acet. 4x and Antimonium sulph. 3x: give alternately when a hacking or whooping cough seems to be coming on.

Coccus cacti 2x, while a most effective remedy for whooping cough is excellent for treating measles.

Constitutionally weak children who have inherited a disposition for tuberculosis and who have chronically swollen glands should be given the following prophylactic medicines:

Calc. phos. 3x alternated with 6x: 2 tablets, three times daily.

Ars. iod. 4x is indicated in thin children who grow fast; to be taken over a period of several months.

Kali. phos. 6x should be given in lung and bronchial complications.

Sulphur 4x should be given when, in spite of packs, the rash does not come out sufficiently.

When the disease has subsided, the child should not be allowed outside in the cold air. Especially in winter the child should be kept in bed for another week or in a warm, well ventilated room. This will guard against any complications.

MUMPS

This is another frequent but harmless childhood disease. It is chiefly the parotid glands that are attacked, but in the case of boys, the testicles may become affected also. Serious complications can ensue when the disease is contracted by a man in his best years. Improper treatment or insufficient care may lead to inflammation of the testicles and if the essential tissue is destroyed sterility will result.

The chief remedy for mumps is Mercurius solubilis 10x; 2–3 drops should be taken every two hours. Aconitum 4x and Belladonna 4x should be alternated every half hour while Whey-concentrate should be used as compresses for the calves of the legs. It is important that the compresses be applied only when the feet are warm. A hip-bath, the temperature of which should be gradually increased from 97° F to 110° F, is also excellent. After the bath the patient should be wrapped in warm blankets. Next, check the bowels. If they are not working properly Arabic plant essence can be given orally or be used as an enema. If the child complains of excessive pain, a warm compress can be applied locally – a few drops of Arnica or Marigold extract to the water will increase the effect. Gargling with a dilution of whey concentrate should not be neglected either.

An old remedy which has proved itself over an over again is hot *St. John's wort oil.* Saturate a cloth with the oil and apply locally. Alternatively the oil can be mixed to a paste consistency with potters clay then applied to the inflamed area and covered with a hot water bottle or heating pad. This will sooth and heal. To complete the cure, take Silica 12x, 1 tablet ever three hours.

COELIAC DISEASE

Coeliac disease is also known as Pancreatic infantilism or Herter's disease. It is characterized by a congenital inability to absorb fats which are split up. With careful diet up to the age of six, normal function may develop by excluding all fats. The treatment should follow along the lines of that used for intestinal catarrh and diarrhea in infants. The principal remedy is the extract of the Tormentil plant, of which 2 to 5 drops may be given spaced out during the day, three to five times. The dose will depend upon the age and the sensitivity of the infant. Start low at first and gradually increase until the stool appears to be of normal consistency. Warm hip-baths or warm abdominal packs prepared with Camomile or Horsetail infusions will prove to be a great help.

The diet should contain plenty of brown rice gruel or porridge to which has been added raw carrot juice. There is a concentrated carrot juice available that is convenient to use and all you need to add to the gruel is ½ to ¼ of a teaspoon. While the illness persists, for adults and children only gluten-free cereals are indicated, therefore rice is advisable in cases of Herter's disease and Multiple Sclerosis. The white flour products, semolina and similar deficiency foods are on the taboo list and under no circumstances should be given to the child. Potatoes steamed in their jackets, mashed and mixed with raw carrot juice are usually well tolerated, but other vegetables, excepting leeks, should not be given until the child is well again.

Among fruits, apples, raw and finely grated and mixed with mashed bananas are permissible. Blueberries can be served always, while grapefruit juice should not be given until the acute stage of the disease has passed. As far as drinks are concerned it has been found that acorn cocoa is beneficial as long as it is given in small quantities. The quantity of food eaten should be kept low. When the digestion has become somewhat normalized (this can be assessed from the consistency and color of the stool) the amount of food can gradually be stepped up. Too much in this case is worse than too little. Should any food cause a digestive disturbance, it should be left out of the diet.

The medicinal remedies and the acorn cocoa can gradually be withdrawn when conditions appear normal. Sometimes, with the return to normal eating, it is possible that a relapse may occur. This has to be dealt with directly by returning once more to the stricter diet. If you wish, add almond milk to the diet as it has proven very beneficial in cases of relapse.

If these suggestions are carried out faithfully and persever- ingly, a complete cure is quite possible. It is good to remember that due to deficient digestion, the food ingested will be only partly utilized and as a result there will be a lack of complete mineral absorption. It is therefore not to be wondered at that children thus afflicted are very prone to fractures of the bones. The disposition to these troubles can be reduced with a preparation of biological calcium. This will serve to replace what was not absorbed from food and act as a part of a supplementary diet.

SORE THROAT (Laryngitis, Tonsillitis, loss of voice, etc.)

It is a fact that incorrectly treated inflammation of the throat can have dangerous consequences that may permanently injure one's health. Careful and thorough treatment of the throat and tonsils will render bacterial toxins harmless and prevent them from spreading through the body. However, it is important to persevere and not stop as soon as the acute symptoms have passed.

The first measure to be taken at the sign of a sore throat is to paint the throat with concentrated whey so it may cut short the case of incipient tonsillitis. The whey will destroy the germs attacking the tonsils and its crevices. This condensed, natural lactic acid from whey has proved superior to the strongest chemical disinfectants and is free from the harmful properties the latter may possess. If this remedy is not handy, the root of the Burnet saxifrage (Pimpinella saxifraga) or the Imperial Masterwort (Imperatoria osthruthiom) fulfills the same purpose if you chew it. Mouth hygiene is so important that even the simplest remedy can be resorted to without loss of time. Gargle with salt water or suck a slice of lemon (unsweetened) for quick action.

In chronic cases the use of special equipment may be necessary. Dr. Roeder's Apparatus (piston-operated vacuum pump used in connection with the modern version of the Hyperaemisation cup can be connected with a special tonsil suction tube) will do much in restoring tonsils to normalcy. Whenever you suspect the beginning of tonsillitis, you should start immediately with a neck poultice, alternating pulped cabbage leaves with clay. Also take Lachesis 12x and a kidney tea prepared from Goldenrod. This will help eliminate the toxins absorbed by the infected tonsils.

The diet should contain a minimum of salt and protein. Sweating should be encouraged, any method of inducing perspiration will do as long as the patient can stand the procedure. Tonsillitis should be recognized for what it is, an infection that needs prompt attention. Many people do not realize how dangerous a sore throat can be. A mother writes: "My seventeen year old daughter had a bad *sore throat* eight weeks ago and she developed an inflammation of the middle ear from it." This is the sort of letter received all too frequently. Heart problems, pericarditis, nephritis, etc. can often be traced to a sore throat that has been neglected. This all goes to prove that the toxins resulting from tonsillitis are far from harmless and that this illness should receive far more attention than it is usually given. In case of tonsil infection, thorough local disinfection will prevent the formation and absorption of toxins and thus avoid later complications. And, to repeat, Whey concentrate can do this better than any other disinfectant. It is not only antiseptic but it also draws the blood to the surface where the strong effect of the whey is most needed. Internally one can combat the disease with a calcium preparation and Lachesis 12x.

If a cough or a catarrh follows the throat trouble, take syrup made from raw fir buds or the narrow leaved Plantain (Plantago lanc.) Kali iod. 4x – 1 tablet three times daily – and Imperatoria to complete the measures to successfully combat *tonsillitis.* When one realizes the simple methods that are at hand for treating this disease it is astonishing that precautionary measures have been so long neglected.

WHOOPING COUGH

Although whooping cough is considered by many to be a minor ailment it can have unpleasant side effects which, in themselves, can lead to some permanent damage. Because of this possibility it is good to give this disease especial attention. There are herbal and simple homeopathic remedies for it and parents should take the time beforehand to acquaint themselves with the most important ones. The herbal remedies may not shorten the course of the disease but can reduce the intensity of the attacks and make the child more comfortable.

First, the bacterial toxins have to be eliminated as in all infectious diseases and physical exhaustion has to be counteracted so as not to invite other complications. Often spasms will diminish after a few days without leaving any unpleasant aftereffects.

TREATMENT

There are many treatments, some of which will be more effective than others. Sometimes it will be necessary to give the little patient a biological calcium preparation and at the same time encourage the elimination of metabolic toxins through the kidneys. A fresh plant preparation consisting of Drosera, Thymus, Coccus cacti, Hedera helix is a remedy par excellent for the treatment of whooping cough and should always be handy where there are small children in the family. The homeopathic's Ipecacuanha 3x and Coccus cacti 3x are equally useful but, as soon as the coughing attacks have stopped, they can be gradually left off. In place of them, Pine bud syrup can be given for a period of time afterwards, as it is good to continue with some medication for a short time after the cure appears to be complete.

Chest compresses should never be forgotten in cases of whooping cough. They can be either a simple compress made from a hayflower infusion or in more severe cases an onion compress. A horseradish compress is more effective; even more so a mustard poultice. A correctly applied mustard poultice or mustard bath, has saved the life of many a child who had already turned blue from a severe case of bronchiolitis (inflammation and gradual blockage of the small air passages in the lungs) and who was frantically gasping for air. Take care that the skin is not exposed to the active workings of the mustard (mustard powder) for too long a period of time. A maximum reddening of the skin is desirable, but blisters should never be allowed to form. If the treatment is applied as described, children can be protected from serious harm.

INFANTILE PARALYSIS (POLIOMYELITIS)

Infantile paralysis is an extremely sinister disease. In actuality it is an illness that lasts only a short period of time. The causative virus is very active and contains strong toxins that in concentrated form can destroy nerve cells and lead to paralysis. The illness itself ordinarily lasts only about two to three weeks. What comes afterwards, paralysis, is the disease's aftermath. It is therefore absolutely necessary to treat the disease quickly. Delay is in no circumstance advisable. It is apparent, from reports reaching me, that it is necessary to remind laymen as well as professional people again and again of the fundamental rules governing the disease's treatment.

Only recently I heard from a father whose son was put in a hospital for observation because it was thought that he might have polio. The doctor in charge let day after day pass, without attempting any treatment, until the first signs of paralysis appeared in the lungs. The boy was placed immediately in an iron lung machine but died within a few weeks, although he had always been strong and a healthy child.

Famous physiotherapists, and above all, Sister Kenny, have proved that immediate treatment can save a life. It is beyond understanding how doctors can still accept the responsibility of delay. It is this very delay that enables the virus to destroy the nerve cells.

TREATMENT

As soon as the first symptoms become apparent it is of utmost importance that the patient should be made to sweat. Use a steam cabinet, tub baths of gradually increasing temperature, hot packs or whatever you choose; the important thing is to produce copious perspiration FAST. By this means much harm can be avoided and possibly the polio itself can be averted. If Sister Kenny's treatment had been given to the boy mentioned previously, he need not have lost his life.

However conservative one may be, it is irresponsible and unprofessional to ignore the excellent results obtained by new treatments of dangerous diseases, even if they are unorthodox in nature. The very first symptoms, and it does not matter whether the diagnosis has been confirmed or not, should galvanize us into action. First symptoms appear flu-like, i.e. excessive tiredness, headaches, aching limbs, lack of appetite, vomiting, etc. These symptoms are sufficient to warrant immediate treatment, the first of which is the inducement of perspiration. If it is discovered later that polio was not the illness in question, you may have gone to some unnecessary trouble. However, you will have no reason to regret it, for the measures taken are sure to have a beneficial effect on a more harmless illness as well.

There is a treatment for polio which sounds unusual but it has achieved remarkable results and for this reason alone it should be considered. Ask your butcher for a bull's testicle, grind it fine and transform it into a paste. Rub the paste into the spinal area several times a day. This external application of fresh hormones has yielded satisfactory results even in advanced stages of the disease. I, myself, have seen it work on patients who already had become paralyzed.

It is, of course, advantageous to assist these treatments medicinally and for this purpose it would be wise to give the plant extract Gelsemium 6x and a Calcium complex. Also, give Nux vomica 4x to counteract nausea. As to the diet, plenty of fruit is indicated so as not to overburden the digestive organs.

Never lose sight of the necessity to eliminate the toxins, not only through heavy sweating but also through the bowels and kidneys. These suggestions have proved themselves in practice and you will find them a reliable help.

Polio epidemics occur periodically and regionally. Hot and sultry weather seems to encourage the development of the virus, for the incidence of this disease is far greater in summer than in winter. In tropical countries it goes on all year round. Research specialists have found that a number of people, especially children, although immune to the disease themselves, nevertheless are carriers of the polio virus. Safe from it themselves, they unknowingly pass it on to unsuspecting victims. However, it is interesting to note that among primitive people very few cases of polio are found and this would lead to the conclusion that our advanced civilization predisposes us to this disease and undermines our resistance to it.

A deficient diet, living in overheated houses and in general, a more or less unnatural way of life, no doubt play their part in producing these effects. How should we protect ourselves from this dreaded affliction? In the same way we should protect ourselves from all infectious diseases: simple healthful living, natural food, plenty of fresh air, light and sunshine. Should a polio threat occur in your locality, paint your children's throats with Whey concentrate which is an excellent antiseptic, and since the virus attack is by way of the nose and mouth it will act as a barrier against it. One final word – the thought that cannot be stressed too strongly – should the infection have already gained entrance, remember, profuse sweating and good elimination of the bowels and kidneys may avert the worst.

INFLUENZA

In this 20th century we have seen the devastating effects of virus influenza which in 1918–1919 killed an estimated twenty million people and more recently under the name of Hong Kong and Russian flu has reached epidemic proportions in different parts of the world. Since its aftereffects can be very serious and because so many do not know what to do when it strikes, the following suggestions may be helpful. It is important that special consideration be given to this disease because negligence can result in a chronic liver condition as well as affect the kidneys, the pancreas or abdominal organs. It is also possible for the myocardium to be affected through conduction disturbances. Skin problems such as eczema may appear. Rheumatism can result in an improperly treated virus flu.

IMPORTANT POINTS IN THE TREATMENT OF INFLUENZA

At the onset of a virus flu we should carefully consider four main points, since they add up to a successful treatment.

1. In the first place we must make use of a physical treatment, through which we assist the body to excrete bacterial toxins. Simultaneously we must watch the condition of the heart, which must be given careful consideration during sweating cures. With this in mind, we may then induce the proper sweating through the use of compresses, a wet pack or a steam bath.

2. Of equal importance is the careful selection of herbal remedies, for these agents make possible an increased excretion through the kidneys and liver and can prevent irritation and inflammation. At the beginning of the flu make use of these helpful flu drops which consist of Bryonia D3, Aconitum D3, Baptisia, Lachesis D10 and Solidago. They have always proved effective in maintaining a milder course of the disease.

3. The question of diet is very important and, while fever is present, the patient should not eat any protein or fat. Going on a liquid juice diet for one or two days has proven to be very beneficial. Grapefruit, diluted blueberry, black currant, orange, grape, cranberry juice alternated with beet juice will be received as a blessing by the patient. The intake of fluids should be in much greater volume than normally to assist the body to fight the disease.

4. After the illness has passed, we must direct our attention to the after-treatment. Even though the acute symptoms have subsided, we should carry through with a physical therapy. Do not stop taking the excreting medication, even if the fever is no longer present. In this manner complete excretion of all bacterial toxins will be accomplished and will prevent their causing temporary or permanent damage elsewhere.

FURTHER OBSERVATIONS ON TREATMENT OF INFLUENZA

Under no circumstances should the fever be reduced with drugs. The reason for this has been given in other chapters. If the patient does not perspire in spite of the increased temperature, the sweating process should be assisted with hot water packs, as mentioned earlier, or with the use of hot Elder flower tea with lemon juice – drink as hot as possible. Goldenrod tea is an excellent stimulation for the kidneys, also.

If the patient is known to have a congenitally weak heart or, should the fever rise to an unusually high degree, give some heart tonic and fruit juice sweetened with honey or some grape sugar which strengthens the heart muscles in the same was as honey.

The body must be regularly cleansed with an infusion of thyme or juniper needles, even though the patient may perspire only moderately. Oral hygiene must be observed in all infectious diseases which means that the teeth and the tongue must be regularly cleansed while the throat should be treated by gargling with a whey concentrate.

Ordinary influenza will benefit from a homeopathic complex remedy, available through Homeopaths. In all infectious diseases, the lungs must work overtime in order to supply the metabolic processes with enough oxygen to burn up the toxins. The sick room should be aired frequently and a cool room is to be preferred to an overheated one. Provided the patient is well covered, it may be advisable to leave the windows open most of the time.

Whenever normal temperature is stabilized for a few days, serve raw fruit and bland foods with a vegetarian diet to follow. For health's sake it is better, as soon as possible, to restore the patient to a natural diet, doing this only when normal health has been re-established.

If you follow the foregoing suggestions, influenza can be quickly overcome and the long prostration and weakness that follows in its wake will be avoided. The lingering aftereffects which many times result from orthodox medical treatment, will be replaced by renewed vigor that bears witness to the fact that nature's own remedies have been successfully supplemented by our own intelligent cooperation.

THE BRAIN

This subject follows influenza because some types of the disease seem to affect the brain or the nervous system in general. When this happens Avena sativa and Acid phos. 4x will be of benefit. Stubborn cases may demand in addition Gelsemium 3x.

The brain is not only a marvelous organ but it is at the same time a great gift from the Creator to man. As a matter of fact, man could do nothing without it; he could not plan ahead, carry out or complete anything. For this gift he should be grateful every day of his life. If a person voluntarily fasts or suffers hunger and deprivation, and as a result loses a great deal of weight, the portion of his weight loss in the spinal cord and in the brain is hardly noticeable. The fact that everything else is affected first shows the importance of the brain as the originator for most processes of life. The walnut serves as a good model for comparison with the brain. The outer hard shell can be compared to the cranium. The nut itself illustrates the cerebrum, while the skin, which can be peeled off freshly picked nuts, may be compared to the membrane or meninx. Between the spinal cord and the brain lies the cerebellum which is the size of a small orange. The brain functions in a marvellous way. If one pictures the control room of a nuclear power plant, an ocean liner, or control panels of a modern jet plane, he can only begin to appreciate the operation of the brain. Everything that takes place, for example, on a plane trip, every change in direction, every fight against the elements, even the take-off and landing, is dictated by the control panel and nothing is done by the pilot without first consulting it, because the control panel is literally the brain of the plane.

In the case of a power plant, the generation of energy, which permits everything to function, comes either from dynamos or nuclear energy which provides the power. In case of failure, the control panel is consulted in order to locate the problem.

FROM IMAGE TO REALITY

It is the blood that supplies the brain with energy. If it contains all the necessary nutrient, nutritive salts and vitamins so that every brain cell receives proper nutrition, then everything will function properly. Not every one of the many million cells has its own function. Our brain is divided into work groups, which are called centers, and up to now more than twenty of these centers have been located. How an entire center can be put out of order is seen in the case of apoplexy, sudden loss of power to feel or think, caused by a brain injury. The attack usually occurs in the inner capsule and not the outer part of the brain, thus not in the cerebral cortex. If the vein on the right side of the inner capsule ruptures, the blood supply to the outer parts of the brain is cut off and the consequences appear on the left side of the body. This change is due to the fact that everything crosses over in the nervous system of the body. Whatever we sense on the right side is registered on the left side and vice versa. If the body is able to repair the damage the paralysis will subside and the ability to speak, which was lost, will return. If the speech center remains disturbed, while the center controlling the connecting ideas functions properly, then the person will find himself in the embarrassing situation of thinking properly, but expressing himself improperly. However, if he writes his thoughts on paper, that he wants to express verbally, this will not be the case.

DISADVANTAGEOUS CONSEQUENCES

If *blood pressure* is either too high or too low it will unfavorably influence the proper functioning of the brain. Dizzy spells or fainting for example may result from too much pressure or lack of blood flow, due to low *blood pressure*. Even though this single most important apparatus, the brain, is favorably located, protected by the cranium, accidents and concussions can cause much damage. Consider the many falls while skiing or engaging in other types of sports. How often does the head or brain suffer a severe concussion or blow without a visible change being noticeable. If the fall is severe enough to cause a tear in the cerebral membrane, the result will be a drainage of the cerebro-spinal fluids and the brain, heretofore practically weightless floating in fluid, will be grounded like a leaking ship. This exerts pressure on various brain centers. The person will feel nauseated, the metabolism center is affected and vomiting and possibly diarrhea will occur. The patient must lie still so that the tear may heal and the brain may once again float on the cerebro-spinal fluid as a repaired ship floats on the surface of the water.

Alcohol and *drugs* may influence the functioning of the brain to the extent that several centers are blocked from performing their normal functions while others are overburdened. Due to this fact the person may lose certain inhibitions and act and feel temporarily as he would not under normal circumstances. Continued and excessive use of alcohol and drugs may result in paresis, an incomplete paralysis that affects the ability to move but does not affect the ability to feel, sometimes called softening of the brain. Complete paralysis may follow especially due to the toxic effects of arsenic, mercury and other metalic toxins which impair and suppress certain processes of the brain and the central nervous system, as in the case of an advanced case of syphilis. The metalic toxins especially may remain inactive in the body for years and come to the surface in very tragic forms during old age.

Meningitis (brain fever) is another disease from which grave consequences can result. Precautions can be taken to prevent it by striving to keep the circulation in good condition. One of the most effective remedies is an extract of Purple Cone flower (Echinacea purpurea). Take 10 drops in some water 2–5 times daily. Dosage can be increased or decreased depending on the severity of the illness. The patient should be kept in a darkened room away from all noise since he will be very sensitive to both. *Meningitis* is a dangerous disease, not only because it can bring lasting damage to the body, but also because it might lead to death.

TAKING PRECAUTIONS

During our productive youthful years, as an indefatigably active person, one often neglects to think about the fact that his central nervous system and brain must still serve its purpose during the autumn of his life. If one desires to be alert and feel well during old age, he must make sure that the apparatus in the control room, the brain, is given more than the usual attention, especially in today's mad pace. How many of us short-change the brain by not getting proper rest and sleep. Fatigue is the great enemy of productivity and it robs us of our ability to reason accurately and utilize our brain power to the best advantage. It is impossible to stress too much the importance of sound and early sleep and let us make sure to help maintain our bodies at peak condition with the help of nutritious foods from natural sources and with proper exercise. By avoiding the poisons found in so many commercial foods and sticking to a natural food diet we will not only contribute to our overall state of health, but have rendered an incomparable service to our brain.

HYPOPHYSIS – THE PITUITARY GLAND

In the same way as a little invisible general commands a large army, or as the important man in the control tower directs and maneuvers jet planes entering and leaving an international airport, so the little gland the size of a dried pea bean serves the body. The *pituitary gland* or hypophysis, weighing only a few grams, was formerly regarded as a degenerated organ.

When, however, the news of its importance spread through the scientific world, and it was discovered that the anterior and posterior lobes produce completely different hormones, a whole new field opened up. Such a small gland has many vital functions to perform. In a way the pituitary gland controls the thyroid, the adrenal gland. Its function is undisputed in regards to the gonad, the organ in which reproductive cells develop, including the ovaries and testes. It has a leading position among the endocrine glands. Its direct link with the central nervous system, especially the area of the Hypothalamus has been the subject of much research since it appears that the pituitary gland influences all vital processes either directly or indirectly. It also appears that, together with the thymus gland, the pituitary determines growth. Since the entire development of the sexual glands and organs are controlled by the *pituitary*, a hermaphrodite's condition may be attributed to an improperly functioning or developed gland. A pregnancy could never run its course without the cooperation of the *pituitary*. The failure of the islets of Langerhans located in the pancreas not only contribute to the diabetic's ailment by producing insufficient insulin but, also, the malfunctioning of the anterior part of the *pituitary* is a contributing factor. No matter how much bile is produced by the liver, the fat metabolism suffers if not acted upon by the hormones produced by the pituitary glands. An abnormal change in blood pressure, too much or too little secretion of fluids, even the triggering of labor pains, depend on a normal function of the anterior part of the pituitary and its secretion of hormones.

Science has not succeeded yet in exploring to the fullest the complex hormone structure of this interesting little gland and this is the reason it is not able to produce these hormones synthetically. It is always a risk to prescribe medicine that has a direct effect on the pituitary, except in small homeopathic doses. Medicines can have a very bad effect or reaction on the patient depending on his sensitivity to the drugs they contain.

As a control center of paramount importance, the *pituitary* should be well cared for. Because of its important functions, it is well protected in an inaccessibly embedded part of the cranium. Taking generally good care of one's health by supplying the body with good nutrition, sleep, proper exercise and deep breathing habits will go a long way towards maintaining the pituitary in good operating condition. Even though we already know a great deal about this little gland, there are many of its secrets that have as yet to be revealed. The instrument panel of a giant jet plane is a complete mystery to the amateur, a radio receiver in a watch case is a technological marvel, and the accomplishments of a miniature calculator never ceases to evoke admiration, but what is contained in the bean sized gland surpasses everything that man has created by a thousand times. Knowing how intricate our body is made, we should have deep respect for it and the organs that function within it. The psalmist well expressed it when he wrote "I shall laud you because in a fear-inspiring way I am wonderfully made. Your works are wonderful, as my soul is very well aware."

THE TONGUE

Just as any one of the other organs the tongue is also a marvelous creation. The singular organization and structure of this muscular organ gives it a flexibility that no other organ in the body possesses. The *tongue*, by manipulating its muscle fibres, can change its shape from flat to broad, thin or thick. The most interesting feature in the structure of the *tongue* is its surface which, when greatly magnified, may be compared to the terrain of the moon. Every elevation and every little crater cavity is equipped with taste buds consisting of elongated cells that join to the sensory nerves. It is thought that four basic tastes are provided by the *tongue* as well as tastes in between. These are sweet, salt, sour and bitter. In these taste cavities mucous membranes are responsible for the presence of a small amount of fluid that enable a taste sensation upon dissolving the substance taken into the mouth.

SENSATIONS OF TASTE

Nerve cells which register the sensation of taste and transmit it to the brain are arranged in a bulb-like manner. The nerve ends may be compared to the roots, while the regulating reaction control represent the different layers of the bulb. Very fine hair like bundles of nerves register the stimuli. These nerve bulbs are called taste buds and an adult has about 3,000 of them. In a comparison with animals, especially the antelope who has 15 times as many taste buds as a human, man's taste sensation is not nearly as acute. If man had as many taste buds as most animals it would be much easier for him to detect or differentiate between poisonous food and healthy nourishing food. Thus animals are more capable than man in distinguishing what agrees with them and what does not.

We note also different taste zones on the *tongue*. If the tip of the tongue is dipped in honey, the sensation of sweetness is immediately apparent. A little further back on the periphery of the tongue the taste of salt is registered and even further back in the same periphery sourness is sensed, while zones registering bitter are found across the posterior section. The center part of the tongue is a neutral area as it does not register any sensation of taste. It is worth noting that the *tongue* is quite accurate as a test organ and this occurs through chemical reaction. Thus a winery is more likely to listen to its experienced connoisseur then to its chemist. This especially holds true in the grading of teas and coffees from different countries. Imagine what it would be like to have no sensation of taste. Certainly there would be no pleasure in eating or drinking, for everything would be tasteless and one would soon lose his appetite for food. Despite its small size, the *tongue* is endowed with many important functions, upon which depend much satisfaction and gratification.

OTHER CAPABILITIES OF THE TONGUE

Even though we know something about the anatomical structure and functions of the *tongue*, we have not yet exhausted its full extent of operations. One of its most important functions is communication. It can be considered the "voice" of the heart to which we may symbolically attribute the ability to feel, think and make decisions. This little organ thus may be a blessing or a curse for ourselves and others. From the Bible we learn that horses and ships are easier to maneuver and control than the tongue. Despite its small size the tongue can incite riots, start wars and bring great calamities on the whole human race. By means of gossip the tongue alienates dearest friends and creates enemies. Envy and hatred make use of this nimble little instrument in sending out its poisonous arrows. Slick as oil, the tongue obeys the voice of temptation, for the chosen victim cannot escape its devastating influence. Many a tongue cannot distinguish between "yes" and "no" thus readily posing a contradiction. Many may pour out the bitterness of the heart through the tongue and thus infect or poison others.

ABOUT THE BENEFICIAL USE OF THE TONGUE

Has the tongue been given the power to speak only in order to cause unhappiness? Certainly not. The apostle Paul reminded his fellow workers to consider everything lovable and well spoken of, for the contrary use of the tongue is the root of grief and vexation. Loving, heart-warming words of advice, admonition, consolation and encouragement should pass the lips, so that this little organ may truly become a blessing. But this can only be if the heart is properly conditioned, if it has the desire to lend a helping hand to the one in distress, and even to overcome hostile attitudes with humbleness of mind. In that case the tongue will become a dispenser of kindness and benevolence. Consider the influence of the tongue each spring when the birds sing for sheer joy as the warm weather ushers in nature's bounty and the soil begins to produce again life-giving foods. Man, too, has the ability to rejoice in song over the things that he has come to appreciate. But the tongue must learn something else. During time of distress, it must keep silent, for its indiscriminate use may cause the betrayal of a friend. Even a foolish man will be regarded as wise if he knows when to keep silent. This did not escape the notice of wise Solomon who in effect said: "Talking is silver, keeping silent though, gold." For many, keeping silent takes greater will power than talking. Is it not strange that such a little organ as the tongue serves such diverse purposes? It makes food and drinks appealing to us, it tells us when something is spoiled, and it helps us to enjoy the means of life. It has the power to express feeling and it can prove to be detrimental or beneficial to each and every one of us. Whether we use it as a positive or negative outlet for our feelings depends largely on the state of our hearts. That is why Solomon advises us to "safeguard the heart, out of it are the sources of life; and out of the abundance of the heart the mouth speaks".

THE TEAR DUCTS

Is it not an ingenious arrangement, in the case of too much emotional stress, that the tear ducts serve as a valve to lessen the inner pressure? How unbearable it would be, even for a child, if it could not release its emotions by crying when a toy broke or whenever some equally frustrating thing happened. It is truly a safety valve that helps overcome emotional stress.

In addition to the excretion of tears when crying, the *tear ducts,* which are located in the upper outer part of the corner of the eye, embedded in a little pocket of the eye socket, have yet another function to fulfill. The tears must keep the conjunctiva and the cornea moist in order to prevent their drying out and bacteria, and other foreign objects, are washed away by the tears.

Even though inflammation of the tear glands occur rather seldom, we often observe the inflammation of the channel which opens into the nose and of the lachrymal sack. If this inflammation is not given immediate attention with herbal packs of Camomile and Eyebright (Euphrasia officinalis) the result may be chronic inflammations or even the formation of abscesses from bacteria. The flushing of the eye with warm milk or Kaslikraut water is a rapid cure for simple inflammation. For those who must work in a dusty environment it is recommended to cleanse the area of the eye with the lids closed by wiping them with cotton soaked in echinacea extract. This prevents dust, dirt and bacteria from entering the eye itself. If the *tear duct* is clogged, it will be necessary to see a doctor in order to have it punctured. If the eyes tend to be encrusted in the morning upon awakening, this indicates a metabolic disorder, which must be treated immediately. It is also wise to refrain from straining the eyes when there is insufficient illumination to read by. Like the rest of the body the eyes need rest at night because they work hard during our waking hours. Even though the eyes are very precious to us, we often neglect to regard them as an indispensible gift and give them the care they deserve. The eyes, amongst the other wonders of creation, are a true miracle and the tear ducts, despite their negligible size and apparent unimportance, are a convincing symbol of a predetermined aid to smooth the unconscious processes of our daily existence.

THE NOSE

Our respiratory organs comprise the nose, the trachea and the lungs. Each of these organs have a very important function, and only a working correlation between them assures a harmless exchange of gases. Instead of being supported by bones, the nose has a built-in cartilage plate. Bone would be too brittle and the danger of breaking too great, especially if one should fall on his nose. For those participating in various sport activities the nose cou d suffer great damage if the cartilage walls were not flexible. To what extent the beauty of the face depends on the shape of the nose becomes evident after a serious accident when the nose is crushed or deformed. Fortunately today, it presents no problem because a mishap of this sort can be easily corrected by plastic surgery.

THE FUNCTION OF THE NOSE

The proper functioning of the nose is of paramount importance to good health. Perhaps not everyone is aware of the fact that the nose serves as a temperature regulator or an "air conditioning unit." If it is very cold outside this mechanism in the *nose* warms the air that we breathe into the lungs and, vice versa, if the air is very hot, a cooling system is activated to make the climate more bearable. Furthermore, the *nose* regulates the intake of too dry or too humid air. Miraculously planned, to the smallest detail, are all these divine provisions and it is indeed astonishing to hear people deny the existence of an omnipotent Creator, despite the many visible testimonies of divine wisdom and creative power. It is only He, who is capable of creating something out of nothing, for only he has access to all his own laws. But these laws cannot become operative by their own powers, neither can they be attributed to mere chance. Let us now see to what extent even a small organ like the *nose* may serve as proof of the above.

First of all, it is a marvelous arrangement that permits the mucous membranes to function in such a way that they keep dust and bacteria from entering the body. We should be careful not to substitute mouth breathing for nose breathing as the nose functions as a screening device protecting us from infections and colds, which are a definite threat to the throat, the bronchial passages and the lungs.

It is interesting to note that the nostrils react to pleasant or unpleasant odors by a simple contraction or dilation of the walls, thus increasing or decreasing the flow of air. Strangely enough the nostrils also react to cold feet, in which case the walls contract, become cold and dry and thus cause the glands to cease to function. As a consequence neither dust nor bacteria are filtered out, which results eventually in a cold followed by a runny nose. Soon the head and the chest are congested. If the mucous membranes function properly they are able to destroy all germs entering through the nose; that is why it is absolutely necessary to cultivate the habit of breathing through the nose at all times.

CORRECTIVE MEASURES
FOR VARIOUS NOSE DISEASES

If one suffers frequently from head colds, it is advisable to inhale from time to time a calcium complex preparation in the form of powder. It is also beneficial to lubricate the nasal passages regularly with a cream containing lanolin. Timely applications may even prevent a head cold from progressing beyond the initial stage. As a rule, when the nose runs freely, we no longer breathe through the nose. Enlarged adenoids may also restrict the proper intake of air through the nose. Even though they are non-malignant growths, their presence can be very annoying. The only effective cure for these growths is Marum verum; failing this, or should they not yield to treatment, surgery would be indicated. Even more bothersome than adenoids is Ozena which is associated with an offensive smelling discharge from the nose. A soothing relief is obtained by snuffing or drawing in of a salt solution containing sea salt to which has been added calcium powder or the salt solution followed by the powder. As an internal treatment, Kal. jod. D 4 and Mercurius solub. D 4 has proven helpful. In the spring often inflammation of the mucous membranes occur and the oral intake of Echinacea extract brings about relief. A more speedy effect may be obtained by soaking a cotton swab stick in a solution of Echinacea extract and swabbing the nostrils. If sores or scales should develop on the inner walls of the nose, apply lanolin cream which will have an immediate healing effect.

A watery discharge of the nose, due to a cold, can be easily stopped. Cut a slice of fresh onion and dip it into a glass of water for a few minutes. Remove, and drink the water in small sips over a prolonged period of time. This will surely cure your sniffles.

A pussy or sticky discharge resulting from an inflammation of the mucous membranes may be cured by slowly drinking a glass of hot water to which has been added 5 drops of iodine. A person allergic to iodine may obtain the same result by substituting 5 drops of camphor instead of the iodine. Again, we would like to emphasize that Echinacea extract taken internally and used externally will bring sure relief.

An inflammation of the sinus passages may cause a great deal of pain. Here again, remedies such as Hydragyrum sulfuratum rubrum D 3 and calcium sulf. D 4 bring speedy relief. With the help of these remedies the rapidly forming pus can be drained and relief can be restored quickly. It is important to bring about immediate relief in order to prevent a chronic inflammation of the sinuses, since this affliction, if not immediately treated may reach a stage where it will stubbornly resist any treatment.

CONSEQUENCES OF INFECTIOUS DISEASES

Toxins, which as a result of *infectious disease,* remain in the system, must be eliminated as they lead only to future ill health. Wrongly treated or neglected *mumps* can lead to an inflammation of the pancreas later on. Suppressed *scarlet fever* may reassert itself in the form of an inflammation of the middle ear. Improperly cared for *tonsillitis* can give rise to inflammation of the heart muscle (Myocarditis) or the endocardium, which in turn, causes valvular defects. The kidneys can suffer too and articular *rheumatism* as well as many other diseases are often the result of toxic infiltrations from diseased tonsils. It is, therefore, important to ensure recuperation through destruction and disposal of the poisons:

1. *SKIN:* Encourage perspiration by applying hot packs, taking hot showers.

2. *KIDNEYS:* Eliminate toxins from the bloodstream by activating the kidneys with Goldenrod or Parsley tea. Also apply Onion poultices and take a kidney medicine.

3. *BOWELS:* Fever tends to dry up the bowels. Simple natural remedies like Linseed tea, Psyllium seeds, Senna pods, soaked figs and prunes, Fruit juice fasting, and enemas will take care that no accumulation and stagnation of toxic fecal matter takes place.

Protein foods, especially of animal origin are always contraindicated in infectious diseases and raw fruit and vegetable juices provide excellent treatment while the fever lasts. Pay close attention to the three points enumerated above to avoid complications that may result from an ineptly treated infectious disease.

POLYARTHRITIS

Polyarthritis belongs to the category of rheumatic-arthritic diseases and it imposes by far the greatest financial burden upon the social welfare and health institutions of the nations. Year in and year out great sums of money are expended in an effort to help millions who suffer from this terrible disease! In my practice I treat many patients for multiple arthritis and I would like to write a few words on this subject.

THE NATURE OF THE DISEASE

Academic argumentation about the real cause of this illness still persists. It is very possible that a microorganism or any of a number of toxins are responsible for it. More often than not, we find in association with arthritis some local focal point which discharges a constant stream of toxins into the blood. The quantity can be very small indeed and the person may remain unaware of the necessity to do something about it, until the body finally reacts at long last with some serious disease. As a rule, various changes take place in the blood and the German and Swiss doctors von Brehmer and Isel have observed some virus in the course of their investigation into this disease. However, no definite solution or explanation has ever been advanced in connection with its etiology.

I have observed that patients suffering from *polyarthritis* usually have a family history of rheumatism in some form or other. There appears to be a definite disposition to the disease and where there is predisposition, the person may be unfortunate enough to get it, even though his way of life and the diet he follows may be precisely the same as another who has not a trace of any form of rheumatism.

Not everyone having chronically suppurating tonsils or teeth sockets will be afflicted with arthritis. You may come down with some kidney problems or some heart affliction while another one is likely to find that his blood vessels harden and arteriosclerosis develops. Someone else may get away with a worse mode of living than we ourselves may be guilty of and yet remain free from this crippling terror. You see, it very much depends upon this disposition mentioned before.

The mysterious thing about the disease is that, without any apparent cause, the joints in any part of the body can become afflicted. The heart too may be affected. There are times when the ailment feels as though it were improving because of a loosening up of the joints and the great relief felt. Then, suddenly, for some inexplicable reason, there is a relapse and a worsening of the condition. These relapses usually occur during the cold seasons, in late autumn and in the wintertime, and so it is that a warm dry summer very often encourages what appears to be a real improvement.

THE REMEDIES OF OFFICIAL MEDICINE

Official medicine has not been able up until now to find any real satisfactory remedy, although the pharmacies and drug stores are overflowing with rheumatic cures. For the most part, the disease was, and still is, treated with salicylic acid preparations. It was thought in recent years that at long last a specific for a hypothetical case had been found, but these hopes were soon shattered. The duration of the disease was hardly shortened and heart complications began to appear as frequently as before. It is now admitted that the salicylic acid preparations merely act as a palliative. It lessens the pain and relieves the inflammation of the joints but not without unpleasant side effects. Gastric troubles follow, head noises begin to make life miserable and the seemingly unimportant dizziness assumes proportions that lead one to believe the patient is drunk. These are additional symptoms brought on by medication that the body has to overcome. Aspirin and similar salicylic preparations are easy to take but they are really not so "effective" (and damaging!) as pure salicylic acid.

Then Schottmueller came along and introduced Pyramidon to combat *Polyarthritis* and what happened? This drug seemed to have even worse effects on the general well-being of some patients. The formation of red and white blood corpuscles was prevented, which gave rise to general anemia, resulting in death for some patients. Sulfanilamides were indicated for the primary infection, not for already established arthritis.

CORTISONE

The great need for a cure seemed to have been supplied by the discovery of cortisone, a hormone derived from the suprarenal capsule and it was acclaimed as the wonder cure. Such enthusiasm about a new remedy is frequent but when it is found not to justify the faith placed in it, it is quickly forgotten.

The reason for the employment of cortisone was based on a theory put forward by a Canadian scientist named Selye. He maintained that the cause of arthritis was to be found in the normal defense mechanism of the body and that cortisone prevents this mechanism from becoming active. According to him, this should cure the disease. When it is administered, pains and inflammations fade away, but what happened? As soon as its action is exhausted and no further dose is given, the old state of affairs returns. Apart from those who have died during treatment, it is known that animal experiments have shown that prolonged medication with *cortisone* tends to atrophy the suprarenal cortex. If the system is given a substance which it should produce itself then the organ which normally does so will degenerate because it has become superfluous. When the medication is later withheld, the atrophied organ will no longer be able to resume its normal function and supply the body with its needs. This will in turn endanger the life of the patient. The same thing applies to the muscles. If they are not exercised they will grow weak and flabby. We have the same evidence of such a thing happening in the case of diabetes. The doctor will admit without argument that insulin is a help but not a cure. Part of the pancreas, the part that actually produces insulin, begins to degenerate if too much of the medication is given. For this reason, a conscientious doctor will prescribe the absolute minimum dosage necessary. The body of a diabetic needs insulin, but not in such quantities that the pancreas is discouraged from making its own. It is obvious that the treatment which produces results without the need for insulin is to be preferred at all times.

HORMONE PRODUCT ACTH

For some time, the American product ACTH has been on the market. It is a hormone produced by the pituitary gland, and in some ways its effect is the same or similar to cortisone. In this case, however, the body is not given the suprarenal hormone direct, but is stimulated by a different hormone to manufacture its own within the suprarenal capsule. Far from degenerating, it is now being overstimulated and grows much larger. The effect of this medicine is not so sudden as that of cortisone, for the suprarenal capsule must be activated first by ACTH to produce a sufficiently high hormone level in the blood to ensure freedom from pain. When administration ceases, no such harmful consequences will be experienced as with cortisone, because ACTH preserves the function of the suprarenal gland. But the question arises: Have we not merely carried the catastrophic effect of cell degeneration one step further? Degenerative changes now take place in the pituitary gland which normally produces ACTH for the body. Since this gland holds a key position in the system's economy (actually it manufactures a considerable number of different hormones) hormone production is thrown out of balance and the resulting troubles may be more difficult to control than arthritis itself. As far as hormone preparations are concerned, however spectacular their effects may be, one must always remember that only one side of the coin is seen at a time, and the other side may look very different indeed. I once had the opportunity to discuss these points with a doctor who had given lectures on this subject and he was frank to admit that he would not use these remedies on himself. There is no denying that there may be justification for their use in certain desperate cases, but let the doctor and patient alike consider very carefully what side effects they might produce and what the ultimate rather than the immediate effect might be. Through careful analysis and patient observations I have made in these matters, I have been led to conclude that all hormone and organ preparations should be viewed with the utmost caution and reserve before prescribing them.

COMBINATION TREATMENT FOR ARTHRITIS

Very good results can be achieved in the treatment of Polyarthritis by careful dieting and natural remedies and by taking the Fango cure (Fango is a natural Italian clay found in the Abano and Montegrotto spas).

The diet should be absolutely natural and similar to the one for cancer and gout. The conclusion about diet is supported by the fact that these diseases do not exist among the more primitive people. It must be our faulty way of eating and living that accounts for the problems that we bring upon ourselves, willfully or unwillfully but, nevertheless, it exists in abundance among the more advanced civilization. Unfortunately this opinion is not widespread and even many doctors who themselves are overstuffed, do not seem to consider diet in the treatment of arthritic patients. A patient came to me and said that her previous doctor treated her but never once mentioned any change of her diet. He told her that diet did not play any part in the treatment of arthritis and that she could eat anything she wanted. Such advice seriously brings into doubt the professional capacity of a doctor who obviously has not kept up with his "homework". He is behind the times and needs a refresher course from time to time to bring him up-to-date with what is occurring in the field of health therapy. Nutritional therapy has yielded convincing proof of the importance of proper diet in treating most ailments and a doctor should not overlook their benefits especially when they can contribute so much to his patient's welfare. For my own part, I am firmly convinced that there is no illness in which proper diet does not play a part. It should be given serious consideration even if it only assumes an minor role in a supporting function.

NATURAL REMEDIES

Goldenrod mixed with other plant extracts is excellent for the kidneys and activates renal elimination. Another fresh plant extract also is good – it contains Petasites hybrid., Polygonum avic., Betula, and Viscum album. To remedy circulation disturbance and venous congestions a mixture of Yarrow, Arnica and St. John's wort oil would be indicated for external massage. Echinacea will subdue and relieve inflammatory conditions. A preparation of the well known Butterbur/Mistletoe combination will make great improvements possible, as well as help to regenerate affected tissues.

Should the breathing be restricted in any way you will find that a preparation using Usnea as a base will help considerably. The remedy is prepared from larch moss and if used in conjunction with external applications of mucilaginous Comfrey root, you will obtain a great deal of relief.

It will be advantageous to alternate with a liniment Camphor and an extract form Eucalyptus and the fresh leaves of Poison Ivy, Rhus toxicodendron, if you are not allergic to it. Packs made up with clay and pulped cabbage leaves are also very good and good results have been obtained from them. To obtain best results alternate them; one night clay and the next night cabbage pack. It has been found that an application of grated carrots is effective.

Biological injections will overcome pain even faster. Homeopathic remedies of comparative low potencies are injected subcutaneously and quickly take effect. Formic acid 12x, Lachesis 20x, Urtica 6x (Nettles), all have proven their worth in this connection. Mistletoe preparations lend additional support to the curative actions of these medicines.

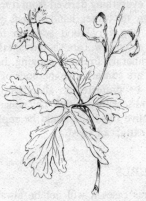

Celandine (Chelidonium majus)

DIET

Follow the diet given under the heading "Natural Foods." Its preparation should be attempted from unadulterated foods only. A vegetarian diet, a large portion of which should be eaten raw, offers by far, the greatest curative diet. Meat and other animal protein foods, with the exception of curd cheese, are according to my experience, detrimental in obtaining good results. If you cannot abstain from meat altogether, it is permissible to take a little beef or veal, but pork, sausages and tinned meats should be completely passed by. Caution should be exercised in regards to fat; they should be of vegetable origin, cold pressed and, naturally, unrefined. Heat will depreciate their health value and for this reason all vegetable fats such as olive, sunflower, poppy, safflower, sesame, coconut, wheat germ and peanut oils should be used in their raw state.

For sweetening, honey (extracted from the comb unheated), grapesugar, sultanas (seedless raisins), or currants must take the place of refined white sugar. The dried fruits can be put through a mincer for ease of use. Raw Rosehip puree prepared with turbinado or fruit sugar fructose is an excellent substitute for jams.

White flour and everything derived from it must be scrupulously avoided. On the other hand, wheat germ taken in limited quantities is a very good addition to the diet. If vegetables are not eaten raw, care should be taken in cooking to preserve their minerals. Pressure cooking, baking and casserole preparation are conservative methods of cooking vegetables and should be preferred to all other methods. Raw salads are very good seasoned with Whey concentrate or with lemon juice and olive oil. Salt should be replaced by fresh kitchen herbs and extract of yeast.

FANGO MUD CURES

In particular serious cases it will not be always possible to avoid the Fango cure, even though all the above suggestions have been observed. Where professors and doctors of Swiss clinics have been hard put to find some satisfactory treatment for their patients, the Fango cure in conjunction with biological treatment has proven most beneficial. Patients who had difficulty in hardly getting around became quite capable of taking up their normal work once more. Should a Fango cure in Abano or Montegrotto become necessary, the financial sacrifice it may entail will be well worthwhile.

If you combine this treatment with the other three already mentioned, under "Arthritis", you will not only favorably influence the cure but at the same time insure it of being permanent. Take the biological remedies with you so you can use them in limited amounts. When taking the cure be careful not to force things. After four or five treatments take a day off and have a bath in the hot springs. Turkish baths are also available in these spas and it would be a good idea to have one turn at each during the Fango treatment. This may prove to be rather strenuous for some people but it will be easier than having to put up with the dreadful consequences of maltreated arthritis.

FURTHER ADVICE ON GETTING WELL AGAIN

If you wish to regain your health to the fullest extent possible, you will have to pay special attention to nature in every way and follow the advice already given. This implies at the same time that you should be aware of the many patent medicines that are alleged to either cure or improve your condition. For a permanent cure, more is required also than just a few injections. It demands much more endurance from both the patient and the doctor. The latter must pay careful attention to the patient's reaction during the various treatments and he will be put to more trouble than normally. The path to recovery may be steep and stony but the important thing is not its difficulty, but the very fact that a way out exists and this will come as a consolation to many.

Those who want to consolidate their cure should continue the natural diet and from time to time take again the remedies previously recommended. This will prevent the trouble from flaring up again. Those who can afford it will want to repeat the Fango cure yearly, at the same time taking the other treatments. This will keep the dreaded arthritis disease at bay and insure your working capacity for many years. Remember there are no magic drugs that will effect a cure and do not expect overnight miracles from plant extracts or baths or Fango cures. It requires patience and persistence to win the battle against this crippling disease.

COLDS AND CATARRHS
DURING CHANGE OF SEASONS

It is not unusual to hear complaints of *colds* when seasonal changes occur. Most people accept them as unavoidable and do nothing about it. Strangely enough it is the women who do least to avoid them. If a woman lives in a temperate climate where winter comes, she should put her vanity aside and forget fashion for the duration, adapting her clothing to the climate. Unfortunately it is difficult to convince a woman to trade her sheer silk stocking for something more practical and healthful such as warm knitted wool stockings.

The seasonal change is the most difficult time for the body for it has accustomed itself, for example, to the warmth of summer and if sudden cold weather occurs the body is unprepared for it. That is where good common sense comes in. We must clothe the body with whatever is appropriate for the weather. Most important of all, keep the feet warm if you wish to discourage colds. It is an accepted fact that warm feet and a cool head are the necessary foundations for good health. The feet are the indicators of the general warmth of the body and as long as they are warm our body will be prevented from getting chilled. People in sedentary occupations suffer to a much greater extent from cold feet because their work does not allow much activity and movement. Exercise improves circulation and keeps one warm. Sluggish circulation makes you feel cold and even overheated rooms do not seem to be warm enough. Overheating does not make up for the lack of exercise and unless the feet are covered with warm stockings and adequate shoes, they will be cold. If you leave an over-heated room inadequately clothed and go out into the cool damp air, the body's vital functions will be lowered and head colds, catarrhs and even pneumonia may result from it.

Never sit down in the morning without having taken some good exercise previously. Do not despise the idea of making your own bed or tidying up your room in the morning or of walking to your work if possible instead of using your car, or of walking to the store instead of hopping in the car. Exercise will increase your circulation, will warm you up, will make you appreciate the warmth of your room afterwards, more than if you enter it already shivering. Brain work is easier after strenuous exercise. The deep breathing made necessary by hard physical work promotes a good circulation and does many other good things for you. You can also encourage circulation by giving yourself a good brush massage in the shower and by deep breathing in front of an open window. Deep breathing purifies the lungs, saturates them with oxygen. This is so important in discouraging the condition favorable to "catching" cold. Where a disposition for the latter exists, eat plenty of calcium containing foods and take a biological calcium preparation in addition. The veins should not be overlooked so that circulation remains unimpaired by physical obstructions such as hardened and narrowed channels through which it must find its way. Heed this advice and you will acquire more resistance to the common cold and similar afflictions.

HOW TO RESIST DISEASE BY TAKING NATURAL ANTIBIOTICS

It is wellknown that those who have anything in the nature of a liver disorder are prone to succumb to all kinds of infectious diseases. Because of this disorder they lack those elements in their constitutional makeup which supplies immunity against various diseases. Effective resistance can be put up, in spite of such weakness, if natural antibiotics are taken.

It is impossible to avoid every sort of infection because we are exposed to it constantly by the food that we eat and the air that we breathe. City air especially is teeming with germs and an examination of one cubic centimeter under a microscope will reveal thousands of germs, spores and bacteria. Insects, such as flies and mosquitoes, are the best known carriers. So even with the utmost care and caution, it is difficult to escape from all the influences, but we can make certain that our bodies resist them. There are certain plants, especially the herbs, which contain etheric oils. Among them are the ordinary culinary herbs that possess antibiotic properties and these are easily available for our use.

THE EFFICACY OF VARIOUS ANTIBIOTICS

The discovery of such antibiotics as Penicillin, Streptomycin, Auromycin and similar preparations which have come into the market has provided us with very potent agencies against bacterial infection and in the case of serious tropical diseases they have been instrumental in saving many lives. Unfortunately, they are being used too frequently for treatment of minor infections and inflammations which very well could be dealt with by simpler means. Too often and too frequent dosing with these antibiotics constitutes a danger which should not be overlooked. In the first place, the body accustoms itself to these substances and gradually fails to react to them in the expected manner. Secondly, the germs for which they are given, develop progressive immunity against them until, finally, the remedy proves useless in its fight against them. The third danger is the harm to the intestinal flora that continued use of antibiotics exerts. As a result of their indiscriminate use digestive disorders are more than likely to result.

Just as certain bacteria in the intestines are necessary for proper digestion and assimilation of food, so plants need certain bacteria to enable them to flourish as they should. For instance, it is impossible to reap a good soya bean harvest if the soil has not been inoculated with the bacteria symbiotically associated with it, or unless the beans have been grown in that particular soil before. No forest could grow without bacteria either. A similar state of affairs exists in the digestive system. That is the reason why *Yogurt* is particularly recommended for all intestinal troubles. It encourages the physiologically normal flora, while it hinders the abnormal one (the putrefactive type) in its development. *Yogurt* is made with a special strain of lactic acid bacilli and these are effective in keeping our insides clean and wholesome by encouraging the growth of the right kind of intestinal flora. If we use some of the various antibiotics previously mentioned, we must expect that they will damage this flora, for it so happens that our best friends in the bacteria world are also the most sensitive to drugs. No wonder then that inflammation of the digestive tract frequently follows the administration of these double-edged remedies. Once the normal barrier against disease germs, namely the "health germ barrier", is damaged the former will gain entrance much more easily than otherwise. Even more conservative methods may then fail, and in a case of a grave disorder, dire consequences may result.

NATURAL ANTIBIOTICS

Those who suffer from liver problems, tuberculosis or cancer have little resistance to disease and the protection offered by antibiotics to their weakened constitution becomes a matter of life and death for them.

As far back as 25 years ago I made some interesting experiments with *horseradish, watercress, gardencress* and even *nasturtiums.* I observed that those who ate these regularly became more resistant to diseases, especially *catarrhs* and infections. At that time, I can remember how some people laughed at the idea of nasturtiums especially having any remedial value as food. It was not known that these particular plants could have such effects. Ignoring the doubting "Thomases" I continued my observations. Having discovered their curative properties, I used them for the benefit of my patients even though I could not offer any scientific explanation for their therapeutic effect. However, modern medicine now recognizes that these observations were not without value and the research work of Dr. Winter, a medical scientist of Cologne, has once and for all time established, for example, the value of *nasturtiums* as an article of diet. The thought of mixing them into a salad no longer seems strange or ridiculous.

Observations showed that the extract from the nasturtium plant was effective in killing insect pests when sprayed upon the afflicted plants. Scientific investigation has proved my contention that it contains substances capable of achieving spectacular results. However, it may very well be that it is not the antibiotic properties of these plants that are responsible for it; they may contain substances with which science is not acquainted and which may prove to be far superior in curative value than those already known to us.

It is not only the nasturtiums that have yielded such valuable results. The common *watercress,* especially the kind that grows along the course of the mountain streams in the Engadine valley of Switzerland, is just as good as nasturtiums. Eat this cress regularly and soon you will acquire immunity to *colds, catarrhs* and infectious diseases. Whether the cultivated watercress produced commercially to a large extent with the help of artificial fertilizers has the same value may be questionable. It is reasonable to assume that the wild growing kind is far superior to the cultivated one.

I have made equally important observations in connection with a little known lichen which grows on larch trees. During my skiing tours I frequently noticed that deer and chamois devoured all the *lichen (Usnea)* within their reach. Investigation has shown that lichen contains considerable amount of carbohydrates. The animals make good use of its food value and, incidentally, of its antibiotic properties which makes them resistant to disease. There is no doubt that *Usnea* clears up *catarrh*. I have seen this confirmed repeatedly. A few times after starting out on a tour I developed a sore throat and a runny nose. As I went along I chewed *Usnea* and found that by the time I arrived home again my cold had disappeared. Such valuable experience led me to investigate this primitive lichen and now I am convinced that its extract has excellent prophylactic properties. If you have a tendency to contract *catarrh* or *colds* try taking this regularly for it is an excellent preventative. Which brings up the question: Why take the risk of using manufactured antibiotics when nature supplies effective and harmless ones? *Lichen* is not likely to have an adverse effect on the intestinal flora and the body will not have to accustom itself to it as it would have to in the case of synthetic drugs. The regular ingestion of salads made from the aforementioned plants can be heartily recommended to everyone, especially cancer patients. Sandwiches can be made from them. Carrot salad can be "fortified" with finely grated horseradish, or the juices can be extracted and taken in small quantities. When your health has been restored and you can once more think of climbing high mountains, do not forget to look for the larch moss. You'll find it on the bark of the larch tree at an elevation of about 5,000 feet. Chew it while you enjoy your hiking.

Another plant which has the same potent effect is Petasites hybridus, the common *Butterbur*. It is of special importance to those suffering from cell degeneration. It should be taken in the form of a preparation as it is too strong to be used in salads. Butterbur is a rather rare plant, usually found near streams in mountain districts. In order to enable everyone to benefit from this plant, it can be prepared along with other plants as a tincture. The mixture may consist of equal parts of the following:

> Petasites officinalis (Butterbur)
> Tropaeolum majus (Nasturtium)
> Cochlearia armoracia (Horseradish)

Nasturtium off. (Watercress)
Lepidium sativum (Gardencress)

Similar ingredients are added to herbal salt, after evaporating sea water. However, foods should be flavored with it after cooking as the heat destroys its antibiotic properties.

THE VALUE OF RAW FOOD

Quite a few of those who once mocked the idea of eating "rabbit food" (raw food) are now beginning to realize that there may be, after all, something to it. The antibiotic properties of food, their vitamin and mineral content and probably many other unknown properties are preserved in a raw food, but are destroyed in cooked food. For the body to receive all the protective substances it needs, everyone should take a certain amount of fresh raw vegetables or fruit and perhaps even cereals daily to effectively resist disease. To comply with this necessity, those who possess a garden should make sure to plant *gardencress, watercress, Nasturtiums* and *horseradish*. Serve these plants finely chopped up in salads, stews, soups or mix with cottage cheese or yogurt or make up a sandwich paste and spread it on whole wheat bread. All who advocate health from herbs and natural foods, especially raw foods, may justify their convictions by the time honored German proverb: "Why seek afar when the good lies so near"!

HEALTH CULTURE –
THE BEST PROPHYLACTIC
AGAINST RESPIRATORY DISEASES –
VARIOUS CAUSES

In my travels I encountered a great deal of *tuberculosis* even in lands which had the healthiest climate. This was particularly true of Greece, a country with an abundance of sun but one which had to fight this disease. In Holland too and in many of the small islands people suffer from lung disorders. Doctors are probably right in blaming the climate of the low lying countries, although there are other factors which include a one sided diet of fish. It is, of course, by no means necessary to have one's lungs affected just because of living in lowlands. Anyone who is sufficiently informed about the cause of the disease can take care to avoid it and thus prevent trouble from starting. This is the wiser course than to cure an already established disease. The following observations can therefore serve those who are well and they will help the less fortunate to improve and even cure their condition.

In the first place, *diet*, as usual, is of the utmost importance. This has been proved by experience gained in every part of the world. People living in the healthiest mountain regions, where others go to be cured, may contract this respiratory disease. Some time ago I met the caretaker of a mountain hut who had somehow managed to get tuberculosis in spite of the fact that he had spent whole winters at a height of over 6,000 feet. The cause was obvious. His diet consisted of too much protein, too much canned foods and too many refined foods such as white flour and white sugar. The bad air in the hut also contributed to his illness; the many skis had to be waxed and the wax was melted by propane fuel adding to the poison already in the stale air. The air was stale because the windows were never opened in the mistaken idea that this would save fuel. Fresh air is an absolute necessity for good health. Some sort of immunization must be resorted to if we are to resist disease for we cannot avoid coming in contact with infection. Research specialists are probably correct in their assertion that it is unusual to find a person in Europe who, at one time or another, has not had a tubercular infection. If one's health has been poor, the infection can easily acquire a strong foothold in the body and be most difficult to dislodge.

Prevention is better than cure and the best prevention is the cultivation of health. Health culture consists of light, fresh air, sunshine, exercise and proper food, to mention but a few of the factors that will contribute in rendering us immune to disease.

AN APPROPRIATE DIET

An abundance of food that contains calcium and vitamins is indispensable. *Cabbage, lettuce, carrots, turnips,* all *greens* and especially *fruit berries,* will go a long way in supplying our health needs. Biologically grown strawberries are one of the best sources of *calcium.* It is equally important to use discrimination in choosing all our other foods. For example, bread should be made from composted or organically grown wheat, rye, graham, soy, or triticale (obtained by crossing wheat grains with rye) flour with the addition of raw wheat germ and bran. If sugar is used at all, it should be unrefined, i.e. raw brown, or turbinado sugar may be used. Honey, grape sugar, raisins, currants and other dried fruits are even better than brown sugar which contains only part of the original goodness found in the raw sap that comes from the sugar cane. To make the right choice among fats is difficult for many brands on the market make "purity" claims but are lacking in the very things the health conscious person is looking for. However, if you abstain from animal fats and most, if not all margarines, and choose unrefined cold pressed vegetable oils you are on the right track. Fresh, *unsalted butter* from *unpasteurised milk* as well as *almonds, walnuts, cashews, peanuts, filberts, pecans* and other nuts are examples of the type of fats that provide the body with good nourishment. Touch lightly the generally used seasonings, especially ordinary table salt, pepper, nutmeg, ginger, cloves and cinnamon. It is better to use the herb type of *seasonings* and there are plenty of easily grown herbs such as thyme, sage, majoram, basil, parsley which are more healthful to use. *Yeast extract* will flavor gravies and sauces better than meat extracts with the advantage of being healthful.

Flatulence (stomach or intestinal gas) can be avoided by not eating fruits and vegetables together in the same meal. Keep them apart. Have fruit and cereal in the morning and vegetables for your midday meal. Stone or pitted fruits such as plums, apricots and peaches are likely to disagree with most people unless eaten in small quantities. Berries or "seedy" fruits are usually better tolerated and also dried plums, better known as prunes. Fried food should be restricted and for those who cannot forego their meat, choose veal and beef rather than sausages and pork. Instead of frying, grilling is by far the best method of preparing meat for the table.

Most people will require a calcium supplement and this can easily be found in the health stores. *Silica* is another important constituent of the blood chemistry and this is supplied by the herb Hemp nettle (Galeopsis). To increase immunity and resistance to *respiratory ailments* a mixture of Petasites off., Lichen islandicus, Usnea, Plantago lanceolata is highly recommended. Its lichen acids combined with the other remedial substances have proved most valuable as a prophylactic as well as a cure for respiratory diseases. The remedy prepared from Petasites and Mistletoe (Viscum alb.) is another effective natural help in combating the disease. Other health promoting herbs are mentioned in the chapter on natural antibiotics.

CARE OF THE SKIN
AND OTHER SAFETY MEASURES

The body's self-healing powers can be assisted greatly by proper skin care and maintaining general body functions in good order. When bathing or showering, the skin should be vigorously scrubbed with a firm bristle bath brush until it becomes a rosy pink color. Afterwards lubricate it well with a skin function oil, either one that contains St. John's wort oil or with the pure oil itself. Lacking St. John's wort oil, second choice would be a good grade of olive oil. Oil should not be applied to the body every day but it is a good idea to apply it once every second or possibly every third day.

To maintain the correct functioning of the body itself, take care so as to avoid cold feet. If they do get cold, take warm footbaths and firmly massage the feet. This will restore circulation. Another important body function that should be given close attention is regular bowel action. In cases of *constipation* a tablespoon of *Flax seed* macerated or soaked in water or a

117

fruit juice of your choice will have a bland though positive effect on bowel movement. *Psyllium*, from the Plantain (Plantago major) is a demulcent and similar to Linseed or *Flax* in its action and in addition to promoting elimination of the bowels, is excellent for soothing intestinal irritation. A regular morning diet, before breakfast, of unprocessed wheat bran in a small glass of water or juice will start the day off right for the constipation sufferer and, incidentally, anyone with diverticulosis (hernia of the lower bowel where small pouches form and push outward retaining digestive substances) will find *Psyllium* and *wheat bran* an excellent way to avoid a serious and painful operation which doesn't always guarantee 100% success. Another debilitating bowel problem is that of *diarrhea* which occurs usually from some borderline food that has been eaten, even something poisonous. Sometimes it may be the result of a drug such as an antibiotic that has been prescribed for some unrelated ailment. The danger of prolonged and untreated diarrhea is the great loss of fluids from the body. It is more critical in young children and, in either case, the faster the counteraction the better, before dehydration further weakens the body. A porridge made from raw oat flakes is helpful in controlling the problem as well as Yogurt, which has a therapeutic effect. An infusion of the Tormentil plant will check *diarrhea* and also strengthen and soothe the nerves. Because of its astringent qualities it is quite effective. And lastly, intestinal disturbances and fermentations often can be relieved and prevented by thorough mastication of the food we eat and we will be doing our stomach a favor by aiding it in its digestive process.

HEALTH THROUGH JOY
AND CORRECT BREATHING

There is no doubt that fresh mountain air has a very favorable effect upon our health and those who are fortunate enough to be able to spend their holidays in the mountains should take advantage of it. Alternately, if you live in a country that isn't "land-locked" the brisk salty seaside air offers other advantages. But mainly, the advantages of the mountains or the seaside are that they get you away from the city air, the smog, smoke and carbon dioxide exhausts of automobiles.

The importance of *correct breathing* can hardly be overestimated and this is one of the preventative measures that each of us have at our own command. If, up to now, you haven't acquired the habit of deep breathing, it can be of immense benefit to your health if you start practicing this successful method of respiration. The development of better breathing helps pulmonary actions, strengthening the lungs and, more important, more oxygen is supplied to the brain. Cultivate the habit of deep breathing and reap its benefits. We all realize that health is not primarily a matter of taking medicines and that many preventative measures are available that are under our own control.

IMPORTANT INFORMATION FOR EXPECTANT AND NURSING MOTHERS

During pregnancy and even afterwards, the mother's happiness is often marred through such troubles as phlebitis (inflammation of the veins), thrombosis and embolism (the presence of obstructive clots in the blood vessels). A few words of advice on how to avoid these problems will undoubtedly be welcomed by all mothers.

There are certain herbs that can be combined with each other to prevent these conditions from occurring and if the problem does exist there is an excellent chance that a cure can be effected. These herbs are:

> Yarrow (Achillea millefolium)
> Arnica root (Arnica montana)

An infusion prepared from these plants is one way to treat the trouble but a still better way is to take them in the form of a fresh plant extract. Combined with the homeopathic anemone remedy Pulsatilla (A. pratensis), this extract is an ideal

119

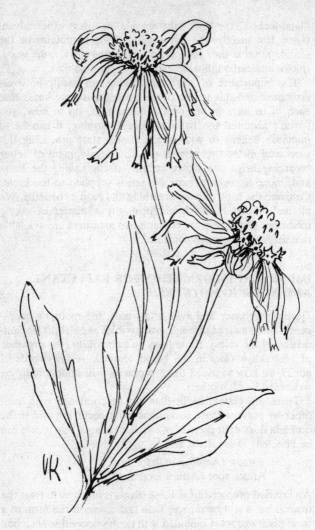

Arnica (Arnica montana)

medicine for pregnant and nursing mothers. It may be interesting to learn about the therapeutic action of each of the aforementioned plants. St. *John's wort* is especially efficacious as a wound healing remedy. It also works wonders in case of injuries to the nerves, when one has to deal with lacerations, crushed fingers or toes, pain resulting from a fall on the coccyx (base of the spine), etc. Brain concussions, injuries to the spinal cord, postoperative pains, neuralgia, headaches also will benefit from this plant.

Another pain relieving herbal extract, *Hypericum* 12, is especially indicated if the mother suffers from pains in the coccyx after giving birth. Take twice daily until the pain is gone, for there is no other remedy under the sun that will cure the pain. Prescription drugs or injections may deaden the pain but they will not cure it.

Yarrow is a typical remedy for the blood. It primarily acts upon and cures such conditions as venous dilation, hemorrhoids, varicose veins, venous congestion in the abdomen and in the legs and is also indicated when there is a rush of blood to the head, frequent and excessive bleeding from the nose and hemorrhaging of the bladder.

Arnica is another excellent remedy for the treatment of veins and it is used in congestive conditions. It has quite an extraordinarily good effect in restoring the female organs after labor and is a reliable remedy for high blood pressure, even when an apoplexy has taken place. Heart troubles or any other kind of disturbance that has its roots in venous congestion, is also benefited by Arnica.

Pulsatilla is a remedy for irregularities in the circulation. It is a sort of hairy anemone and is very potent, almost poisonous. For this reason it should not be taken as an infusion but only as a homeopathic potency. The other three plants mentioned are quite safe to take as a tea and are part of our herb healing treasures.

For *morning sickness* during pregnancy there are simple remedies such as Nux vomica 4x which disperses as a rule the unpleasant nausea almost immediately. If this should prove ineffective try Ipecacuanha 3x or Apomorphinum 4x. Why endure the discomfort and unpleasantness of morning sickness which rob the mother-to-be of the joyful anticipation and expectancy of a child when harmless homeopathic remedies can smooth the way so easily. For a complication free pregnancy it is further advisable to take a calcium complex and the extract prepared from Aesculus hip. (Horse chestnut).

THE MOTHER'S MILK

All arguments to the contrary, *mother's milk* is the only natural and perfect food for the baby. Nothing is so important for the infant's well-being in later life. This is proven over and over again by infant mortality statistics which show that artificially fed children have a ten times greater death rate than those who have been breast fed.

Most important for the baby are its first days when circumstances may decide whether it will live or die. Even in animals we note how nature does not tolerate any interference without unhappy results. Any farmer or country person knows how difficult it is to raise young animals without their mother's milk, how the best and most promising ewe sometimes dies when it is given cow's milk or milk from any other animal that is not the mother. There is a time and place for everything and for every new born creature its *mother's milk* is essential to the healthful process of life. The calf must have cow's milk, the lamb must have sheep's milk and babies must have their mother's milk. This is the only physiologically and biologically correct way to develop the human body, its bone construction, its nervous system and its organs and tissues. And psychologically, it can be said, there is no substitute for breast feeding that will give the feeling of security and that will lead to a well adjusted child. With the alarming rise in crib deaths, recent statistics have verified that none of these deaths have occurred to babies who have been breast fed. While authorities have been unable to pinpoint the cause of the crib deaths it is more than a casual coincidence that the infants who have died were artificially fed. Why risk an untimely death when you know what is best for the infant.

Mother's milk and especially the very first milk, called colostrum, contains enzyme-like elements, biochemic salts and vitamins which cannot be found in any other food in the same quality and proportion. It also is the source of certain immunizing agents and Alexine, that protects the baby from infection. This is the reason why very young breast fed infants are absolutely immune to certain infections. What a wonderful protection for them!

The argument that suckling a baby damages a mother's health and beauty can be discounted immediately because there are sufficient proofs to the contrary. It is well known that breast feeding stimulates the entire glandular system of the mother, that utilization of the food and its vitamins is at its best during this time and that the reproductive organs fall back into place much more easily in nursing mothers than in those who renounce their birthright to breast feed their offspring. There is no doubt that a psychological rapport and harmony are permanently established between the mother and the child. In this way they both profit by a mutual relationship from this natural function, as is always evident when we refrain from interfering with the natural laws of creation.

For normal development and resistance to disease in later years, the foundation laid by breast feeding is of the greatest importance. Experience and medical statistics prove that breast fed children overcome infection and disease much more easily than artificially fed children and with less complications than artificially fed children of a similar environment.

Mothers are sometimes unhappy and nervous when the flow of milk does not appear on the very first day, but it should be remembered that this would be quite unnatural as the baby should not receive any food during the first 24 hours of life. At the beginning the very nutritious and somewhat laxative colostrum must not be held back from the baby on any account, because it helps in the elimination of feces or waste which accumulated during its prenatal life.

When the colostrum ceases to flow, the normal milk comes in. If there is not enough milk to satisfy the baby, a few drops of Urtica (Nettle) extract per day will help the flow. This herbal remedy will increase the milk in quantity as well as quality. *Read also the chapter on Crusta lactaea.*

CALCIUM AND SILICA DEFICIENCY

It can happen that some time after the baby is born, a mother develops signs of glandular trouble, defects in the lungs or even tuberculosis. As a rule the disease is dormant, or at least the disposition for it. Great demands are made upon the organism during pregnancy and this may give rise to the manifestation of an inherent weakness. The growing fetus requires great amounts of *Calcium* and if the mother does not take care to enrich her bloodstream with sufficient quantities of natural minerals, nature will not starve the embryo but will draw from the reserves of the mother thus weakening her bones, teeth and tissues. The saying that each child costs the mother a tooth is only too true. Easily assimilated *Calcium* in the form of raw, finely grated carrots, red and white cabbage, lettuce, sauerkraut and the like, should be eaten daily and if for some reason this is not possible, do take a good calcium preparation, not derived from milk, but from plants. In addition it will be necessary to give attention to the *Silica* requirements of the body. Infusions or extracts from Horsetail, Galeopsis and other *Silica*-containing herbs will supply this mineral. *Vitamin D* is another necessity, for if it is lacking, *Calcium* will not be utilized by the body however much we may ingest of it. *Oranges, codliver oil* and various emulsions contain plenty of D and liquids and tablets are available on the market which can supply daily needs.

Another important point to consider is the efficiency of the kidneys and the skin. If these channels of elimination are in any way obstructed, accumulations of uric acid and other metabolic waste matter may prevent assimilation of calcium and other vital elements.

As fundamental as it is, many overlook the necessity of eating slowly and chewing the food thoroughly. Food well masticated and salivated is half digested – remember that! Getting back to calcium for a moment, it has been observed that lack of it causes disturbances in the glands with internal secretions resulting. The lack of calcium also affects the lymph glands in a similar manner. Flatulence, internal fermentation and putrefaction then take place and poison the system. All these points have to be considered and if care is taken to avoid or observe them – as the case may be – you will have fairly good assurance of escaping illness. It is impossible to evade every infection but a bloodstream plentifully supplied with calcium and silica can deal with them easily. If you are subject to catarrhal afflictions, if your teeth are bad, if your glands are chronically swollen and if you succumb to every infection you happen to come in touch with, then you will want to take to heart the health message revealed here. As the old saying goes: "an ounce of prevention is worth a pound of cure", or stated more directly, prevention is better than cure and for this reason counter all suspicious symptoms with appropriate measures.

VARICOSE VEINS

When the veins degenerate and no longer function properly the circulation becomes congested and varicose veins develop. This happens quite often during pregnancy and right after giving birth. Whenever this occurs the problem should be straightened out at once, for neglect will slowly but surely cause further trouble. Neglect brings on thrombosis and embolism. If a good pregnancy is desired, an easy labor and a trouble-free post birth, look after the veins!

In order to get rid of varicose veins quickly, a strong hypertonic saline or sugar solution is injected into the afflicted veins, which cause them to shrivel up and cease to function. Each calf possesses two inner and two outer principal veins and each thigh, one of each with smaller branches. If one of them is put out of action, the other will have more to do and in time, will degenerate. How can one vein manage to do the work of two especially when the work was too much when shared by two veins? Eventually the second vein will go out of action too and the circulation will depend on the subsidiary veins. These can expand a little and become stronger, but not enough to save the circulation from being impeded. True, temporary relief is obtained from these drastic measures but, sooner or later, the circulation will get worse and worse. Among the elderly it is not uncommon to see ordinary or senile gangrene which can be traced back in many instances to previous interference with the venous system. Indeed, even young people can be affected. The danger of embolism and thrombosis is accentuated by meddling with the blood vessels.

TREATMENT OF VARICOSE VEINS

If you meditate on the significance of the blood, the Bible's assertion, ". . the soul of every sort of flesh is in its blood" will become clear to you. Goethe's reflection in "Faust", "Blood is a very peculiar fluid", expresses a similar thought, namely, that blood is life or the life is in the blood. Not only is the development and proper functioning of our bodies dependent upon our blood, but also our perceptions, feelings – in fact – our whole attitude and outlook towards life.

We have often heard about hormones, the glandular secretions that greatly influence the functions of the body. They also directly affect our emotional state and even go so far as to form our character. Thus, it has been clinically proven time and again that character, as we know it, can be altered completely through a pathological change in the quality and quantity of hormone secretions. Such thoughts make us feel very uncomfortable about taking a blood transfusion.

If the blood is to fill its task properly, it must contain all the minerals and vitamins the body requires to maintain itself; and the circulation has the important task of carrying these elements to every cell. And even if the cells receive everything they need, they would still be unable to exist, unless the circulation attends to another aspect of their existence – the carrying away of the metabolic waste products. This is accomplished by the part of the circulatory system known as the venous system.

If you are moderately well acquainted with bodily functions, you will know that the arteries carry the nutrient laden blood to the cells, while the veins carry it back after the cells have taken what they need. Thus arteries and veins are complementary to each other. Everything in creation is so arranged that normal function and activity can take place.

Disturbances in the venous system are much more frequent than in the arterial system and women, especially, suffer from venous congestion. When people complain of *cold feet* it is usually a sign that the blood circulation is malfunctioning. Two factors may be responsible, lack of exercise or insufficient clothing. Cold feet can lead to diseases of the abdominal organs and, not infrequently, the kidneys may suffer. Young girls are easy prey to disease because they ignore the fundamentals of adequate clothes preferring nylons to cottons and woolens which give the most protection in bad weather. Unfortunately they are more interested in fashion than in matters of health. Is it any wonder that the menstruation is accompanied by cramps and other unpleasant symptoms such as chilblains? Many have to go to bed for part of their menstrual period and a psychosomatic dread is gradually built up during their teenage. All this is due chiefly to venous congestion and an impaired circulation. If the consequences of neglect are to be avoided, these problems have to be dealt with promptly. Alternating hot and cold footbaths and similar measures complemented by herbal remedies and a more sensible way of dress will prove to be the answer to these problems.

NATURAL REGENERATION OF VARICOSE VEINS

It is imperative that people should be warned against this harmful treatment of varicose veins. Why must dangerous methods be employed when the opportunity to regenerate the veins by natural means exists? When varicose veins appear, the body is in need of a good calcium preparation, i.e. Calcium-Complex; also a plant preparation made from the horse chestnut, the plant extract Aesculus Hippoc. (Horse chestnut). An extract made from Yarrow, St. John's wort and Arnica (Hypericum Complex) is also very good for this condition. The veins may be regenerated in a really wonderful way by means of these three remedies. Pay attention to the natural diet too. In this way you can either prevent varicose veins from developing or you can regenerate them to such an extent that they will not give you any further trouble. All this advice is especially important for expectant mothers because it is not only helpful to the circulation but also prevents complications during confinement. The remedies mentioned will exert a beneficial influence upon the venous system and remove congestions so that there will be no danger of thrombosis.

Other organs of the body should be, like varicose veins, regenerated rather than done away with. Why should we be given a certain number of veins if they were not necessary to our well-being? There is no doubt that every anatomical change in our bodies through surgery has its repercussions. Unfortunately, it only becomes obvious after the damage is done. It is extraordinary that we should have more confidence in human knowledge and ability than in Creation itself.

Once it was considered the fashion to remove the appendix whether it was diseased or healthy and surgeons used to brag about how many they had extracted in a year. It got to the point where only one in ten children could expect to reach adult age with the appendix intact. Fortunately, today, the profession is more enlightened and such short sighted decisions have been abandoned so that an appendix is removed only when absolutely necessary. Tonsils were another organ that doctors yanked out with consuming passion if a youngster complained of having a sore throat frequently. But these organs can be treated and regenerated long before they are beyond repair. Really there can be no excuse for neglect because each of us know our physical weaknesses and if we become aware of something wrong and delay taking care of it, we have only ourselves to blame. It is imperative to give immediate attention to slight physical signals, and with persevering care and patience, using the remedies that are available, results will be rewarding.

Anyone who suffers from varicose veins should treat them perseveringly and by natural means. Do not expect a miracle – an immediate cure – for it took time for them to become diseased and it will take time for them to cure. Healthy veins play such an important part in our bodies that any attention we give them to ensure their proper function will be well justified.

OPEN LEG ULCERS

Those who suffer from open leg ulcers usually are unaware that it is wrong to attempt healing them over without, at the same time, improving the general condition of the blood-stream. Even though a good natural ointment is used, it is better not to try to heal the ulcer too quickly. If the secretions with their metabolic toxins cannot drain away freely before the blood has been purified, it will give rise to increasing discomfort. This has been confirmed by many whose leg ulcers have been healed prematurely. It is an important principle of "nature" curing that the body uses just such open leg ulcers and similar afflictions, as safety valves, through which it can drain off material which cannot otherwise be disposed of. If this valve is closed, the toxins will saturate the body and cause such conditions as vertigo, general weakness, etc. The remedy can be effected only by encouraging the venous system to function properly by stimulating the kidneys. As was mentioned before, a remedy complex especially suitable for the veins contains St. John's wort, Yarrow and Arnica. If in

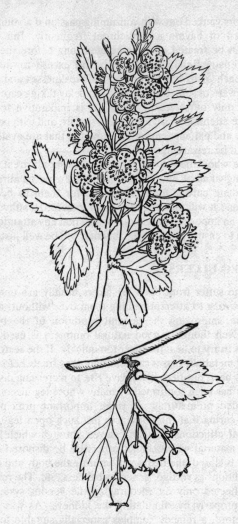

Hawthorne (Crataegus oxyacantha)

addition to these, an extract from horse chestnuts is taken together with a biological calcium preparation, do not be surprised if the ulcers once more begin to discharge and we at once feel better. Sooner or later this internal medication, designed to purify and vitalize the bloodstream, will cause the ulcer to heal naturally. There need not be any fear of unpleasant consequences, such as occur when the healing process is forced. If the patient is constipated, relieve the condition by giving Psyllium seeds and well soaked prunes or figs. This relieves pressure on veins due to excess straining to pass stool.

If *high blood pressure* is noted, very often by a feeling of faintness, Mistletoe, Hawthorn and Arnica are well known remedies that have a regenerating effect on the arteries. It may be that the heart requires strengthening too, but this has to be assessed on an individual basis.

Appropriate diet cannot be overlooked to successfully create the preconditions for any healing process. By now, this need hardly be emphasized since all natural remedies should be complemented by correct diet. In this particular case the diet should consist of very little salt and protein. All meats should be reduced to a minimum, or better still, altogether eliminated until complete recovery has been achieved. Pork, sausages of all kinds, eggs, cheese, white sugar and flour and canned foods are to be avoided. Eat plenty of steamed vegetables, raw salads and corn products.

HEMORRHOIDS

Hemorrhoids, more commonly known as *piles,* are distended veins in the colon and are very much like varicose veins. Whenever you observe blood in your stool, it is almost certain that it comes from piles, although it could be an ulcer in the colon wall. Continued use of aspirin prescribed by many doctors for strengthening the heart will also produce lesions which show up in the form of a bloody stool. To assess the diagnostic value of blood in the stool correctly it is important to know that light colored blood, i.e. blood that LOOKS like blood, comes from some lesion situated in the colon. Blood from higher up in the large intestines and the stomach can no longer be recognized because the action of the digestive juices transform it into a dark mass.

A fairly unmistakable sign of piles is the feeling of welts or ridges within the anus that swells especially when the stool tends to be hard. This condition can be conteracted with Millefolium, the fresh plant extract from Yarrow, applied externally.

Hamamelis virginica (Witch hazel) and Calcium fluoratum, applied externally have produced good effects on such cases. But the best remedy of all is Hypericum-Complex. For local treatment and palliation use suppositories containing cocoa butter and Hamamelis. Tea made from the Tormentilla plant and nettles are equally beneficial. Spurge (D. laureola), although poisonous if taken internally, used externally will rid the pains. The best way to use it is to pulp the plant and apply it as a poultice to the anus. Sponging the anus with cold water will help prevent piles once they have been cured.

LEUCORRHOEA

This frequent ailment is popularly known as "The Whites". Many women suffer from it badly and very often it occurs regularly, at certain intervals. Unfortunately many doctors belittle this problem and advise, "don't worry about it", and think that this will settle the whole matter. However, investigation of the effects of Leucorrhoea more closely reveal that it constitutes a drain on the vitality of the sufferer and that it undermines the nerves. The question arises as to how to cope with the problem.

Normally, the mucous membranes of the vagina and internal genital organs secrete lactic acid which prevents the development of harmful bacteria. If this production of lactic acid is insufficient, inflammation of the reproductive organs will develop and a mucous discharge occurs. Knowing how efficient natural lactic acid is as an antiseptic and disinfectant, it is possible to substitute concentrated whey and use it as a douche because it will work wonders! Since there is usually a deficiency of calcium salts as well, it would be wise to take some kind of calcium preparation in addition to the douche. Sitzbaths prepared with herbs, such as Camomile, Juniper, Goldenseal, will complete the treatment against Leucorrhoea, but you must remain in the bath for a minimum of a half hour and more desirably an hour at a time and keep the water at a constant temperature of about 98° F. Again, it cannot be stressed too much, the importance of getting busy right away at the slightest suspicion of a problem existing.

WEIGHT CONTROL

A thought that formerly existed was that thinness was due to an insufficient intake of food and eating too much resulted in getting fat. Yet there are people who eat a lot and remain extraordinarily thin, and others who eat very little food and put on weight. Everything, they say, turns to fat!

Progressive research has shown that disfunction of the glands, which discharge their hormones directly into the bloodstream, is partly responsible for both excessive corpulence or thinness. The glands primarily responsible for this are the Pituitary, the Ovaries, Testicles and Thyroid. Over-function or imbalance usually leads to thinness while sub-function of any of them leads to corpulence. It has been observed that removal of the ovaries, or a disease that leads to their sub-functioning, causes the person to put on weight. Getting fat after the change of life confirms this fact. A typical example is the inhabitant of a southern climate. How slim and supple the Italian or the Latin and South American girls are in the early prime of life. But as soon as they approach the change of life, usually at a much earlier age in hot countries, the glandular secretions diminish and they become plump. If the older generation is stout and comfortable, it can be traced to the insufficient functioning of the internal secretory glands and, more than anything else, the sluggish action of the ovaries. In

133

this case the Sitzbath and other measures which stimulate the ovaries would be of immense help toward reducing corpulence.

Pituitary obesity is not as easy to deal with as is its ovarian relative, because this gland is less amenable to corrective treatment. There are, of course, glandular preparations on the market which do act on the pituitary but, as with all other similar remedies, their administration is a delicate undertaking. And neither do these preparations always produce positive results with the pituitary. The ovaries, as previously mentioned, are more easily treated by special preparations on the market.

The simplest expedient that can be recommended, especially one that stimulates the functioning of the ovaries, are various foods that contain Vitamin E. The most important of these is wheat germ. There are people who won't eat wheat germ for fear of getting fat, because it has been recommended to thin people who wish to gain weight. Women need not worry about this, for wheat germ and its Vitamin E only regulate the function of the ovaries – stimulating their function in the case of fat people and reducing their function in the case of thin people.

Apart from that, it contains other valuable nutrients like protein, phosphates, and natural sugar. All these have a good effect on the body without endangering an abnormal weight rise. Thus, anyone suffering from obesity should not hesitate to take wheat germ, for it will not increase weight but oppose it.

There are those who fear to take any food rich in vitamins because they are afraid they might overdose themselves. This fear is only justified where synthetic vitamins are concerned, for indeed they can overdose. Such a thing cannot happen with natural vitamins from organically grown food. Being an integral part of organic compounds they are never too concentrated.

The body uses only what it can, while any surplus of certain natural vitamins is stored up; others are passed off. For the reasons mentioned above, synthetic vitamins never can equal natural ones. As the Book of Books expresses it: "Human folly brings the wisdom of the wise to nothing." We may be able to analyze matter but when it comes to achieving a biologically synthetic equivalent, we fail. There are always hidden forces which defy analysis which are essential to the life process. Thus, it is much more desirable to turn to natural biological sources because creation is orderly and harmonious and if we keep within its guidelines, we cannot go wrong.

Recently, artificial vitamin preparations have been fostered by their manufacturers; before that, blood salts ruled the scene. But fortunately, far seeing researchers like Drs. Hahnemann and Schuessler found that various minerals are required only in the most minute amounts and can only be assimilated in triturated form (ground into a fine powder.)

At one time it was believed that gold could be made artificially; indeed, an artificial man was considered a possibiity. Our age has become less ambitious in that it merely attempts to produce a tablet or pill which contains all the nutrients the body requires and thus make artificial nutrition possible. Before too long it will be abandoned and the same fate will overtake synthetic vitamins. They can never replace or even equal those forces which the Almighty has put into the plant kingdom. A return to natural principles will prove much more profitable than all the speculative theories the human mind is capable of conceiving. In this way, the natural way, the problems of obesity, glandular disfunctions and metabolic disorders will be more effectively solved.

DANGEROUS AND SAFE REMEDIES FOR OBESITY

Fat people must never let themselves be pursuaded to take a reducing preparation. If the person does not know the contents of whatever reducing pill he is taking, he should make absolutely certain it does not contain iodine. This is a dangerous element and should be used only homeopathically with the greatest of caution. One should also be very skeptical of any highly touted weight reducing remedies as these can seriously damage the body and result in ill health. Most of the claims are highly exaggerated and while the medication may partially accomplish its purpose, the directions do not say in what condition, physically or mentally, you may end up. For the sensible person, there shouldn't be a shred of doubt that a safe way to reduce is by means of a suitable diet and a well planned exercise program. While counting calories may not exactly be to your liking, it is the only basic way to achieve the wished for results without doing any serious harm to your body.

In many cases it is true to say that when a woman puts on weight, the ovaries are partially to blame; it is the case after there has been a hysterectomy or change of life. The Pituitary has been often blamed but seldom justly. In any case, avoid drastic action in reducing so as not to run the risk of permanently injuring your health. In the case of women, Sitzbaths to stimulate the ovaries are excellent. Also a homeopathic preparation, Ovasan 3x in combination with a suitable diet can give very good results. The diet should consist of a little protein and one should avoid all white flour products as well as white sugar. Keep to a natural diet as far as possible and take plenty of fruit and vegetable juices, especially carrot, grapefruit, grape, and orange juices. Experience will tell which juices suit you best, for some acids, though harmless to people in good health, do not always agree with someone not quite so well. Also, stick to reasonable quantities of the juices and do not go overboard. Use reasonable care and caution.

All chemical reducing pills should be completely avoided, for these are dangerous not only to health but to life itself. Ingestion of many of the preparations on the market has ended in tragedy. If you feel you must reduce, take only natural remedies.

TAKE CARE OF YOUR EYES

A recommended treatment for the complex mechanism we call the eye would be out of place here. Instead, here is a simple piece of advice using prophylactic principles, that will do much to preserve your eyesight. It will help you use nature's basic laws.

It is a fact that excessive brain work causes eyestrain. The more natural and free from stress we are in our daily lives, the better it will be for our eyes. It might be added that the poor nourishment derived from present day packaged foods contributes to the development of eye problems also.

All this can easily be changed. How can this be done? The answer is simple. Formerly when we were not so eager to work overtime by artificial light, and got plenty of rest, there were not so many painful, weak and tired eyes as there are now. Let us therefore try a most extraordinary remedy. Let us turn back the wheel of time and try living for four weeks without electric light. Let us renounce the convenience of modern lighting. Let us refrain from switching on the light. Your painful, burning, overtired eyes, which no longer can do their work properly, will thank you for this. In order to be well armed against the tyranny of custom, carefully plan your day so that when it gets dark, you will not be tempted to turn on the light. Use your evenings for relaxation and recuperation in preparation for that sleep which ushers in the end of the day. Try to do this for four weeks. In experiencing this temporary new way of life, one will appreciate why the Creator has given us the bright light of the sun by day and the gentle soothing moonlight by night. If you make full use of the night for rest, you will wake cheerfully with the first gleam of day, without feeling tired and sluggish. What you had intended doing by artificial light, you can do with far less effort in the full light of day. It is quite astonishing how this compliance with nature's laws gives one a facility for work and at the same time renews the energy of overtaxed eyes. The unnatural burden of artificial light, which year after year we impose on our eyes, will no longer bother us if we establish a daily rhythm which follows the coming and going of daylight. The natural order of things has been established by our Creator and the more we set ourselves against it, the more our eyes will suffer. Indeed, in time it will be hard to imagine a contemporary person without spectacles. Immersed as we are in the fast pace of life, in the atmosphere of artificiality, we have lost touch with the natural rhythm of life.

How would plants get along, if day and night they had to live in a constant stream of light, without a chance to regenerate themselves in darkness? Their cells would rebel and their natural functions would be impaired. Why then should not man conform to the harmony of the natural laws? Why should he not use and enjoy to the full the priceless wonder of the early morning hours instead of missing out on them? Why should he lie in bed, while the sun shines radiantly outside, while he is trying to recover the hours of sleep lost the night before? Why does he create this restless night for himself, instead of sleeping quietly during those hours before midnight building up strength for the next day's work? If we could only reorganize our time our eyes would indeed benefit enormously. When light fades, let us put aside our work, and when daylight comes once more, take it up again, strengthened and refreshed. Not only our eyes, but our whole bodies will benefit from this natural way of life. Give this routine a try in the spring or summer. In winter it is quite normal to wake up with the daylight, but, unfortunately, at that time of the year we are tempted to continue our working day far into the night. In the spring, then, let us start our good resolution, to give our eyes the natural daylight in the earliest hours of the morning and in the evening to give them a rest rather than work under artificial light. It is true that the pace of modern business and the hurried rush of everyday life may preclude taking the time to do this, but we must remember that once the eyesight is damaged it may be irrecoverable.

SIMPLE REMEDIES FOR EYE PROBLEMS

It is a proven fact that carrot juice has a very favorable effect upon the eyes on account of the Vitamin A it contains. Any measure which improves the circulation in the supply of blood to the eyes will be assisted by a carrot juice diet although, in itself, good circulation will do much to restore normality. As supporting factors in the treatment both Hypericum and Calcium complex may be taken while the kidneys will benefit from Goldenrod and Galeopsis and will supply the organism with sufficient Silica.

Since liver disorders, constipation and overtiredness can also be the causes of eye troubles, be careful to see that both liver and bowels are functioning properly. The liver can be restored to good working order by taking Chelidonium 2x, Podophyllum 3x or Chelicynara. Very often the constipation will disappear after taking these. Avoid the use of prepared foods from the grocery market and cut down on salt and protein. If you feel you are overworked, make sure to get to sleep at least two hours before midnight. Oat extract (avena sativa) will tone up your nerves and strengthen you generally. In the case of a blocked tear duct, external treatment with clay packs prepared with Horsetail tea will benefit the eyes. If you have conjunctivitis make up an eye bath from Eyebright (Euphrasia officinalis) and Marigold tea.

INFECTIOUS SUPPURATION OF THE EYES AND MOUTH

Infectious eye and mouth suppuration (discharging pus or festering) can be cured in a short time, if one follows the treatment described by this mother who writes the following:

"Our little one is better. The eye and mouth suppuration stopped within five days of our starting to use your remedies. The child was pitiful, but now is romping around happily. Our treatment was as follows: Before meals we gave him Solidago and a cod liver oil preparation with orange juice and then an easily assimilated calcium preparation. After the meal we gave him Hepar sulph. 4x and Lachesis 12x. The eyes were bathed twice daily with well diluted Hypericum Complex and twice a day we put an onion compress on his neck. We could soon notice improvement in his condition. We put St. John's wort

oil on his sore lips and dusted them with calcium powder.
During the day we gave him fruit juice to drink and also an
infusion of Horsetail (Equisetum arvense). Several times we
made use of clay packs made with Horsetail tea, medicated
with a few drops of St. John's wort oil which were applied to
his eyes.

We were indeed thankful and happy that this dangerous
infection has now gone. We continue to give the child Solidago
(Goldenrod), cod liver oil preparation and the calcium."

As a rule such troubles are simple to heal if the body is given
the right help. It is better to take no action than to treat
anything incorrectly. Attempts to suppress the symptoms by
destroying the causative germs with drugs undermines the
natural powers of resistance. The same foolishness is displayed
by those who treat plant diseases by spraying them with
poisonous chemicals which not only kill pests but weaken the
plant's own defense against diseases. No wonder farmers who
grow on a commercial scale are forced to increase and intensify their spray programs from year to year. No man by himself
can heal – that must be left to the self healing powers of the
body to accomplish. Let us hope that this truth becomes, once
again, more widely recognized.

THE CAUSE AND TREATMENT OF HEADACHES

Pains caused by headaches should never be treated with drugs.
It is better to try and discover their causes and remedy these
because no other approach will give permanent results. Many
times headaches are caused by intestinal or digestive disturbances. Putrefactive processes develop gases which enter the
liver through the portal circulation and from there, find their
way into the bloodstream proper. Once these gases have
affected the blood nothing will stop them from affecting the
delicate brain and nerve cells. Abdominal diseases and over-
work can lead to headaches. Another possibility is the existence of a spinal lesion or what is popularly known as a slipped
disc. It almost goes without saying that such a condition

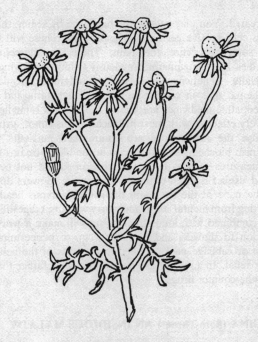

Camomile (Matricaria chamomilla)

requires the services of a chiropractor who is trained to work on structural changes in the spinal column.

There are two other factors that should be considered in regards to headaches. Headaches may be caused by an allergy to certain foods. It may be necessary to eliminate foods, one by one, that are suspect, until the cause is discovered. The other cause can be attributed to nervous tension which, according to some authorities, accounts for a large percentage of headaches.

Whatever the cause, a headache per se is never an illness, only a symptom or an outward manifestation of an illness. Taking drugs and antidotes are useless because the cause must be treated. You may relieve the headache by seeing that the nerve cells receive certain biochemic salts. These will lessen and sometimes cure the pain. There are homeopathic remedies like Sanguinaria canadensis (Bloodroot) which are especially beneficial in cases of migraine headaches. Biochemic salts in combination with Sanguinaria and other homeopathic medicines are known as Complex remedies and are very effective with most headaches. This is not surprising because the medications are natural cell nutrients which replenish biochemical deficiencies in the bloodstream. Physical measures such as bowel elimination should not be neglected. Relief is often obtained from warm showers directed on the nape of the neck and the spine. Nervous headaches resulting from mental strain and worry will upset digestion and that combined with loud street noises will make it worse. In addition to showers and a relaxing cup of peppermint tea, onion or cabbage packs applied to the back of the neck will bring relief. In any case use natural remedies rather than try over-the-counter drugs.

ANGINA (Sore Throat) AN INSIDIOUS MALADY

It has been observed that many times the toxins of an untreated angina may cause very unpleasant side effects, more severe at times than the actual illness. These toxins may, in fact, bring about an inflammation of the middle ear, rheumatic fever and arthritis. The toxins may also be responsible for a partial paralysis of the cardiac valve which leaves the patient with a permanent cardiac defect. This was brought to my attention not too long ago by one of my patients. She was a healthy woman and had given birth to her children without any complications until the day that a neglected angina put a tragic end to her health. The doctors share my belief that her cardiac defect was a direct result of the presence of angina toxins in her body. Unfortunately, to further complicate matters, her stomach and intestines were adversely affected by the allopathic drugs she had been taking. Today, this formerly vigorous and healthy woman is a very sick person.

From this case history let us learn not to overlook an angina or to neglect it as if it were of no importance. If we do neglect it, we are permitting it to take its destructive course. It is important to understand that angina may have a more drastic effect in a low pressure system, that is at the beginning of a warm air current. Remember to stay indoors during bad weather. The fact that a lymphatic person or someone suffering from a calcium deficiency is more susceptible to this type of sore throat points up the need for having a source rich in calcium in the diet. It is also recommended to support this by taking a calcium complex.

EFFECTIVE COUNTER MEASURES

There are many natural remedies that have proven dependable in the treatment of sore throat. Right from the start one should take Lachesis D-10, five drops in a little warm water three times a day, a solution of lactic acid 15 % to 20 % strong. Soak a small, soft brush in an undiluted whey solution and paint the throat with it. Rapid attention to developing angina will avert more serious problems. As additional treatment take Echinacea extract three or four times a day to help increase resistance to the disease. If the bronchial passage becomes infected it is wise to take a few drops of Imperatoria ostruth (masterwort) two or three times a day.

Do not neglect to treat a sore throat externally as well. A pack made of cabbage leaves or grated horseradish mixed with whey or curds is a great advantage in treatment. Pure horseradish may be too strong so mix two third grated carrots or curds with one third horseradish and you will still have a mixture that is strong enough to do the job.

A proper after-treatment is indispensable for the total excretion of all toxins. This can be achieved by taking a complex, the main ingredient of which is Solidago virg. (Goldenrod), a remedy that stimulates the kidneys. Steam baths are helpful, too to speed up the excretion of toxins. The diet should be low in protein, but high in anything that may give strength and energy. Never let up on the treatment of angina as the effort will well repay the burden it may entail.

HAY FEVER

It is certainly miserable to suffer from *hay fever* while those more fortunate enjoy the flowering beauty of the plant kingdom. Once this malady surfaces it is rather difficult to banish it. In order to effect a permanent cure, it is necessary to begin an appropriate treatment no later than February. Thus it is imperative to counteract hay fever before the trees and flowers begin to blossom.

A treatment consisting of ten homeopathic injections of formic acid and herb complexes has brought about proven relief. In order to assure permanent success of the treatment it must be repeated at the beginning of the following year. And during the entire year do not neglect to take Calcium complex. Furthermore the nose should be lubricated with a biological cream containing lanolin and Vitamin E. This prevents the mucous membranes from drying out. At the same time one can take Galeopsis, Kal. jod D 4 and Arsen album D 4.

Of special benefit are two to three teaspoonsful of honey mixed with fruit juice. The diet should consist of natural foods and by all means stay away from any bleached products such as white flour, refined sugar and products made from it, animal fats and any ready cooked packaged foods. A teaspoon of bee pollen also is an excellent treatment for hay fever.

BENEFICIAL TYPES OF FOOD

It is of paramount importance to have a diet rich in calcium. As far as vegetables are concerned of prime importance are carrots, spinach, celery, parsnips, rutabagas, lettuce, endive, turnips because they are high in calcium. So too are all kinds of fruit. Add to the diet plenty of figs, raisins, Brazil nuts, walnuts, pecans, sunflower seeds, almonds and pine kernels. When you leave home for a trip or to go shopping for a day, take along a jar with a mixture of nuts and dried fruits. It will satisfy your appetite and fill you full of energy. As long as the snow is off the ground it is possible to harvest parsley and watercress to meet Vitamin B-12 needs. This presents no problem in tropical countries where the harvest is a year round thing. But, if one lives in a temperate or northern clime, it would be a good idea to sow watercress seeds in flower pots and raise them behind a sunny window so that plenty of this healthy vegetable is available during the long cold months. Other foods of equal importance are those containing large amounts of Vitamin A and C. Vitamin A is found in many fruits, vegetables, nuts and seeds and it is highly concentrated in codliver oil, and the liver of different animals. Since some people cannot prosper on organ meats, vegetables offer the best bet. A partial list of those vegetables high in Vitamin A are: Spinach, parsley, carrots, lettuce, endive, watercress, gardencress, cabbage, beets, asparagus, peas and beans to name a few. Vitamin C is found in abundance in the citrus family as well as in tomatoes and many of the green leafy vegetables.

ADDITIONAL AIDS

Much benefit may also be derived from the natural calcium supplements contained in such foods as milk and milk products, whole grains and unrefined cereals. Unquestionably, the body needs calcium more than any other mineral if for no other reason than to keep the skeletal bones healthy and strong. However, it is well to remember that calcium needs acid to maintain it in solution and properly distribute it to different parts of the body. Two natural products containing calcium are Ursenea and Lachenmoss. They effectively strengthen the mucous membranes. To combat susceptibility to catarrhs and coughs, a mixture of crushed larch buds with honey and other ingredients will be found to be an excellent remedy. As a preventative measure in taking care of the throat, try Echinacea extract and *whey* since Echinacea counteracts infection and gargling *whey* cleanses the mouth and throat. If the throat infection has already progressed, it is advisable to apply undiluted whey to the inside of the throat. A very severe catarrh or even bronchitis may be cured with Imperatoria (Masterwort). We often recommend to people who like to take hikes through the forest, although we suspect this is mostly a European custom, to chew fir or tamarack (larch) buds, which have a preventative as well as a healing effect.

STRANGE LAWS OF IMMUNITY

Life in its constant flux and change presents us at times with rather unusual questions. Is it not strange that, while infectious diseases in our part of the world are on the decline, the death toll from metabolic disorders and other ailments of an advanced civilization show a sharp increase? Could we possibly interpret this as something resulting from our decreased resistance? The question though remains: What exactly makes us so vulnerable to metabolic disorders? While all this is somewhat puzzling, if we carefully review what experience has taught us, we may yet find the answer.

During the time I spent in the Amazon area, a measles epidemic took the lives of thousands of Indians living in the jungle. In Switzerland and most of Europe, and America too, it is practically unheard of that a child or an adult, for that matter, dies as a result of measles. Why is that so? The bacteria are just as toxic as ever but nature has a way of manipulating things more skillfully than man. The layman as well as the physician should familiarize himself with these biological laws and their conforming adaptability and learn to respect them. Thanks to the miraculous generosity and benevolence of our Creator, the laws of nature, given time, serve as an effective counterforce to any attack of this sort. In the beginning the bacteria cause widespread disaster among people and take numerous lives, but a few generations later, a degree of immunity has been reached and later on the illness has only negligible consequences. This is the history of tuberculosis, which only 60 years ago was a major cause of death. Diphtheria and other infectious diseases likewise have lost their frightening effect during the past 50 years, due to immunization provided by inoculation.

LAWS WE ALL SHOULD OBSERVE

By looking at the plant kingdom we can see a certain conformity to natural law with respect to the assimilation and creation of forces of immunity and defense. Proof of this is DDT which, only eight years ago, killed all but two species of insects in our country. Today there are about 40 species that are immune to DDT. While I was staying in California I observed that it was necessary to increase the strength and toxicity of the insecticides continually in order to obtain the desired results. The detrimental consequences were that millions of birds and bees died while the insects became immune to the more deadly doses of poison very quickly. A friend of mine told me that an industrial firm in Guatemala had started using a very potent insecticide that could completely wipe out the entire bee population destroying the honey harvest completely. When the biological processes of nature are so disturbed by chemicals, it is bound to affect whole segments of the human population deliberately.

As a result of the aforementioned conformity to natural law, we may presume that in 50 years from now the Indians in the Amazon area will no longer die from measles, since by then they will have developed the immunity which we have already. As long as the Indians remain primitive and can avoid the detrimental effects of an ever encroaching civilization, they will not have to worry about many of our illnesses either. The ever increasing number of deaths resulting from diabetes, cancer, heart failure, multiple sclerosis and other diseases in our advanced society will continue to be negligible if nonexistent among the Indian tribes of the Amazon.

147

Many physicians, biologists and nutritionists are aware of these dangers, advocating the return to eating natural unprocessed foods as a protection against modern diseases. A warning and an appeal has gone out to change our life style if we want to enjoy a long and happy life and enjoy good health. Notably among them is the famous specialist Dr. Joseph Evers who treats thousands of people suffering from multiple sclerosis. Dr. Ever's book, "Gestaltwandel des Krankheitsgeschehens" is so impressive that even a healthy person, after reading it, will change his life style without delay. Every person can learn from the clear and logical arguments of this experienced researcher. In his book, Dr. Evers proves to us that nature has a greater share in increasing our life span than scientific research does.

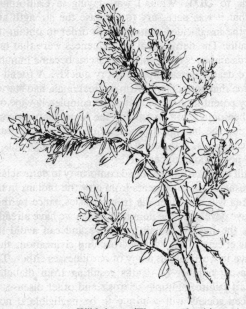

Wild thyme (Thymus vulgaris)

ASTHMA

Difficulties in breathing are one of the many signs of *asthma*. There are three different kinds which we must recognize in order to select a correct method of treatment. They are asthma nervosum, bronchial asthma and cardiac asthma. The symptoms must be carefully analyzed and considered to carry out an appropriate treatment.

ASTHMA NERVOSUM

If our nervous system is very sensitive and tends to be spasmodic and we suffer from asthma, we often attribute it to a weakened nervous system. It becomes evident, therefore, that in order to effect a successful cure, the nerves must first of all be treated.

BRONCHIAL ASTHMA

Bronchial asthma is different from the above mentioned asthma in that it is mainly caused by certain climatic conditions. A change in locale generally provides the desired effect and cure. Living by the ocean, where the air contains a large percentage of iodine, usually has a positive influence and asthma attacks will disappear. High altitude often proves to be equally beneficial. An elevation of 900 meters (2,800 feet) generally suffices although sometimes an elevation of 3,600 to 4,500 feet may be necessary to overcome the problem. The third alternative is the hot, dry air of the desert which, in many cases, has helped to relieve asthmatic discomfort.

It is also possible that spasmodic contraction may be a reaction to certain pollens in the air. Sensitivity to these pollens is also the cause of hay fever. If our financial situation permits us to move to a different climatic zone, we should by all means do so, since a cure can almost be guaranteed if we combine change of climate with appropriate natural remedies. Although financially able, sometimes a person may find it difficult to uproot himself from familiar surroundings and leave relatives and friends for a strange place. But one must face the fact that asthma, in many cases, will only respond favorably if this is done. Once the person has moved, if attacks do not recur within a year or two, he may want to reconsider moving back to his former home. As a rule, once the asthma has been cured it is not likely to return again even if the person returns to his former area. It is more difficult to obtain a successful cure, however, if bronchial asthma is a result of an old, improperly treated lung ailment. In this case it may be necessary to remain in the new location where benefits have occurred.

PHYSICAL APPLICATIONS
AND TREATMENT WITH DRUGS

Drugs used in the treatment of bronchial asthma are mainly of an anti-spasmodic nature. It is interesting to note that a patient, who has been promised a cure, does indeed feel better after simple novocaine injections. This also is a form of psychotherapy which leaves the patient favorably disposed toward the treatment. Another substitute for novocaine is formic acid.

Strong asthma pills, taken over a long period of time, are not recommended even though they may bring about the desired relief. These pills contain extracts from an African plant, Ephedrin plus Atropin, an extract from thorn apples, as well as other strong ingredients. While the body may react favorably to these strong remedies, a complete cure is hardly ever obtained while one, at the same time, runs the risk of becoming dependent on these drugs. In this case, homeopathic remedies are more advantageous and dependable. The following ones have proven excellent, depending on the particular need of the individual: Arsen alb. D-6 – D-30, Nux vomica D-6 – D-20, Zinc valer. D-3, Antimon sulf. aurant. D-4 and a Belladonna preparation of high potency.

Among the herbal remedies, a preparation containing an extract from Petasites off. (Butterbur), taken in the form of a syrup, seems to be most effective. This anti-spasmodic herbal remedy is extremely reliable and has an amazing positive effect without any side effects even when taken over a period of time. Lately we have come to recognize as very beneficial a phyto-therapeutic remedy Khellin, derived from Ammi visuage. In more popular terms this preparation is known as Khella. It is absolutely harmless and when taken in conjunction with a Petasites preparation, it is very effective. Both of these herbal remedies may also be recommended for the treatment of emphysema and bronchitis when accompanied by spasmodic coughs.

In addition to herbal treatments and positive psychological orientation, physical therapy has its place in the treatment of asthma. Of importance are foot baths alternating between hot and cold water, massage hip-baths, as recommended by Louis Kuhne, brush massages, mustard packs and chest mud packs.

CARDIAC ASTHMA

Even though cardiac asthma has the same characteristics as bronchial asthma, no abnormalties of the bronchial passages can be detected. Cardiac asthma is the result of a cardiac weakness. If the left half of the heart is affected this means an accumulation of blood in the lung. In case the right half is affected, it is the result of poor blood circulation in the lungs, which in turn causes a decrease in the exchange of gases.

The facial skin of a person suffering from cardiac asthma has a bluish hue to it. Another sign is difficulty in breathing when engaged in the slightest physical activity. As soon as the cause of this problem has been established, one should begin a treatment with cardiac remedies und drugs that influence the vascular system. Instead of digitalis which tends to accumulate in the body, it is recommended and quite helpful to take Convallaria known as Lily of the Valley, in conjunction with Scilla maritima (Squill). In order to strengthen the moyacardium a Crataegus (Hawthorn) preparation with Cactus, Valeriana, and Avena sativa has proved to be very helpful. Medicine that is stimulating to the general circulation, such as Horse chestnut (Aesculus hipp.) taken with a calcium preparation also has a positive influence on recovery. In any case it is advisable to diagnose the cause of the disease and then proceed to treat it according to its medicinal requirements as well as using different forms of physical therapy.

NEW FUNCTIONS OF CALCIUM

We all know the importance of *calcium* as a structural component for our bones and teeth. A low calcium level indicates a calcium deficiency. The effect of this deficiency is especially dangerous in pregnant women, and generations ago it was an accepted belief that this was the price a mother-to-be had to pay for bearing a child. But more serious is the fact that a calcium deficiency in the blood may bring about tetanus-like conditions with cramping and spasmodic contractions.

Calcium, though, is not only a composite mineral, but also a union of components which aid in the elimination of harmful metabolic sediments, especially acids which are excreted with the urine. Let us look at oxalic acid, for example, which plays a part in the formation of kidney stones. When combined with calcium it becomes oxalic acid calcium which is a substance that can be disposed of by the urinary organ. Scrofula, a form of tuberculosis characterized by the enlargement of the lymph glands, can be avoided if a proper balance of calcium is maintained in the body. If the calcium level in our blood is normal it can protect us from the harmful effects of radio active strontium 90. This discovery, while new to many of us, is reassuring since it is not very difficult to influence our calcium level positively and thus keep it normal. Reasons for maintaining a safe level of this vital mineral should be sufficiently clear and convincing so as to never forget its importance to our health.

Whole kernel foods, raw vegetables and dairy products are all excellent sources of *calcium*. Unfortunately our body is unable to assimilate calcium contained in water or calcium in any other inorganic form; that is why organic calcium of plant origin is to be preferred to all other forms. If, in spite of what one considers to be a proper diet, he still suffers from a calcium deficiency, then it is important to take a biological calcium complex.

INFLAMMATION OF THE EAR

An earache should not be taken lightly as serious conditions can develop from it. First of all apply a poultice to the neck, an onion one will do. Give up using chemist's ear drops, adopt a fruit diet and avoid all highly seasoned and heavy foods. Syringing may be done with infusions of Plantago major (broad-leaved Plantain), Camomile, Marigold or Lemon balm.

If throbbing is felt deep down in the ear, if the pain gets worse at night, Calcarea carbonica 6x (Calcium carbonicum) will help to relieve it. The patient should receive competent treatment for, at this stage, inflammation of the middle ear can develop with serious effects. Pus, instead of escaping through the ear drum might break through the thin bone wall and discharge into the cranial cavity producing a very dangerous situation.

Improperly treated infection of the middle ear can result in meningitis. Serious problems of the ear are created by scarlet fever, measles, whooping cough, diphtheria, influenza, tonsillitis, etc. because they scatter their toxins throughout the body and the ear becomes susceptible. If complications, consequences and relapses in such diseases are to be avoided, elimination of the toxins is of utmost importance. Improper treatment can lead to loss of hearing by affecting the auditory nerves.

Pulsatilla, Belladonna, Sulphur and Mercurius solubilis, homeopathically potentized, are generally indicated remedies for treating inflammation of the middle ear. At the first sign of inflammation Hepar sulph. 12x is very effective and if there is danger of septic infections Lachesis 12x can still save the situation. In cases of protracted discharge, Silicea 12x taken alternatively with Causticum can help considerably. Should there be a tendency to a relapse, recourse to an occasional dose of a constitutional-building remedy Baryum carbonicum is very desirable. Anyone with a tendency to ear problems should take the fresh plant extract from the broad-leaved Plantain (Plantago major) for a few months at a time as a preventative measure. This is one of the best remedies for ears and will also sharpen the hearing.

SUPPURATION OF THE MIDDLE EAR

When children complain of earaches – inflammation of the middle ear – very often insufficient attention is given to it. The child complains, has perhaps a slight runny discharge which then changes to pus. We put the child to bed and think our duty is done. Unfortunately the correct treatment has been overlooked. The reason so many people are hard of hearing and in some cases deaf in one ear is because this childhood condition was neglected. Ear infections can affect the brain and the eyes, too, may suffer from chronic infection of the ears. Neighboring organs as well as those in different parts of the body, can also be harmed. Therefore no time is to be lost in treating the ear when the first danger appears.

When the suppuration of the middle ear has become a chronic condition, the following directions will help give the patient alleviation. Place an onion poultice behind the affected ear and if relief isn't forthcoming change to a mustard poultice. This will draw internal accumulations of matter to the surface. This is particularly important in connection with inflammations of organs of the head. Inflammations can be drawn away from the ears, eyes and nose to the neck or shoulders. Internal remedies are 5 drops of Belladonna 4x every two hours and 2 tablets of Ferrum phos. 6x every two hours arranged in such a way that every hour one of these medicines is taken. For as long as the ear discharges and suppurates Hepar sulph. 4x is effective, and when there is no more pus, Silicea 12x will in most cases clear up the problem. Follow up with one drop of St. John's wort oil and one drop of the extract of Plantago major once daily into the ear.

When there is a nasal catarrh and pharyngitis, which is an aftermath of the ear problem, take Cinnabaris 3x and put 5 drops of Plantago major tincture on cotton flannel and place it in the ear. This will bring about a healing of a chronic inflammation so completely that the hearing will be quite normal once more.

The auditory nerve together with the complicated interior anatomy of the ear can be permanently damaged by bacterial toxins and the little bony structure can be actually suppurated out. When this happens, no treatment can restore the hearing apparatus to normal again. Never lose time starting immediately on an intensive treatment whenever problems with the ear begin to manifest themselves.

Another problem which results in *deafness* is called otosclerosis. This is the name given to the type of hearing loss that results when the stirrup bone (the stapes) becomes locked, preventing the transmission of sound waves through the hearing nerves. The diagnosis is readily made in conjunction with hearing tests. In this case there is no disease involved but a physical impairment. Today it is possible to regain your hearing again by means of an operation called "Stapedectomy with Prosthesis". In this procedure the locked bone (the stapes), which is about the size of a small grain of rice, is removed and replaced with a teflon-wire prosthesis the average length of which is 4.75 millimeters (there are 25 millimeters in an inch). The surgery is very delicate and therefore performed under a microscope. Since it is the motion of the stapes that stimulates the hearing nerve which passes the impulse to the brain, this operation has restored normal hearing to hundreds of thousands of people. This is something to consider if it is found that impairment of hearing is due to a physical cause instead of a diseased nerve.

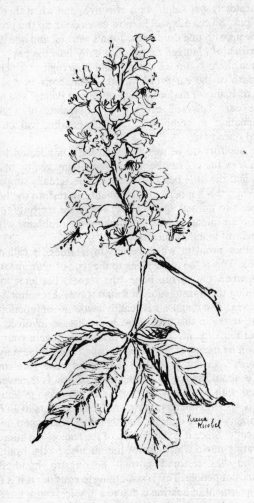

Horse chestnut (Aesculap hyppocastanum)

SUPPURATION OF THE ANTRUM

If you just think of how suppuration of the *antrum* comes about, you will be able to see how quite simple remedies can deal with the cause of this problem. For the most part, such an inflammation originates in the nose, especially after head colds, sore throat, influenza, scarlet fever, etc. It can, of course, come from neglected and chronically suppurating teeth. When this happens the secretions of the local circulation becomes congested, normal functions can no longer be sustained and the body must find another way out. The leucocytes and lymphocytes now appear on the scene to avert the danger. The body has various possibilities of defense and if the normal way of dealing with infections is not open, other measures are instituted. And suppurations of *antrums* or *sinuses* is one way of preventing worse developments. You can usually recognize it by its one sided nasal discharge which has the consistency of thick pus. Acute throbbing and pulsating pains in the upper jaw or forehead, depending upon the cavities afflicted, accompany the abundant discharge. In case of chronic *sinusitis* (the inflammation of the cavities of the head) the pain may be absent but besides the one sided discharge hoarseness may exist. Merely syringing the cavities will not get rid of the causes. In addition to specifically acting natural remedies, other eliminating measures must be employed. An onion compress, while not very pleasant, is without doubt simple and effective and better than many drastic treatments. Chop an onion finely, place it between two pieces of gauze and bind it around the neck at night before retiring. The two homeopathic remedies Hepar sulph. 4x and Cinnabaris 3x (4x for children and delicate patients) will help eliminate the pus and heal the affected part. The foregoing makes syringing unnecessary and superfluous. A chronic case can be helped by hot compresses placed over the affected part and is especially helpful if the problem has resulted from a cold.

UNPRETENTIOUS REMEDIES FOR NEURITIS

It is true that repeatedly applied compresses of plain hot water will soothe the pain of neuritis. Still better effects are produced by herbal poultices, well heated before application. One can, of course, put the herbs in a linen or cotton bag, immerse it in hot water, wring it out and apply it quickly. This is a more intensive treatment. Other alternatives are slightly warmed St. John's wort oil poured on a piece of cotton or woolen cloth and applied. Another method is to mix potter's clay and hot water into a paste and apply, not forgetting to place a hot water bottle or electric heating pad on top of it, to prolong the heat and intensify the effect.

An old, very simple, though perhaps not very pleasant method has shown its worth. Soak a piece of cloth or gauze in hot paraffin, lay on the inflamed part and cover with wool. This is easily done on the back, arms and legs. This is a simple, inexpensive treatment. Anyone living in rural areas where lamps are used instead of electricity can easily use this paraffin method of treatment. Take care to leave the compress on the affected part until the skin appears red as the paraffin can burn and blister. The use of formic acid has proved very successful, especially in cases of neuritis and sciatica. If a patient knows where there is an ant heap, he should take his painful leg there and let the ants work on it. Later, having wiped off the insects he will really benefit from this "treatment" which equals an injection of formic acid. Otherwise, a direct injection of formic acid is the alternative. This will in most cases relieve the neuritis. If yours proves to be a very stubborn case you can combine both these treatments and confidently expect quicker results. It is to the patient's advantage to rid himself of toxins. Especially in the spring in a temperate zone, a blood cleansing can be accomplished with bitter herbs to be followed by a juice fast diet so that the impurities can be disposed of more readily. After the juice fast start on a natural diet so as to avoid absorbing more poisons which may start up new problems.

PERIOSTITIS (Inflammation of the fibrous membranes covering bones)

Just a little hurt, a cut or a torn skin. Such a thing can happen so easily at home or in the fields. What to do! Let the wound bleed freely and you will be able to forget all about it. So I thought when I injured my left foot some time ago.

Such things were always happening and no further trouble resulted. I naturally thought this time it would be the same. Within two days, however, the foot became inflamed and the first signs of blood poisoning could be detected. Two clay poultices made the symptoms disappear; but instead of continuing the treatment as I should have done, I did nothing further. From time to time, especially at night, I noticed a dull pain which seemed to deepen. After more than a week it got so bad I could not bear it any longer. *Periostitis* had evidently set in. Clay poultices no longer helped. In fact, I could no longer bear the poultices which formerly gave relief. Soaking the foot in a herb bath now did nothing towards relieving the pain. After two terrible nights I decided to apply the exanthematic treatment (Baunscheidt or Pyronex treatment) and after about two hours the pain had completely disappeared. The inflammation was drawn to the surface and the pain was eliminated. How much simpler is such a treatment, compared with the allopathic method where pain-killing drugs are prescribed and surgical treatment is recommended. Only someone who has experienced relief through natural and reliable means can appreciate how wonderful it is to draw from nature's storehouse the wide variety of remedies available.

STRAINED LIGAMENTS AND SINEWS, ANKLE SPRAINS, ETC.

There is a way to restore to normal in the quickest possible time the various *sprains* and *strained ligaments* that one experiences in his lifetime. One of the ways is as follows: Beat until stiff the whites of 4 or 5 eggs. Add Eucalyptus or

Camphor leaves but before adding put them through a mincer two or three times until they are transformed into a paste. Or if you do not have a mincer, use a pestle and mortar and grind the leaves into a powder, and add about 1 ounce to the egg whites. If neither of these leaves is available then use very finely chopped pine buds or needles. Mix the ingredients thoroughly into the beaten egg whites, spread the mixture on a piece of cloth, and bind loosely over the painful part with an elastic bandage. The hardening of the egg white will provide a firm and strong dressing. If necessary renew the dressing every other day. When the pain has subsided, massage the affected part with Comfrey tincture after which cabbage poultices can be applied. Pulped raw potatoes, curd or similar remedies can also be used for poultices. Usually this treatment brings results within three or four days. In cases of bruises and strained ligaments or muscles, warmth is always a necessary part of the cure.

GOITER AND IODINE SALT

Dr. Eggenberger of Herisau started the idea of *iodine salt* and it is partly due to his initiative that it was first introduced in Switzerland. Thus it spread to other countries as people realized the important role that this new product plays in avoiding certain forms of *goiter*. Admittedly, iodine salt is good for anyone whose thyroid gland is under functioning and it can do no harm. But to people whose thyroid secretion is excessive, iodine salt can lead to an attack of Basedow's disease (exophthalmic goiter). Experience show that if such people take the slightest amount of iodine, they get palpitations. These unfortunate people think they have some form of heart disease and run to the heart specialist to find out what is the trouble. In every case, because of lack of a warning on the salt package, they have been harmed by what appeared to be a harmless salt. It is quite incomprehensible how the introduction of this salt can be considered or offered as wholesome for everyone. It should be recommended only for those suffering from goiter. It is, of course, an undisputed fact that a *deficiency of iodine* leads to the development of *goiter,* for there is no doubt that the thyroid needs iodine. But it can be found in the foods we eat in sufficient quantity and can be easily assimilated without having recourse to a manufactured product.

If, for example, you throw away edible skins from fruits and vegetables, the outer layer of cereals (bran in particular), in short, anything that is part of the whole food, then you will sooner or later have a mineral deficiency which includes lack of iodine, which ultimately will encourage the development of goiter. Instead of using *iodine salt* it would be far better to eat foods in their natural state and avoid white flour, refined sugar and most canned foods, all products of civilized feeding. The introduction of *iodine salt* is partly due to the fact that those who lived in land-locked countries or in the vast stretches of the middle west in the United States (commonly known as the "goiter belt") apparently need more iodine than they normally get through the food they eat. To augment their iodine intake *sea salt* should be on the table at all times. On the other hand those who live near the sea do not seem to suffer from goiter or other thyroid disturbances. In coastal areas more fish is consumed and fish fresh from the sea has a high iodine content. Sea salt contains iodine in such combinations and proportions that has all the advantages of a seasoning and none of the disadvantages of a manufactured product because it is produced by nature and "nature does it better." If herbs are added to *sea salt,* then you have the perfect seasoning and flavoring for all your foods.

If you have a garden, another way in which you can avoid the possibility of having a *goiter* is to enrich the soil with iodine, for the amount of *iodine* in the food your garden produces will depend largely on the amount of *iodine* in the soil. Therefore, feed the soil with bone meal and other iodine containing mineral fertilizers. The plants growing in such soil will absorb the iodine and thereby satisfy the bodily requirements. This natural, biological solution is much to be preferred to the orthodox medical way of taking *iodine*.

Iodine belongs to those medicaments about which one cannot establish generally valid rules. In the same way one cannot say that alcohol is harmless because most people drink. Consumed in moderation many show little sign of damage to their health, while others who are more sensitive are easily affected adversely by drinking. For example, wine taken in moderation is said to help digestion. The apostle Paul once advised his companion Timothy to "take a little wine for your stomach" when Timothy had complained of indigestion. It is therefore necessary to know ones own nature, for individual sensitivity and disposition will determine the final effects. One cannot arrive at the conclusion that if certain things are harmless to one person they are harmless to everyone. If you are sensible you will consider your individual nature and reactions and let this be your guide. For some with alcoholic tendencies, for example, abstinence may be difficult but if your health is at stake it may be the course of wisdom to make the necessary effort.

POSTOPERATIVE TREATMENT FOR GOITER

An operation for *goiter* should not be considered a complete cure necessitating no further treatment. On the contrary, postoperative treatment is necessary so as to eradicate the cause of the disease. To have recourse to iodine remedies is, according to Basedow, absolutely wrong. Instead, choose foods rich in *iodine* and use *sea salt*. Eat plenty of bran, watercress, sea weeds and other iodine rich plants. In addition homeopathic and botanic medicines can be used whenever indicated. Similarly cabbage and clay poultices can be applied to the affected area to produce strong effects by leaving it on for prolonged periods of time.

162

TREATMENT FOR ANGINA PECTORIS

There are different kinds of *angina pectoris* that come from this extraordinary illness which produces heart cramps. It is caused by a deficiency of blood supply of the heart muscle, which in turn induces oxygen starvation. The serious symptoms do not appear at once, but increasing instances of cramping heart pains with a feeling of tightness across the chest – so-called "cardiac insufficiency" – should warn that immediate action must be taken. The newest treatment with hormones has yielded comparatively good results. There are, however, various homeopathic and herbal remedies that should not be overlooked in the treatment of this disease. Correctly employed they are invaluable. Consider the good effect of Tabacum 6x has on acute and serious cases; or 12x potency in chronic conditions. The cramping heart pains which induce fear, dizziness and nausea, the hesitating pulse beat and the cold sweat will be relieved by Tabacum in the potencies mentioned above. It works well in nicotine poisoning, thus proving the homeopathic principle: like cures like. Whenever a constriction of the coronary arteries is produced and with it the symptom-complex of *angina pectoris*, Tabacum 6x will greatly improve the condition.

Imminent collapse, with cold sweat on the forehead and a cramp which travels far down the legs, invariably requires the use of Veratrum album 6x.

Heart hormones are very effective in cases of genuine *angina pectoris* in which dilation and gradual loss of tone occurs. The heart is actually regenerated by their use.

Arnica 30x given as an injection (alternatively, 10 drops of the attenuated tincture in a glass of hot water can be sipped during the day) acts especially well in arteriosclerotic conditions of the heart and blood vessels. Five to ten drops of the Crataegus mother tincture as a daily dose will strengthen the heart generally while Galeopsis (Nettle) mother tincture and Cactus grandiflorus 2x will be found very effective, if asthmatic symptoms manifest themselves.

If the patient has a high color, slightly bluish, and the veins are somewhat dilated Naya 12x would be indicated. If the blood pressure is high, use Visca drops, an extract from mistletoe. Correct breathing, a slow sustained expiration, can very often stop an attack at the beginning and afterwards blood can be drawn away from the heart by bathing the arms. These arm baths have a remarkably good effect and they are to be recommended for incipient attacks. A warm bath with an infusion of lemon balm added will have a calming influence on the nervous system. After the bath massage the body well with a natural skin functioning oil for relaxation of the nerves and a general feeling of tranquility.

The proper functioning of the bowels, as with all illnesses, is especially important here. For gentle though positive movement use *Psyllium seeds* pulverized or a preparation of *Flax* or *Linseed* – both are good herbal *laxatives*. As regards food, a diet rich in natural fruit sugar, but meager in protein and salt, is recommended for *angina pectoris*.

AN OLD COUNTRY REMEDY

Generally speaking, bad heart cramps are relieved only by strong medicines, usually Amyl nitrite or Trinitrini. There is, however, an old, exceedingly simple remedy which is quite easy to come by. It relieves cramp pains and leaves no aftermath or complications. It is good for a cramp in asthma cases too. This is an old peasant remedy which has been in use for centuries but now, alas, it is almost forgotten.

Take fermented cider, the older the better, heat it until it reaches the boiling point and quickly remove it from the fire. Soak some towels in the hot cider and place them as hot as they can be borne on both arms, covering each arm completely. The heat plus the fruit acids of the hot cider will decongest the heart circulation, soothe the blood vessels and the nervous system and relieve the cramps. This simple method can be augmented by putting a hot linseed, hay flower or lemon balm compress on the heart.

Cramp-like conditions brought about by angina pectoris or other similar causes follow the course of the sympathetic nerve. Very often they begin in the pit of the stomach near the sternum and move up to the neck leaving a feeling almost amounting to strangulation. Such distressing conditions will be relieved in a remarkable way if the suggestions made above are followed.

ATHLETE'S HEART

Sports of all kinds, if carried to excess, can endanger the heart. There is a great difference between the pleasure of movement, the joy taken in playing the game, and the slavish pursuit of a competitive sport. If you force yourself beyond your endurance and strength, you must not be surprised if your heart muscles become distended. This takes place when it loses its elasticity. At all events, one can help such a condition, and to a certain extent, regeneration is possible but the old proverb: "prevention is better than cure" speaks for itself.

Most sportsmen have strength and resistance but they must not make the mistake of thinking that they possess an unlimited amount of resilience or ability to spring back from over-exertion. Thoughtless waste of any of our potentialities will be followed by loss of fitness. Why sacrifice so much to sport and have to pay a big price for years to come? Physical fitness programs are excellent if one knows the limitations of his body. Why dash with abounding strength into overstrenuous sports and come out with chronic ill-health? Many will think that I am painting a pessimistic picture but this is not so. How often do we hear of famous sportsmen or athletes reduced to physical wrecks unable to climb without loss of breath, suffering from weak pulse, low blood pressure and ear and head noises? There is nothing wrong with being devoted to sports but be careful to not over-devote. To heed this warning is difficult for those who have already given up their "body and soul" to this demanding taskmaster. The passion for winning in competitive sports consumes a terrific amount of strength

165

and energy and places a severe strain on the heart, sometimes destroying it. There is no doubt that physical fitness programs properly set up can be a great benefit to young and old alike and all of us should have as our goal, to promote good health, a regular planned exercise schedule. There are many different *exercises* that definitely help tone the muscles, control weight and strengthen the heart and among the most popular are *walking* or *hiking*, then *bicycling, jogging, tennis, skiing, swimming, weight lifting, calisthenics,* etc. Whatever sport you engage in do it in moderation in the beginning, gradually increasing the pace to the point where you get the most benefit out of it. Don't run to win – run to exercise and you will be better off both physically and mentally.

CALCIFICATION AND CALCIUM REMEDIES

There is quite a wrong idea extant about calcium remedies, calcification, and above all, *calcification* of the arteries. Quite often a patient is heard to say, "I can't take Calcium-complex as I'm suffering from hardening of the arteries and it obviously would not be good for me to take any more calcium." This is naturally a very wrong idea. Biological preparations like Calcium-complex have absolutely nothing to do with calcification. On the contrary, someone who is suffering from hardening of the arteries *can* take such a biological calcium preparation without further ado, for it can be easily assimilated. It can be used to repair worn out parts of the body and is never deposited. The word "deposit" in this case is used in the sense of arterial deterioration or degeneration whereby the elasticity of the arterial walls suffer. First of all, fatty substances called Lipoids, are deposited on the lining of the blood vessels and later the calcium. According to some research workers, the thickening takes place as a natural necessity so as to strengthen the walls of the arteries. It is thought that the body, as a defense measure, deposits calcium when the veins have lost a certain elasticity and stability and thus cannot respond any longer to conditions of pressure. Other researchers, however,

166

are of the opinion that it is just because of these deposits in the vessels, the so-called *Arterio-sclerosis*, that they become brittle. In any case, it is a sign of age which appears due to a disturbance in the general metabolism brought about, probably, by an excess intake of protein. But, no matter what one does, he can never make the calcium in his food responsible for the pathological process of *calcification*. The skeletal system of the body contains reserves of calcium which would be quite sufficient to calcify our entire system of blood vessels, yet in practice, such contingency never arises. As far as possible Naturopathy treats *Arteriosclerosis* with remedies that restore elasticity to the vessels. The blood pressure will thereby be reduced, for it previously had to rise because of constriction, compelling the heart to exert greater pressure to keep the circulation normal. Arterio-complex, a combination of Arnica and Crataegus extracts, Visca drops, a Mistletoe preparation and wild Garlic wine have produced excellent results, At the same time care should be taken to reduce the salt and protein intake to a minimum. Fresh fruits and vegetables and especially unpolished rice should frequently figure on the menu, because these will gradually normalize the condition.

If at any time it becomes necessary to take Calcium-complex, remember that this medication has a good rather than an ill effect on hardening of the arteries. This should reassure the patient who is frightened away from a good calcium preparation. He must now realize that such a preparation is not in any way associated with the sclerosis of the arteries and helps rather than hinders a cure.

CALCIUM

There has been a lot said and written about the importance of *calcium* for our bodies. Without calcium, neither our bone structure, nor our teeth, nor the greater number of our body cells could exist. It is therefore necessary that we should eat plenty of calcium containing foods.

Calcium also plays a great part in defending our bodies against infectious diseases, especially diseases affecting the respiratory organs. Children who are calcium deficient are prone to infectious diseases, quickly develop swollen glands and in general health are usually below par. Their bodies are constantly engaged in an unequal struggle to keep up their physiological functions. Nature provides us with a good example. Meadows that are short of lime always have a quantity of moss growing in them. If, however, you give them a dressing of this mineral, you neutralize the acidity of the soil lacking lime and there is a certain parallel in the human body for where there is a calcium deficiency all sorts of diseases and especially infectious diseases will thrive. Since this information has been known for many years we find all kinds of calcium preparations on the market. But all those phosphoric, carbonic and lactic acid combinations of calcium have failed to fulfill their purpose. Man has remained deficient in this element.

About 25 years ago I debated with a well-known chemist in Davos, Switzerland, who had great experience in the manufacture of calcium milk and other calcium preparations. He declared that he was swamped with orders because it was generally known that calcium milk played an important part in the treatment of lung diseases. Yet he said this remedy is of little or no use, for in order to be assimilated, the calcium would have to come from the vegetable kingdom. Now this was a professional man from the "old school", but he could think biologically. It was his sincere conviction that strengthened me to resolve to obtain calcium from fresh, green nettles. I can say that I succeeded in producing a calcium preparation from this plant which the body can readily assimilate.

A fortunate association with other triturated biochemic calcium combinations has led to this Calcium-complex which has given thousands exactly what could be expected from a natural biological calcium preparation. But nobody should depend on any of these preparations, for the purpose of this book is to make you aware of the possibility of helping yourself without them.

I should like to show you how I would go about overcoming a calcium deficiency, first of all in these children who are born with it as well as any adult who suffers from it.

Infants should be given a natural diet, including plenty of liquid in which unpolished rice has been cooked, for there is much nutritional value for small children in this. Naturally, for the infant there is no substitute for the mother's milk and no woman should pass up the wonderful privilege of breast feeding her baby. As soon as the child starts on supplementary foods, natural rice is the best foundation. Then carrot juice, which is rich in calcium and minerals and easily digested, can follow. Later, almond milk with fruit juices added, can be introduced. Be sure to obtain tuberculin-tested milk whether it is cow's or sheep's milk. Unfortunately it is impossible to rely on the absolute cleanliness of milk and whether it has come from tubercular-free cows or not. Judging by the way some of these wretched cows are imprisoned continuously in stalls, it is not surprising that they are unhealthy. Good milk can only come from cows living on pasture and under natural conditions. Sheep's milk is better for small children because of the healthy outdoor life they live and is richer in calcium and vitamins and of greater nutritional value. Goat's milk can be given for a time but not permanently.

It is important that growing children, even adults, should avoid white sugar and white flour and that their food should be eaten in the same condition that their Creator gave it to them. In such food they will find all the vitamins and minerals in the right proportions and combinations – you simply cannot improve upon nature. Always have in mind: "back to natural foods, away with artificial products" that human greed for gain has imposed upon us. While the manufacturer profits, the body is damaged. The damage does not show it from one day to the next. The consequences of deficiencies, chemical additions and other aspects of food sophistication may take a long time to manifest themselves, but sooner or later people fall victim to them. Whether it is cancer, increased susceptibility to infection and disease, or a debilitation of the body, the possibilities are always to be reckoned with. This is brought about by man's lack of resistance, which depends on a healthy body fed in a natural way.

SAUERKRAUT WITH CALCIUM POWDER

Perhaps in different parts of the world, not all my English speaking readers will be well acquainted with *Sauerkraut* and I will briefly discuss it. Most country dwellers among you will know that cattle are often fed on "silage" during the winter months to replace the field grazing. The silage is produced by stamping the freshly cut grass into a huge concrete container or pit. The stamping will expel all air from the grass and this is very important. It is only by the exclusion of air that the desired lactic acid fermentation of the grass can be obtained. When the container or pit is filled with the grass to be used as silage, it is weighted down, sealed up and left to ferment. If all the pre-conditions of the desired kind of fermentation have been met, the grass will turn to silage within 4–8 weeks. Well, *Sauerkraut* is basically silage, but in place of grass, shredded white cabbage is used; the addition of salt, herbs, buttermilk, etc. serves only to flavor and to encourage formation of lactic acid rather than any other kind of fermentation. Sauerkraut is widely used on the continent and most country-folk prepare their own supply for the winter months when there are few fresh vegetables available.

When preparing *Sauerkraut* be careful to use very little salt but do not hesitate to use such plants as marjoram, thyme, juniper berries and, of course, mustard seed, which are very important to the preserving of the Sauerkraut. *Sauerkraut* made from white cabbage is very rich in calcium and possesses great curative value when eaten raw. The calcium content can be increased by adding ground eggshells or washed oyster shell powder in the proportion of 1 level teaspoonful to 1 pound of *Sauerkraut*. This powder can be mixed with the shredded cabbage in the same way as you would do with the herbs, etc. The resulting fermentation will turn the mineral *calcium* of the shells into easily assimilated *calcium lactate*. If you prepare a small wooden barrel of Sauerkraut every autumn and enrich its calcium content in the manner suggested, you will find that by eating it regularly, in two years there will be no calcium deficiency in your family. If you buy it from a health food store instead, mix one of these two powders in it and let it stand for another day before eating it raw. This latter way of taking calcium is not quite so effective as the former way but it is still better than medication with commercially prepared calcium. A small quantity of eggshell or oyster shell powder can be mixed with your salad dressing, if you prepare it using lemon juice, as this acid will dissolve and change the lime of the shells and assimilate it better.

NETTLES

Another excellent source of calcium is the nettle. Gather young *nettles* in the spring, chop them very fine or put them through a mincer, then mix them into a salad. They can also be sprinkled over potatoes or other dishes that one would normally garnish. No one would even notice that it was not one of the other garnish greens. Put it in soups just before serving, or on spinach, always making sure never to cook the nettles. Thus you will be sure of eating something that contains first-class calcium phosphate, Vitamin D and other important minerals.

Some time ago I gave this information about nettles in my monthly "Health News" and later heard from many Bernese (Swiss canton) country women who were delighted with the way their children responded to *nettles*. They said the children were rosy cheeked and healthy and seemed to have increased their resistance to disease by taking *nettles* as recommended. Why don't you adopt this simple inexpensive method of increasing your own calcium intake? Why buy expensive preparations when there are other more valuable garden produce

171

available for just the preparing! This is an investment in good health and when you prepare the nettles yourself you know it is fresh, pure and natural. Isn't it worth the trouble? Of course, because it is a sure investment in prevention.

IMPORTANT FACTORS IN THE TREATMENT OF LUNG DISEASES

Rest, light, air and sun are recognized factors in the cure of *lung diseases* and their value has been proved beyond doubt.

"Lift your eyes unto the hills whence cometh your help" are the words I found written over the entrance of the Sanitarium in Arosa, Switzerland. They illustrate clearly our dependence upon natural forces for healing. They are at the same time an honest admission by orthodox medicine that it is primarily air, the climatic conditions of the mountains especially, that provide the curing of lung diseases.

Another factor must, however, not be forgotten and that is nutritional therapy. The body must be supplied with material in which it is deficient before it can attempt regeneration. Foods rich in calcium and vitamins are indispensable and among these, raw, freshly pressed juice of carrots, grapes, oranges, grapefruit, etc. take the first place. These juices should be taken in little sips, not a whole glass at a time. In this way if anyone has a low tolerance for fruit acids or for those who are not used to natural drinks, there can be no unpleasant gastric disturbance.

Plenty of fresh vegetables should be served daily and salads should not longer be made with vinegar. Use lemon juice.

Concentrated protein foods must be reduced, while natural culinary herbs, which stimulate the appetite, are much to be preferred. Easily assimilated calcium in the form of Calcium-complex and Silica, which is found in Galeopsis, will produce wonderful results. In this connection I must mention Usnea, the moss found on the larch trees. The animals of the forest make good use of its lung strengthening properties and we should use it for combatting weakness of respiratory organs. If you cannot chew the moss, take an infusion of it instead. These are, in a sense, not medicines, but nutritional plants and bear out Hippocrate's principle that "food should be medicine and medicine should be food." In reality, remedies from the plant kingdom really belong in the category of curative foods.

Don't forget our old friend codliver oil that has many benefits. If you can't stand it plain, take the emulsified with orange juice and you will like it much better.

The lung patient needs to be influenced psychologically too, as the mind acts upon the glands and a morose or fearful state of mind will thoroughly upset the glandular secretions. The cultivation of a constructive and hopeful outlook will greatly contribute to the well-being of the patient while a negative mental state may very well retard progress and possibly prevent the success of the cure.

Skin function, too, should be encouraged by giving the body a daily friction bath with a brush, after which the skin should be oiled with a good skin function oil. And don't forget the bowels! They need special attention. The same can be said for the kidneys. It is a precondition for the cure of almost any ailment, that these eliminating organs function properly.

Patients who take to heart this advice will surprise their supervising physicians by the increased rate of progress they will make during their rest cures. It cannot be otherwise, for whenever we assist the inherent healing power of the body by eliminating existing deficiencies and weaknesses progress is bound to come.

SPEEDY HEALING FOR SHINGLES (Herpes Zoster)

Shingles are no easy disease to treat and they often take a long time to disappear. It is therefore good to know of the excellent results that can be achieved with the natural modes of treatment combined with homeopathic medicines. Employing the latter medicine, the following may be given in the form of injections: Formisoton 6x and Rhus tox. 12x. To be taken orally: Mezereum 3x (Spurge Olive). To stimulate the kid-

173

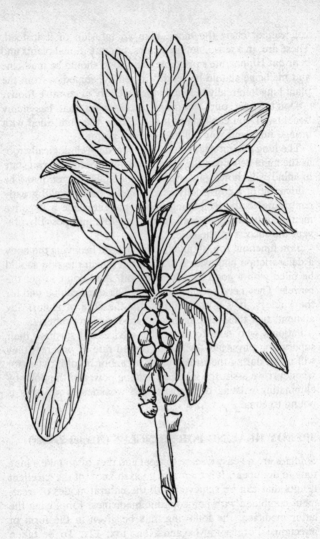

Daphne (Daphne mezereum)

neys, drink Goldenrod tea and an infusion of Rosehip kernels. Locally, dab with Extract of Lemon balm and Marigold. Attention to the diet is important. Cut down on salt and concentrated proteins such as cheese, eggs, meat and fish. Eat plenty of fruit and wheat, millet or barley flakes. Also plenty of vegetables and raw carrot juice. Any organically grown cereals are permissible. Exact observations of these suggestions will shorten the duration of this complaint considerably.

INSOMNIA

If you suffer from *insomnia* it will first of all be necessary to eliminate the factor responsible for it. You may have been drinking strong coffee for years. If this is the case, gradually wean yourself away from it by using a cereal or fruit coffee. It may be difficult at first but the palate will gradually adjust itself to the new taste in a surprisingly short time. In the end you will be taking a harmless drink that will permit you to rest through the night undisturbed. If you have cultivated the habit of "robbing the refrigerator" before going to bed, you should try to break this habit because a full stomach before retiring is not conducive to a good night's rest and is usually responsible for bad dreams. Our last meal of the day should precede bedtime by 3–4 hours. After the evening meal, instead of plopping down to watch TV, take a short walk and take deep breathing exercises. These will help digestion, benefit your health and go a long way towards insuring a good night's sleep. The common sense approach is, after all, the best approach.

A good sleeping draught is Lemon balm, the effect of which may be increased by the addition of hops. The homeopathic remedy is Avena Sativa (extract of oats). These, taken together, have an excellent sleep inducing effect and ready-made preparations are available on the market. Valerian is often prescribed but its effects as a sedative are narcotic. However, a drop added, the two drinks mentioned will have a calming result.

Mountain guides in Switzerland know of and use another good remedy. It is Marmot oil and a teaspoonful of this taken daily will induce sleep. Since it is not too palatable it is best taken in gelatin capsules. Do not forget that the habit of going to bed early conserves health and energy.

STOMACH DISORDERS

We frequently blame the stomach for all sorts of troubles when, very often, the liver is at fault. If the acids of fruits or fats cannot be digested and cause discomfort, it is a sign that the liver is not functioning as it should. Once the liver has been restored to its normal function, the stomach will perform its task perfectly and the former distress will disappear. To accomplish this, exclude from your diet temporarily fruit and fat acids and concentrate on unpolished rice. This is very easily digested and will not affect the liver in any way. Thus, it provides an excellent basis for the diet necessary. Add to your diet, millet, buckwheat, or whole wheat. Salads are good too, but prepare the dressing with *whey* concentrate instead of vinegar, which has a bad effect on the gastric mucous membranes. Indeed, vinegar is very often the cause of liver disorder or secretion problems in the stomach. It makes itself evident by a burning sensation which comes from excessive gastric secretions.

If you wish to get rid of this burning quickly, take a little wood ash in warm water. Put the ash in a cloth, suspend the cloth in warm water and let it soak for a few minutes, then drink the warm water. Charcoal is also good as a neutralizer and may be obtained in any drug store. It may sound unpalatable to suggest raw potato juice diluted in water but it works very well. Dry rolled oats, well chewed, will also neutralize acidity. Centaury infusion extract counteracts heartburn and heals at the same time. Milk, on the other hand, has a good effect on the symptoms only. In these various ways, heartburn, which has evidently come about through some mistake in the diet, can be readily cured.

STOMACH ULCERS

Fasting has proved to be a good remedy for *stomach ulcers* but, of course, one must have adequate reserves of strength to embark on this course. Drinking raw cabbage juice and carrot juice are equally beneficial and raw potato juice can be called a specific for the same condition. Here are three marvelous remedies at hand which can be grown in your own garden. Of course there are other remedies such as Hamamelis but when you have available home garden remedies it is hardly necessary to go out and buy the more expensive kind.

If you have difficulty in taking the raw vegetable juices, just put them into soup after it has been cooked and allowed to cool a little. The concentrated taste of the raw vegetable is lost in the soup but you will still get the benefit of them. Condensed Bilberry (also known as Whortelberry or Cowberry) and Licorice juices have proven to be excellent. Take 1–1½ ounces of these thickened juices daily, keeping them in the mouth so that they become well salivated. Since ulcers often result from nervous disorder make sure the person is free from worry and in quiet and peaceful surroundings.

GASTRIC AND INTESTINAL POISONING

There is every reason to consider this subject more closely, especially today, when use of chemicals on the farm and in food manufacturing is constantly on the increase.

Anyone who has lived in a tropical or subtropical climate knows how dangerous it is to eat fruit that has not been thoroughly washed. To be on the safe side it is better to eat fruits that can be peeled such as bananas, oranges, pineapples and mangoes. A cucumber salad made with unpeeled cucumbers can actually endanger life in the tropics. The possibilities of poisoning greatly occupied my mind when I myself fell victim to it. I had been in search of certain herbs and while in the woods, I crossed a clearing in which there grew wonderful specimens of Belladonna. As the ground just there was very steep and slippery, I involuntarily held on to the strong plants.

177

Later I came upon some large poison lettuce which I broke off and examined more closely. Shortly afterwards I found some strawberries under a luxurious growth of herbs and, forgetting I had not had the opportunity to wash my hands, I began to eat the luscious, tasty and delicious fruit. On my way home I picked some Rhus-toxicodendron – a poisonous plant – and held it in my hands. I remembered all this later that night when I awoke with violent abdominal pains. On the whole, I am not particularly sensitive to poisons and I usually am not sensitive to Rhus-tox because the worse it can do is cause a rash even if one is allergic to it. I had also eaten vegetables raw, bought from a store, and this could have contributed to the disturbance. Whatever the cause, the results were very disagreeable.

SUCCESSFUL TREATMENT

Intensive diaphram breathing eased the pain considerably, but it returned and awakened me continuously. In the morning I tried to get some relief by going out into the open air. While out there I collected some giant dock leaves which I put on my abdomen to ease the pain. For a short time I experienced relief, but later in the morning it started up all over again. The bowels acted well but I passed very little water. This surprised me but I should have realized that the body was keeping back the liquids so that it might eventually help to empty the bowels. And so it was. A violent diarrhea set in and continued all through the morning. Everything poured out but in be-tween I tried to get on with my work. At the end of five hours I had to give up. I took sips of Lachesis 12x, Echinacea 2x and clay. Later I took Belladonna 4x in the hope it might do some good since I had handled the Belladonna plant the day before and this could have been to blame for my condition. The various remedies did do some good and towards midday I was able to vomit. Strangely enough I brought up the lunch from the day before. Such sluggish digestion I hadn't noticed before. Unfortunately, by now I was much too tired to con-tinue looking around for a remedy to relieve the nausea although Nux vomica 4x and Ipecacuanha 4x would have served me well. I had overworked considerably during the previous week and this probably contributed to my feeling of utter weariness. I now began to get cramping pains in my heart so I took some heart tonic and within five minutes the heart had calmed down. As the bowels were quite empty and the medicine which I continued to sip did its work well, I soon was quite better. Deep breathing still caused some slight intestinal soreness, but my otherwise healthy body had triumphed over the poison.

SPECIAL POINTS TO NOTE

Many people would become fatally ill from poisoning, especially if they were constipated at the same time. It is therefore of utmost importance to empty the bowels immediately to get rid of the toxins. If the bowels do not function and it is impossible to vomit, then the body is forced to deal with the decomposing material in some other way. If it cannot render it harmless, a very serious condition might result and under certain circumstances could prove fatal. It is ignorance or carelessness on one's part if he does not take steps to move the bowels when the first sign of poison becomes evident. If after taking a remedy the patient should vomit, then an enema should be given immediately. Do not worry about vomiting up a laxative, for the stomach is being cleansed through it and this in itself is of value. If the bowels are helped to function, hardened feces will dissolve, even if there has been constipation. Dragging, cramping pains will be a sign that things are beginning to move. The body will do its part if only we give it the proper help. Frequent diarrhea is a symptom of poisoning and failing a response to remedial medications an enema is very necessary. If the heart is in good condition, take a good heart tonic.

After the bowels have been properly cleansed, it is best to fast for a time. Hunger will soon tell you when your stomach is again ready to receive food. Start with light cereal gruels and

179

in case the liver is still a bit sensitive, sip raw carrot juice. After two or three days clay mixed with water should be taken; then fast a second time for a little while, providing your heart can withstand it.

As soon as the feeling of hunger returns, proper meals can be enjoyed once more. If a fever occurs, do not be concerned as this is an indication that the body is fighting the disease. The only good thing that can be said about such an emergency is that it provides an opportunity for thoroughly cleansing the body, although we wouldn't want to recommend it as a standard method for doing so. One must not take medicines which suppress symptoms and impede natural functions, for such a course would prove detrimental in the end, even though it may be the easiest course. If we are to avoid mistakes we shall have to accept nature as our teacher.

INTESTINAL PARASITES

In the temperate climates it is the worms which have to be considered. When whitish pieces, looking like bits of noodle about ¼ inch wide and 5–10 inches long, are found in the stool, you can be sure it is part of a tapeworm. When the *tapeworm* has grown to its full length, it casts off a piece from the end, which is the egg-containing, reproductive part, while it continues to grow at the other end. Such a tapeworm can produce hundreds of thousands of eggs, which in agricultural areas finds its way into the cess-pit. If people, as they do in many areas, make use of the cess-pit for manure for their garden, the worms can be spattered onto the vegetables in heavy rain. This constitutes another possible source of infection. If this manure is used for meadows, the cows and the sheep stand a good chance of getting infected too. There are various kinds of tapeworms, the best known being from cattle, pig and fish. You can also get trichinosis from insufficiently cooked meat, especially pork and fish. Another dangerous *tapeworm* is Taenia Echinococcus (dog tapeworm). If a dog which is infected with tapeworms as much as licks your hand or face it is very likely you too will become infected. If ever a dog licks you be sure to immediately wash your hands or face thoroughly and make sure your children do the same. It is a very bad habit to let dogs lick you and it is much better to take exaggerated precaution than to have to combat the serious complications which a dog's tapeworm brings with it.

The danger in this case is not simply just having worms in the intestines; the eggs too must be considered as grubs develop, and these bore through the intestinal walls and are thus carried by the bloodstream to various parts of the body. Hydatid cysts then form in sizes from a pinhead to that of a baseball. You can readily appreciate how dangerous this can finally be.

Other intestinal worms should not be considered as a harmless evil. On many of my lecture tours, I have become increasingly aware that in most places there is a real plague of worms. At least half the children have worms, usually Oxyuris vermicularis or Ascaris lumbricoides and these can spread in the same way as a tapeworm. The damage these worms do, unfortunately, are not nearly enough realized. The poisonous metabolic excretions of the worms become absorbed and change the blood picture, which is responsible for the discomfort. Usually children, deficient in calcium are more likely to be hosts to worms and with infection of the blood the dangers multiply.

The Ascaris lumbricoides not only produce toxic infection but the larvae developed from the eggs penetrate through the intestinal walls into the lungs where they continue to grow. The patient may think that he is suffering from a very obstinate bronchitis, not realizing that the problem is entirely due to worms. From the lungs, the worms work their way back through the respiratory passages into the digestive tract from which their eggs emerge 70–75 days after the initial infection.

Even now, the travels of these worms are not ended, for when fully developed, they are not only to be found in the intestines, but sometimes even in the nose and mouth, to the disgust and horror of the infested person. They have also been known to bore their way into the bile duct causing jaundice, or right through the intestinal wall, which may give rise to a fatal peritonitis. They may increase by several hundreds and block the intestinal canal posing danger to life.

I could continue with the story of the dangers to which worms can expose us, but perhaps by now you have been convinced that worms are not a harmless eventuality that can be ignored.

Getting rid of *tapeworms* is not as easy as you might think. I once got rid of one for a young boy. The worm had withstood all the doctor's chemicals and drugs and he wanted to send the boy to the hospital for further experiments. However I succeeded in eliminating the *tapeworm* through the following procedure:

Diet: Plenty of vegetables, fruit and raw carrots; no meat, bread, potatoes and nothing containing flour. Lunch: Lentils, carrots, onions, garlic, cooked together in a pan and later seasoned with raw Sauerkraut; and in the morning before breakfast he took a handful of de-husked pumpkin seed, a handful of unsweetened cranberries and chewed them well. An hour later he drank one to two cups of tapeworm tea without sugar and occasionally he drank garlic milk.

Recipe for *tapeworm* tea: ⅙ oz. powdered Aloes, ⅔ oz. Black Alder bark, ⅔ oz. Senna leaves, 1 oz. Valerian root, and slightly more than 1 oz. of Peppermint leaves. Mix altogether and infuse for 10 minutes in boiling water as you do with ordinary tea.

When you get rid of the *tapeworm,* make sure that the head is there too; if not you must start the treatment all over again in two, or three weeks time. If nothing happens the first day, continue treatment for yet another day. An enema with garlic milk can be very advantageous. Constipation at such times must be tolerated on no account. If it exists take a laxative. In stubborn cases of tapeworm, ½ a teaspoon of Kamala powder should be given daily. Once the tapeworm has been passed, it should be burned. The disposal of Oxyuris vermicularis and Ascaris lumbricoides worms can greatly be facilitated by "worm granules" derived from the tropical bush Carica-Papaya.

I know many worried mothers will say when they read this: "I can't possibly give my child any more worm medicine because he was so completely upset by the last one." This remedy is happily different from all others, in that it expels the worms without having any ill effect on the body. Ordinary worm medicines poison, kill and so dispose of the worms. But worm granules made from Carica-Papaya does not work like this.

The effective substance is not a poison, which would be bound to hurt the body to some extent, but a ferment, a protein digesting substance, which actually digests the living tissue of the worms in the intestines. Thus, the intestinal wall is not in any way damaged; it remains just as unaffected by this plant ferment as by its own ferment.

However, there is another kind of protein which is digested by this ferment and for this reason one should abstain from all meat products. You see, if the proteins you take in your meals use the worm killing ferment for digestion, it will not be available for digesting the worms and that is the reason you take it in the first place. Not only should the patient abstain from meat but also from eggs, cheese, fish, etc. for they too are protein foods. If you observe these hints, the results will convince you that worm granules from Carica-Papaya takes the first place among harmless and reliable worm remedies.

It is possible that, a short time after you think you have gotten rid of the worms for good, you will notice them again. This does not mean that the worm treatment has been ineffective, but, that through carelessness there has been a further infection. Eggs deposited by the worms near the anus either get into the bed or, through scratching, get under the finger nails and thus into the alimentary canal, where the trouble starts all over again. Or possibly the microscopic eggs are shaken out of the bed when it is made, joins dust in the bedroom and are breathed into the body to begin production again. Worm larvae have actually been found on top of a bedroom bureau, so cleanliness cannot be over-emphasized. The room should be dusted daily with a damp cloth and the bed linens changed frequently. Diet is most important to the cure. However, we may indulge in one optimistic thought: not everyone succumbs to an infection of Oxyuris larvae, for the natural resistance of the body and good digestion do not give them a chance to develop.

THE MYSTERY OF OUR BLOOD

The Bible tells us that the "soul is in the blood." The chemist also senses the mysterious action of the blood when he claims that the blood is very special. He was aware of this long before his assertion was supported through the findings of various research experiments in our modern times. It was the declaration recently made by a well known scientist that made me stop and think. He claims that the condition of a person can be determined by looking at his blood. According to his theory, a single drop of *blood* reveals everything about the health of the person. Research though has not found a proper diagnostic method to utilize this assertion. Scientists must first search and find it before they can properly evaluate it. The method of blood crystalization already leads us one step ahead. This method certainly merits our attention. No doubt other methods will be discovered and the time seems near when most illnesses such as cancer, gout and many others, may be detected in their early stages long before the usual symptoms become observable. Even though the *blood* has been sub-divided into groups, and the RH factor has been discovered, we know already that the texture of our blood may be either coarse or fine. Just as the skin shows either large or small pores, there are many singularities of the blood, for example, differences in its content and structure that remain to be revealed.

If the exploration of the *blood*, this truly mysterious red river of life, had progressed beyond the present stage, there would hardly be 20,000 cases of death due to blood transfusions a year in the United States. In the future, it is very likely that surgeons, having been educated to recognize the great risks involved in transfusing human blood, will make better use of plasma or blood substitutes.

Hepatitis, a much feared inflammation of the liver, with infectious jaundice resulting from transfusion, should here be mentioned. The prevention of serum hepatitis is a problem that up until now, has not been solved. Considering that even the medical director of an American blood bank expressed much concern over the risks involved in transfusions and that many surgeons, due to unsatisfactory experiences, prefer to work with substitutes, is it any wonder that the patient should be able to express his personal preference and make his own decision?

How could we humans possibly know all the secrets of blood, not having had a part in its formation? But to Him that created it, it is no mystery. He denied the consumption of blood to the survivors of the great deluge and this became the basis of law even for his own people. It was again stressed as binding upon everyone by the original church during the life and times of the apostle Paul. The principles of this law are still valid and binding down to this day.

If we take a closer look at those various laws, we find that they are not only of educational value, but are also beneficial to our health. Their careful observation can be only for the protection of the individual. The person who refuses blood in any form, for whatever reasons, will get more and more support and approval for his conviction as research progresses.

THE LYMPH(ATIC) GLAND, THE WHITE BLOODSTREAM

Even though the lymphatic vessels are longer than twice those of the red blood corpuscles, our knowledge of the white blood corpuscles is still very modest. The lymphatic veins, much finer than those of the red bloodstream, are distributed throughout the entire body. Contrary to the red bloodstream, the lymph stream flows only in one direction and the fluid is returned to the venous blood stream after its task is completed. The body can be divided schematically into four parts in the form of a cross, starting at the belly button. Each of these four fields corresponds to a lymphatic network, with a center located at the right and left side of the groin area and in the armpit region. Smaller centers are also located below the lower jaw, at the right and left side. Leading to these centers, the lymph glands form little nodes which reach maximum size in the center itelf.

FUNCTIONS OF THE LYMPH STREAM

The lymphatic system is responsible for keeping the body fluids, the blood fluid and the brain fluid in order. The total amount of fluid accounts for 60 % of our body weight. In addition to this, the lymph cells have another vital function. Like the county police, they must destroy all invading organisms that enter and endanger the cells. We are referring here to bacteria, which are more or less vicious or perilous, depending on the species. For example, if we suffer an injury or a rusty nail penetrates the skin, millions of bacteria enter the body. The fine, outer lymph vessels are not strong enough to successfully combat the intruders and the bacteria continue their journey into the nodes of the centers. The centers then call up their defenses and the vessels expand and we feel a swelling in the area of the groin or armpits. This can become as large as a chicken egg. If the lymphocytes, phagocytes, other circulating white blood cells, and whatever name the defense mechanism may have, cannot handle their job, the lymphatics, a closed system of tubes, becomes swollen. It takes on a reddish color and becomes very sensitive to pressure. This condition is called blood poisoning or toxemia, even though the toxins are still contained within the white bloodstream of the lymph. If all toxins and bacteria were passed on to the red bloodstream, one would not be able to survive one's childhood because of the many poisons that would enter the body. Connected with the lymph system are also the *tonsils* and the *appendix*. They too, have the job of cleansing the body and destroying the germs. Both serve as important filtering systems, which never should be removed except for valid reasons. Their removal constitutes a weakening of the forces in the fight against bacteria.

In the event that cancer cells escape during a smear test or an operation, the lymph generally harbors them with the intent of destroying them. If they are not successfully destroyed, these gigantic cells begin to grow and multiply, and the result is the much feared lympho-granuloma, or cancer of the lymph. That is why surgeons remove all lymph vessels and nodes during a cancer operation, especially in cases of breast cancer. The lymph has another function to fulfill, namely to absorb emulsified fat and return it in small quantities to the bloodstream. All so-called antibodies, which insure immunity against infectious diseases, are formed in the lymphatics, which explains the importance of a properly functioning lymph. Certain disorders of the heart, the kidneys and the vessels can be attributed to a partial failure of the lymph system.

SUPPORTIVE TREATMENT (HEALING METHODS)

Plenty of exercise and proper intake of fresh air are great for our lymphatic system. Mountain, sun and ocean air have an excellent effect on the lymph.

A proven botanical substance, extracted from the subtropical Echinacea plant, is recommended especially for the lymphatic system. Echinacea, taken internally and used as an external application, brings about relief quickly in cases of swollen lymph nodes and toxemia. For external use the freshly squeezed leaves can be made into a pack, or a cotton swab can be soaked with the tincture. If the condition is an acute one, take 10 drops of tincture with a little water every hour. Because of its excellent effect Echinacea should be kept in the medicine cabinet of every home.

INTERESTING FACTS ABOUT THE LYMPH

Without the lymphatics, also called the white bloodstream, man would succumb to incessant bacterial attack in no time. The leucocytes are the police force of the body. Their function is to destroy invading germs that enter through ruptures in the skin caused by cuts or injuries. At the same time the white blood corpuscles are actively involved in repairing the destroyed parts of the cells. The lymph network can be compared to that of blood vessels, the latter much longer than the former. The mucous membranes, especially those of the intestines, also have an extensive tightly woven net of lymph vessels.

THE SPLEEN

Even though we do not know much about the efficacy of the spleen, it is a fact that it is the largest lymph gland of all, located to the left side of the stomach just opposite the liver. Despite its location it has nothing to do with the digestive system, nor is it connected in any way, or related in function to any other organ. The spleen is connected directly to the bloodstream and not to the lymph. It could therefore be located anywhere else in the body, the only logical explanation for its actual location being that there is ample room for it. To this day, the spleen is still puzzling the scientists. One could go on living after the spleen has been removed, but the production of white blood corpuscles is so minimum, that one could not survive an attack of micro-organisms as violent as in the case of malaria, for example.

THE CIRCULATING CELLS

Lymphocytes and leucocytes are circulating cells; they leave the lymphatics as well as the bloodstream and move about between the walls of the cells, which is made possible by their minuteness. Whenever and wherever they are needed they are ready to attack. It is truly astonishing to note that there are more circulating cells in our body than there are people on earth. While an accurate count cannot be taken, they number in the billions.

CORRECTIVE MEASURES

Despite its excellent organization, the lymph often needs support. For example, a *calcium and vitamin deficiency* creates a difficult problem for the lymphatics. Protuberances, notably in the groin area of children, and at times on the neck, behind the lower ear, can be attributed to this deficiency. Lack of calcium and Vitamin D is marked by susceptibility for colds and catarrhs, angina and other infectious diseases as well as the loss of appetite, irritability and fatigue. In most instances relief can be brought about by a proper diet. In particular, sweets, bakery products and snacks must be avoided and the same goes for refined food items prepared with white flour, refined sugar and highly processed oils. Eat more vegetables and salads. Take a Vitamin D complex with Nettle-calcium. Calcium should be given to children as a prophylactic measure long before any of the above symptoms ever appear.

Horseradish has a most favorable effect on the lymph and is one of the best remedies available. Often the most stubborn disorders of the lymph disappear when a teaspoon of horseradish is taken daily. If it tastes too strong, mix it with cottage cheese or finely grated carrot.

TUBERCULOSIS AND CANCER

When the lymph system is working properly, it is impossible for *tuberculosis* or *cancer* to develop. In the case of cancer, the proper functioning of the liver is essential. That is why special attention should be given to both the liver and the lymph. Long before tuberculosis can be diagnosed, careful observation will disclose the presence of painful lymph nodes when pressure is applied to them. These early symptoms, observable years ahead, certainly warrant our special attention. In order to keep the lymph in good condition one must have adequate amounts of oxygen and sunlight. Dark apartments, facing away from the sun should be avoided, since they favor a natural environment for breeding germs that cause tuberculosis.

This malignant disease of the lymphatic glands, also known as Hodgkin's disease, afflicts more men than women. As early as 1832 Thomas Hodgkin described it in detail, but to this day its cause is unknown. The disease begins with a fever and it is termed by some scientists an infectious disease. The virus responsible for it has not yet been identified. Other scientists consider it a type of cancer and treat it with x-rays and cobalt rays. As a rule, the success of this type of therapy is of short duration. In cases where only a few nodes are affected by the disease, their removal is recommended until a better method can be found to deal effectively with the disease.

A switch to a natural food diet consisting of plenty of raw vegetables, cottage cheese (or curds), horseradish and *wild rice* has proven very beneficial. The disease is often accompanied by anemia. This can be counteracted successfully by drinking daily one tenth of a liter (about 5 ounces) of carrot and beet juices and, in addition, Alfavena. Petasite preparations taken with Colchikum D-4 have brought good results.

THE CAPILLARY SYSTEM

Only a few people know that the capillary network of the human body consists of 100 million meters of blood vessels. This would be two and a half times the circumference of the earth if all the tiny vessels were put together in one long line. It is not enough to be familiar with the structure of these tiny vessels, but we should also know their functions. The exchange of metabolic waste material and the passing on of carbon dioxide from the arterial to the venous blood system, and many other functions known and unknown to us, take place in the capillary network.

The body as a whole and the capillary system in itself can be adversely affected and harmed by mistakes in our diet or, for that matter, an unsuitable way of life. A diet rich in uric acid producing foods, such as meat and eggs, if used as substitutes for vegetables and fruits, cause a degeneration and dilation of the capillary network to a degree that when magnified, they have the appearance of small varicose veins. Too much alcohol consumption has the same effect on them. Chemicals, absorbed from medicines and nicotine, may alter the vessels and adversely influence the nourishing of the cells and thus disturb the entire metabolic process. This astonishing physical work of art in our bodies is of no benefit to us if we do not respect and value it and deliberately interfere with its function through improper diet or drinking to excess. Defects of the capillary system cause a degeneration, slackening and aging of the muscles and nerve cells due largely to improper diet. If we do not realize the importance of guarding our health until we are old, we are like the person who wasted all his fortune when young. In his old age he lives in poverty while contemplating the bygone luxury of his youth. We can compare youth to the 7 fat years referred to in the Bible. We should act wisely, just as Joseph did, storing up good health in order to be able to, figuratively speaking, live off of the "savings" during the "lean" years of advanced age. By adopting a healthy normal way of life in our youth we can insure good health in advanced age.

FUNCTIONS OF THE CIRCULATION

In order to illustrate the function of the blood circulation, let us for a moment consider the postal train travelling from Basel to Lugano and back, making stops right on schedule to unload on the way to Lugano and picking up mail on the way back to Basel. Imagine the confusion if the train did not keep its schedule. At each station we can see the postmaster looking for the postal train und trying to calm down the people who are waiting in vain for their mail to arrive. Such a mix-up could be very upsetting to everyone.

We can draw an analogy between the train and the circulatory system. Let us compare the train on its way to Lugano with the arterial network, which has the job of supplying the cells with nourishment to complete the process of feeding millions of cells. Minerals, vitamins, enzymes, amino acids, sugars, fats and even oxygen are being transported by the arterial network on a strict schedule. Suppose that something interrupted the schedule and the cells failed to receive the various substances transported by the network, what would happen to the body? There would be a general break-down resulting in serious illness and possibly death. The more we learn of the unusual function of different parts of the body, the more we can appreciate how wonderfully are the works of the Creator.

Every little cell, like a factory, needs raw materials and fuel. Only if it is supplied with all its necessities on schedule during life's span, can it be expected to perform as marvelously as it does. Lack of quantity and quality of raw materials forces the cells to find a make-shift solution. It is only under the most trying conditions that the cells look for short-cuts and thereby suffer in their performance. A case in point is shown when the body resorts to construction of gigantic cells, known as cancer cells. The cell itself is not guilty, for it fights and resists as long as possible to the point where failure can no longer be avoided.

We must, at all cost, assure that the mail trains of our artery system can keep their schedules by stimulating the circulation through exercise und proper breathing techniques. And above all we must provide the raw materials at the proper time in proper quality and quantity.

Thus far we have spoken of only one of the functions. Not only must the supply be considered but, like every manufacturing plant, we must concern ourselves with the waste products the body produces. They must be promptly disposed of to enable the body to function efficiently.

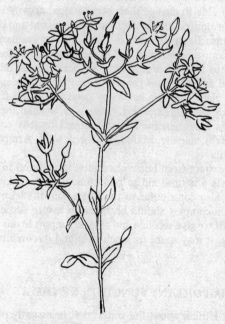

Centaury (Centaurea minus)

The train on its way back to Basel may be compared to our venous system, which is responsible for returning all "ashes" and waste products, carbon dioxide, uric acids and others. These waste products are being recycled in the liver or eliminated with the help of the kidneys. If this process of transportation is obstructed, problems will arise, since the accumulation of waste causes tension and pressure. The train may be derailed and the mail may be scattered, which means in terms of our body, the formation of varicose veins.

HELPFUL HINTS

What can be done to counteract this condition? Some people may be able to change their occupational activity in order to avoid prolonged endurance, especially in cold and damp environments. Being sensible in choosing our garments is most important; the abdomen and the legs should be covered sufficiently to insure warmth and high heels should definitely be avoided as they throw the whole body out of balance.

The plant kingdom has many good things to offer to keep the body running smoothly. Many girls, woman and expectant mothers have benefited from a famed remedy consisting of four herbs, namely, Milfoil, St. John's wort, Arnica roots and Pulsatilla.

An extract from horse chestnuts, in addition to the above herbs, is a natural aid to body function. Since mineral deficiency also contributes to the formation of varicose veins, a Calcium-complex should be taken to assure successful treatment. If we give sensible and natural support to our circulatory organs, it may spare us much pain and discomfort at a later time.

THE IMPORTANT FUNCTION OF THE ARTERIES

When I think about the traffic that incessantly passes every morning and every evening over the highways leading to and from cities like New York, Los Angeles, etc. I realize that the expression "traffic arteries" is justified and appropriate. If for some reason those arteries were paralyzed, as they have been in the past, from snow or torrential rains, these cities would also become paralyzed. The importance of arteries in our own bodies, by comparison, need a free flow of traffic in order for them to survive. Even the most humanly perfect body, possessing a perfect muscuar structure, a well organized arterial traffic, will begin to decay or degenerate as soon as our intelligent well-trained brain is damaged by sclerosis or hardening of the arteries. The anatomical structure is much like a cable, made up of different layers, the inside being a smooth tube. This tube is covered with other layers that consist of elastic, loosely woven threads, but still tensile and connective. This artery tube can withstand a pressure of about 20 atmospheres (a unit of pressure equal to 14.69 pounds to the square inch).

This knowledge provides us with some understanding of how our artery system functions. In the same manner as the heart, the arteries are supplied with blood through a network of veins, the so-called Vasa vasorum, which is built into the inner walls of the arteries. Furthermore, the walls of the arteries have their own network of lymphatic vessels and nerves. The farther removed the arteries are from the heart, the more branched out they become, and consequently their total cross section becomes proportionally larger, causing pressure to decrease and the walls to become thinner. A cross section of the capillaries, at the very tip of the arteries, is about 50 times smaller in diameter than the finest human hair.

THE ARTERIES IN THE BODY MAKE-UP

Dr. Hoorne, a Dutch scientist, once said that the body is made up of veins. It was he who discovered a system of making the blood vessels visible by injecting a red colored fluid into them. Peter the Great, who happened to be visiting Holland at that time, was intrigued by the experiment and wanted to take the first preparation home with him. Unfortunately, though, it had spoiled when it arrived in Russia because the sailors had consumed the alcohol from the glass that contained the preparation.

Considering that every one of the billions of cells in our body has access to the uninterrupted flow of the artery system is truly miraculous to contemplate. It takes the blood only one second to reach the venous capillary loop from the arterial one. It is at this moment that the metabolic process takes place, where oxygen is withdrawn from the blood and carbon dioxide from the tissue is permitted to enter. At the same time the nutritive material from the blood enters the tissue and the metabolic products from the tissue enter the blood stream. Having fulfilled its function, the blood now flows back to the heart via the venous system.

The circulation of the blood between the heart and the lungs and back to the heart again takes about six or seven seconds. The circulation through the heart, which supplies the myocardium by way of the coronary vessels, takes place in about three or four seconds. Blood supply to the brain takes eight seconds and to the tip of the toes, about 18 seconds. One blood cell, in the course of a day, can make about 3,000 round trips. Day and night the cells are moving about incessantly. It seems that nothing in this world is more fond of travelling than our blood cells. Beginning at the heart, a cell reaches the loop of the capillary with a swift motion. The farther away it gets, the slower the motion becomes because of a narrowing of the canals. At last it disposes of its load, as an express messenger would do, and begins immediately its return trip through the venous system. Due to physical stress, cold weather, excitement or fever, the blood cell speeds up its pace. Depression and psychological upsets, however, cause a slow-down. Billions of cells then are improperly nourished and illness may result if the situation is not remedied by means of positive psychological influence. This is an example of how psychological depressions may lead to physical infirmities.

NARROWING AND HARDENING
OF THE ARTERIES

A hardening of the arteries may have terrible, and at times, incurable consequences. The victim literally degenerates physically and mentally. To this day more civilized people, especially in Europe, the United States and Australia die of diseases of the arterial walls and the number of fatalities is increasing. The length of our life is often determined singularly by the condition of our arterial walls. *Arteriosclerosis* begins with a small alteration, which looks like a flat sore or ulcer. This sore then develops into a growth of the connective tissue, causing a calcium deposit in the arteries. Consequently the opening of the artery becomes smaller and smaller, losing more and more of its elasticity, eventually becoming hard and brittle. The result is that blood pressure increases, leading to thrombosis or embolism of the brain or a cerebral hemorrhage. A cardiac dilation or a hemorrhage of a blood vessel near the heart, as well as a shrinking of the kidneys may occur.

WHAT COULD BE RESPONSIBLE
FOR ALL THIS?

1. A diet high in fats, especially animal fats, which promotes an increased formation of cholesterol in the blood which is eventually deposited on the artery walls.

2. Nicotine is another factor contributing to a narrowing of the arteries, especially where the coronary vessels are concerned.

3. A diet abundant in protein, such as derived from meat, eggs and cheese. A diet too rich in these foods may lead to such a condition.

4. Too much consumption of alcohol is harmful to the capillary walls and thus may contribute to the advancement of the disease.

PROPHYLACTIC TREATMENT
AND PROPER MEASURES

1. A diet consisting of wild rice, curds and salads may have miraculous effects, if adhered to consistently. By lowering the blood pressure in a natural way, it becomes unnecessary to take any radical remedies. This natural treatment makes it possible to regenerate the blood vessels right from the beginning. As we can see from diet experiences in Asian countries, rice bran positively influences the regeneration of the arteries.

2. Plants rich in natural iodine, such as sea plants, contribute largely to the prevention or cure of this disease. Such sea plants can thus be processed for use as a seasoning or food.

Other medicinal herbs or spices beneficial here are watercress, all other kinds of lettuce, horseradish, garlic, Allium ursinum (leek) and small quantities of extracts from the Rauwolfia radix (root) or a mixture can be made of Rauwolfia and Mistletoe.

3. Plenty of oxygen is necessary and this means taking long walks through forests and mountains or on the seaside. Strenuous walking and deep breathing are an excellent tonic. If arteriosclerosis is already diagnosed, avoid higher altitudes. Low pressure and less oxygen could lead to a stroke.

For those who spend most of their time sitting in an office this advice is especially indicated. If one does not wish to be considered a fragile, elderly gentleman who has to be led to his office, he should give careful consideration as to how he spends his time away from the office, making sure he doesn't spend it at a bar instead of outdoors.

ADVANTAGEOUS PREVENTION
OF POSSIBLE HARM

One does not have to be a fanatic in order to admit that modern, civilized man is living rather dangerously. Just think of all the conveniences we gain from technology in our modern times. They bring with them less activity in the outdoors and cause pollution of air, water and food. Our indulgence in refined food products does not exactly contribute to maintenance of good health either. The arteries degenerate as a result of many disadvantages of our life style; signs of old age appear much too early, decreasing our productivity and sometimes bringing an early end to our lives. The average increase of our life span, due to reduction in infant mortality, does not change this picture either. It is not a question of reaching a high age by artificially maintaining ourselves through the use of drugs or other things foreign to our bodies. It is much better to live to a ripe old age and still be healthy and vigorously active with full possession of our minds. Our life style and the way we eat should be dictated by the laws of nature and not by those of society which, at best, contribute very little to our physical well-being.

ARTERIOSCLEROSIS, CORONARY THROMBOSIS, HEART ATTACKS

While I was spending some time in the Far East, I paid special attention to the occurrence of the above illnesses. It was quite evident that among the people living in the countryside of Japan, Korea and the Philippines, heart related diseases seldom occur. If they do occur it is usually among urban dwellers who have a higher standard of living, that is to say, they buy more factory made foods and have a high cholesterol diet. In all these countries of the Far East the country people eat very little fat, generally not more than 50 grams (a little less than two ounces – 28 grams = one ounce) of fats and oils a day. These 50 grams consist of mainly home-made highly unsaturated fats. Another advantage to their health is the habit of eating rice to meet their need for carbohydrates. This is known to keep the arteries young for a long time. Among these people for whom rice is a daily staple, it has been noted that coronary vessels, especially the arteries, are in much better condition than in those who live on a higher economic scale. The benefits derived from a regular consumption of sea plants, such as *seaweed*, is still a secret which may offer many answers to our questions in the future. It is the custom in Korea, Japan and many Chinese provinces to eat rice served with thin leaves of pressed *seaweed*. During our stay there, we adopted the custom, and although I do not know if it was psychological, I must say it made us feel very healthy!

If you are concerned about preventing these three diseases, or if you are a victim of any, you should consider carefully the following rules which are basic to preventative as well as curative treatment.

1. It is of paramount importance to minimize the consumption of protein and fats; especially animal fats should not be eaten. Rather, substitute natural oils such as sunflower, poppy seed, corn or safflower oil.

2. *Wild rice* should be the foundation of the *diet*.

3. Raw vegetables and curds should supplement the rice *diet*. Make it a point to have on the table every day fresh salads, prepared with fresh whey and natural oils.

4. Take your Vitamin E from wheat germ oil and include in your diet any dishes made from sea plants.

5. Instead of regular cheese, eat only mild, white cheese, curds or cottage cheese, sometimes called Farmer's cheese. If it is difficult to part with the old meat eating habit, eat very little of it and infrequently. The same holds true for eggs, which should never be eaten hard-boiled.

6. Salt should be used very sparingly if at all. Try sea salt with a mixture of herbs as a substitute for seasoning.

7. It is of the utmost importance to provide the body with enough oxygen. Take long country walks at a good pace to stimulate deep breathing. If it is not possible to do this on a daily basis, at least use the weekend for that purpose. Instead of spending time looking at television or behind the wheel of a car, get out and exercise your legs, and your heart will benefit also.

If we try to live according to these seven rules, our life span should be considerably lengthened assuring us of health and vitality during our most advanced years. By obeying nature in a simple way, she will reward us in turn.

PREVENTATIVE MEASURES FOR EMBOLISM AND THROMBOSIS

Women especially suffer from clogging of the blood vessels, which often occurs after surgery or just after having given birth. Generally, the clogging occurs sometime between the third and the eighth day following surgery or delivery. In such cases a physician will give an anticoagulant injection which dilutes the blood and promotes dilation of the vessels. More interesting and helpful though is a later prophylactic treatment, which should be taken by everyone who shows a congenital tendency toward embolism or thrombosis. This is of special concern to people with varicose veins.

PROPHYLACTIC TREATMENT

Of utmost importance here is to take proper care of the intestines, because intestinal disorders such as insufficient bowel activity or retention of fecal matter causes the blood to become saturated with metabolic toxins. A liquid *diet* of juices once a week usually has a favorable influence on regularity. Our diet should be made up of natural, untreated, unrefined foods which, by themselves contribute greatly to the correction of irregular bowel movements.

Secondly, it must be remembered that sweating cures have an important place in the treatment of *embolism* and *thrombosis*. This, of course, is easy for people who engage in strenuous physical activity. But sweating can also be brought about by mountain climbing, hiking, digging a ditch, gardening or weight lifting. If profuse sweating is induced, one should be sure to change moist clothes frequently. Since some people

201

are unable to induce perspiration through physical activity, they should give serious consideration to a sauna bath at least once a week.

Thirdly, it is important to take certain medicinal herbs. For example, *pregnant women* should not wait until shortly before delivery to take the herbs but should take them months ahead of time in order to improve the condition of the blood and to bring about a positive influence on the whole vascular system. Recommended is Hamamelis, an extract from the so-called Indian miracle plant. As early as the Middle Ages women knew that embolism and thrombosis could be prevented by taking Arnica, Milfoil, St. John's wort and Pulsatilla. In Switzerland and other European countries these four herbs have been combined into a preparation that has proven helpful to hundreds of thousands of pregnant women during the past 30 years. Many women have reported that serious complications at the time of delivery were prevented because they had been taking this preparation during *pregnancy*. They reported easy deliveries without any kind of complications, which had not been the case for them before, when they had not been taking the preparation. A very well qualified and experienced mid-wife once told us about a perfect delivery which, according to her, could only be attributed to the fact that the mother had been taking the preparation during her *pregnancy*. We must not overlook the importance of Calcium complex because of its favorable effect on the vascular system. A fresh plant extract from horse chestnuts should not be overlooked either. Careful attention to these prophylactic remedies will overcome complications and make for a more successful and easy delivery.

THE CALCIUM PROBLEM IN OLDER PEOPLE

Many times older people have raised the question as to whether it is advisable to take calcium preparations or even to eat foods high in calcium. It is known that in later years the potential danger for arteriosclerosis and the hardening of other body tissues is greatly increased. On the other hand, it is an indisputable fact that during old age calcium is being withdrawn from the bones and deposited in vessels and tissues. This causes the bones to become brittle and porous and the tissues, blood vessels and scar tissue to accumulate calcium deposits. Looking at the surface of this argument it would appear advantageous to cut back on calcium intake. But it has been proven that a diet low in calcium, surprisingly enough, even promotes the loss of calcium from the bones.

How can this problem be solved? Calcium is a basic mineral which compounds easily with acids. If during the latter part of life the body accumulates certain acids (oxalic and other acids), which should have been eliminated with the urine, the body compounds these with calcium to form calcium salts. By reducing them to an unsaturated state they are rendered less harmful. If we do not permit a deficiency to develop in the mineral metabolism, and if we see to it that the calcium level remains normal, we can be sure that there will be no abnormal decalcification in the vascular system and tissues, even during old age. This is why it is so important to continue taking calcium preparations even before reaching advanced age. The perennial question that now comes up is: What can be done to prevent premature aging?

FAVORABLE PROPHYLACTIC MEASURES

An older person, first of all, needs plenty of oxygen, which simply stated, mean plenty of exercise and deep respiration in the outdoors. It would be beneficial to engage in some light sport. Golf is an excellent sport if one doesn't get lazy and ride the electric cart all around the golf course. If this is not possible, light work in the yard or garden is good exercise. Taking long walks through the forests or some hill climbing will provide enjoyable and pleasant exercise.

An older person should also eat foods high in iron, which assures proper oxidation in the blood and normalizes the metabolic process of burning up energy. This can be achieved by simply adding to the diet plenty of raw vegetables and salads. This is easier to do during spring when many kinds of cresses and lettuce and the tender leaves of spinach are available. Do not forget the freshly sprouted shoots of the nettle plant which are of astonishing value. There are many alternatives to assure that the daily requirements are met.

The glands should be stimulated to provide for sufficient internal secretion. Daily brush massages and showers, alternating between hot and cold water, are of great value. But it is wise not to get chilled. Refrain from using the cold water if there is a chance that this might happen. It is also important to get plenty of sleep, especially in the hours preceding midnight. It is a good idea to cultivate the habit of "early to bed, early to rise" as this promotes a sense of well-being. When one is exhausted and overtired and goes to bed late, sleep does not come easy. As a supplement to the mineral content of our diet we will find *Kelp,* a sea plant preparation, very wholesome and fulfilling a need. As previously stated, it does not affect one adversely to eat foods high in calcium and to take biological calcium in addition. We may also want to stimulate the function of the kidneys in order to insure proper elimination of uric materials by taking Nephrosolid, a natural herb preparation.

RECOMMENDED DIETS FOR HYPERTENSION, ARTERIOSCLEROSIS AND OTHER SIGNS OF OLD AGE

It is important to determine whether *hypertension* can be attributed to a kidney disease or whether it is caused by the diminishing elasticity of the arteries. If it is not a question of a kidney disorder, but one of the arteries, this may be easily corrected through a rice diet, as this is effective with practically all afflictions resulting from *old age. Wild or brown rice* is more beneficial than the ordinary processed kind. Two commercially prepared rice packages, "Uncle Ben's" or "Avorio" may serve as a compromise because both of these brands still retain many of the important minerals found in wild rice.

It is not easy for a European or, for that matter, an American who is used to potatoes, to stick constantly to a rice diet. But, since we have irrefutable proof of what a rice diet can do for Orientals, in this particular instance, we would do well to imitate them if we want to eliminate the worries of high blood pressure. Make a heroic effort to substitute rice for potatoes. The reason rice is of such importance in this diet is that it serves to restore the elasticity of the arteries. Curds are also good as a supplement because they supply the body with protein and can be very tasty when served with vegetables and salads.

A doctor in the United States recently helped many people suffering from *hypertension* by means of a diet similar to the one we have suggested. With this treatment the high blood pressure disappeared, but with it, also a considerable amount of money. If you can adhere to the diet for four weeks, and make an extra effort not to revert to your old eating habits, you will begin to notice improvement. It takes a little will power and certainly encouragement from the family members, but having the incentive to overcome the problem will make you glad that you adhered to the diet.

BREAKFAST

Even without meat, eggs and cheese breakfast can be considerably varied from day to day. We can prepare an excellent substitute coffee, get some pumpernickel, whole kernel bread or rye crisp, butter and honey or jam (without additives), etc.

A *Muesli,* the famous Swiss breakfast food, made from berries, fruits in season, flaked oats and other cereals, is a wonderfully refreshing way to start the day. All these foods besides being nutritious are very tasty and refreshing.

Instead of having fruit every morning, we may want to, for the sake of variety, drink cereal coffee with a roll spread with butter or curds, covered with slices of radishes in springtime, fresh seasoning herbs or tender leaves of lettuce. During the tomato season we may add this wholesome vegetable to our breakfast. Or, make a tomato salad with *whey* dressing. At certain times of the year when horseradish and the various kinds of cresses are available, they too may serve as very refreshing additions to the morning meal. This diet may be quite different from the one you have been accustomed to and may not be exactly to your liking in the beginning but be a little daring and try it anyhow; it will help your problem.

MIDDAY MEAL

The meal we eat at noon is the most essential part of the treatment, which indeed it can be, if prepared according to the following instructions. Prepare *rice,* curds (cottage cheese) enriched with horseradish, and a salad of four or five different fresh vegetables, not forgetting to add some garlic or leek. If you are afraid of the strong aftertaste of the garlic, be assured this can be easily corrected by eating parsley after the garlic.

If the *rice* dish is varied, it will not become tiresome. For example, it is possible to prepare a tasty vegetable rice dish, as is done in the Far East. One of the most favored rice dishes is rice with zucchini. For variety there are the following: rice with tomatoes, rice with egg plant, rice with mushrooms, rice with soy beans, etc. To all these dishes add creamed curds or cottage cheese with herbs and don't forget the salad.

For the sake of variety we may want to prepare a *sweet rice* dish with berries and almonds or other nuts, and eat this with a fruit compote made from fresh fruit. Finish it off with cereal coffee.

The *rice* should be cooked so that the kernels are separated. To cook it so that the grains do not stick together, bring the water to a boil and slowly add the rice so that the boiling does not stop. This will cause the rice grains to burst quickly and cook separately. Be sure not to overcook it as it will lose its taste and become starchy. To increase the taste of a rice dish add a chicken bouillon cube, chopped parsley and a little grated cheese and bake in the oven.

BUCKWHEAT

Years ago, *buckwheat* was more popular than today. Since this cereal dish, just like rice, provides excellent relief from high blood pressure, it should appear on our table regularly. It may be prepared in the same way as rice and may be used as a substitute for rice along with curds and salads. One method of preparing buckwheat is by cooking it in a vegetable broth to which has been added homemade tomato stew and finely chopped herbs. If chilled it can be served with tomato and lettuce. Another variation is to mix buckwheat with onion, garlic and majoram, let it get cold and then fry it slowly.

THE ART OF PROPER SEASONING

When suffering from hypertension it is important to consider the type of condiments used. The diet should be very low in salt. The proper use of the different condiments is an art and should be carefully studied by every cook. Food should never taste dull if the appetite is to be stimulated. Instead of salt, the following spices are to be recommended for health reasons: horseradish, parsley, majoram, thyme, paprika, curry (if used sparingly). Garlic and onions are especially helpful in enriching the taste of rice as is also the use of herbal sea salt.

DRINKS

If we want to add to our vegetable dishes a suitable drink, we should choose something that contains lactic acid such as diluted *whey* or any of the vegetable juices such as carrot, celery or tomato juices. It should be remembered never to make a practice of taking a drink while there is food in the mouth as this prevents proper mastication of the food and also prevents the pre-digestive process to take place in the mouth.

DINNER / SUPPER

It is advisable to take only a light meal at night and particularly refrain from eating any hard-to-digest foods in order to insure good rest. We should eat some fruit and full kernel bread, spread with butter or perhaps a little jam and a cup of cereal coffee. Or in lieu of that, a dish of *Muesli* with fresh fruit added makes an excellent end-of-the-day meal.

If vegetables rather than fruit are preferred, make a dish of cold buckwheat and serve with any salad. Or, as another idea, make some fresh vegetable soup accompanied by a roll and a mixed salad. In order to avoid fermentation, it is best never to mix vegetables and fruit at the same meal. This may be a habit difficult to break but observance of this rule will promote better digestion and prevent gastric disturbances.

NORMALIZATION OF BLOOD PRESSURE WITH THE HELP OF WILD RICE

It is a proven fact that a *wild rice* diet assures normal *blood pressure* and this equally applies to regulating low as well as *high blood pressure.*

Not long ago I received a letter from a friend in Germany to whom I had recommended a wild rice diet and he was very enthusiastic about the excellent results he had obtained. He remained on the recommended *diet* for 10 weeks and found that, not only had he lost weight but that his blood pressure had gone down from 230 to 190. This alone was a success in itself. He followed this up with a two week restful vacation, which again resulted in a further drop of blood pressure, this time to 170. This patient is 63 years old and it is especially interesting to note that he obtained such excellent results without the use of any prescription drugs – simply by following a *diet* of wild rice, curds and salads. If he remains on this diet he will experience a further reduction in blood pressure and with it, the elasticity of his blood vessels will once again be restored.

Even though my friend did not have to make use of any additional medication, it would not be wrong to supplement a diet of this kind with certain preparations which would make it more effective. Considerable success has been obtained with an extract of Mistletoe, which helps to lower the blood pressure. In the same category are Crataegus (Hawthorne) and Arnica, both of which have positive effects on the arteries. If blood pressure decreases, it means not only the reading of it has gone down but a genuine rejuvenation of the vascular system has taken place, due to a restoration of the elasticity of the vessels. If we realize the grave consequences of *high blood pressure*, it is well worth the effort and endurance to carry through this recommended diet to rid ourselves of it.

LOW BLOOD PRESSURE (HYPOTENSION)

While high blood pressure is given much attention in many books and periodicals and successful measures have obtained excellent results, much less is known about *low blood pressure*. What causes it? Where does it come from? and What can be done about it? are all too frequently asked questions. Yet, these questions are not as yet adequately answered even in the literature of advocates of natural methods of treatment. A person suffering from hypotension may be subject to *dizzy spells* or even occasional fainting at high altitudes of

1,500–1,800 meters (5,000–6,000 feet). Every little exertion may cause an imbalance in the blood circulation or the normal heart activity. A change in locale is often necessary to permit the patient to live in a lower altitude. In 90% of all cases, symptoms appear as a result of improper activity on the part of the *gonad* glands, the organs in which the reproductive cells develop. In a woman the *ovaries* do not function correctly and in a man it is the male sex glands that function improperly.

WHAT KIND OF RELIEF CAN BE OFFERED?

As soon as medication is given that stimulates the glandular activity, normalization of the blood pressure will result. One should abstain though, from taking strong hormone preparations, which force blood pressure up too quickly. This influence generally, is not a lasting one and it may even cause certain side effects. It would certainly be better to stimulate the gonads indirectly with an iodine-potash preparation containing organically bound iodine from marine plants. Although all kinds of algae can be used, *Kelp,* however, is most appropriate as is also Rauwolfia root which is grown in India and Ceylon. When suffering from hypertension, extracts from roots are used to bring about a decrease in the blood pressure but when given in homeopathic doses of D-6 or stronger potency it has the opposite effect – it normalizes low blood pressure. This very interesting observation first made by Dr. Hahnemann, has been mentioned before in connection with other areas of treatment. For women, a very good homeopathic remedy regulating the function of the ovaries, can be highly recommended. It is called Ovasan D-3 which is free of all side effects.

The plant *Hyssop,* which was already in use during biblical times, has proven very helpful in the treatment of low blood pressure. Recalling the biblical occasion, God's divine request to Moses, made at the time of the celebration of the sacrifice of the Pashal lamb, is known to all Bible readers. At that time the Jews were asked to paint their door posts with the blood of the lamb. For a paint brush they used a bundle of hyssops. Even to this day the Samaritans use hyssop to prevent the curding of blood of the sacrificial lamb. The juice in the hyssop plant actually does have blood coagulating properties. In the 51st Psalm, hyssop is mentioned in connection with spiritual cleansing. This plant, one of its kind, indeed possesses strange powers and its benefits in affecting blood pressure favorably by acting on the *gonad* glands is undeniable.

OTHER REMEDIES

In order to increase *low blood* pressure it does not harm to drink red wine from time to time. Or, some may prefer to eat pollen which helps to increase low blood pressure due to its stimulating effect on the gonads. *Bee pollen* is very wholesome and in severe cases of low blood pressure the pollen may be eaten in its pure form. But a warning should be given to those with high blood pressure. If bee pollen is taken in quantity it could provoke a stroke. The person who has reason to believe his blood pressure is high should use extreme caution in taking bee pollen. Once I observed a case of a person, suffering from *hypertension,* who had taken a considerable amount of pollen. It would have been fatal if immediate counteracting measures had not been administered in time. It becomes clear from this example that, if improperly used, the effect of natural remedies may not always be harmless. We have another substance that increases blood pressure; raw *carrot juice.* People with *high blood* pressure must abstain from drinking carrot juice while those with low blood pressure will experience excellent results. It is important not to eat carrots whole or as a salad, since they are not effective in that form. The healing property is only contained in the pure juice. This applies also to *beet juice.*

While not generally recommended, if we feel *dizzy* at a high altitude, we can alleviate the problem by drinking a strong cup of coffee. This applies in case of *low blood pressure.* If one lives in a coastal area and has low blood pressure, oysters are excellent food for stimulating the function of the *gonads* and regulating blood pressure.

A downward vascillation of *blood pressure* is generally accompanied by a lack of vitality and energy, observable in persons who are physically below par. It is therefore not sufficient to simply treat the symptoms of dizziness, but it is of utmost importance to affect a positive influence on the over-all condition of the person in order to regain lost strength. This is much more desirable than to force ourselves with one last effort to attend to our daily duties and chores. If the *gonad* glands do not function properly, the result is not only a loss of sexual potency, but a loss of general vitality and energy. This translates itself into a lack of desire to work and a lack of creativity in physical, mental and artistic fields. A condition like this should never be permitted to exist unless one has already passed the years of active involvement in life, which is to say he is about ready to die.

GANGRENE

Gangrene is a term associated with the death of tissues due to loss of vascular supply, generally observable in older people. The condition requires immediate attention without the slightest delay. If neglected, the skin of the legs or foot turn a blue-reddish color, it becomes shiny and hard and makes the patient very uncomfortable, especially at night, when the patches begin to burn to the extent that there is no relief, except by exposing the legs to cool air.

The symptoms usually appear in older people, but have their beginning in early adult life. The disease can be the result of having been exposed repeatedly to cold and moisture. It is also possible that gangrene can result from untreated frostbite. This is dangerous because the cells and vessels of the feet suffer permanent damage. *Gangrene* can be the result of the process of varicose veins drying up. Prolonged standing or sitting is harmful to an older person because of a slowdown in

212

the blood circulation of the veins. Having a job where lots of moving around is required will make one feel better and at times the pain will subside altogether. Even though the disease cannot be cured completely, it is possible to influence it with the help of natural preparations to a degree that the person may go without serious complications for many years.

A recommended treatment is to add 5 drops of Arnica D-1 to a little water and to make this into a wet pack. This external application should be alternated every other day with the taking Echinacea extract and Lachesis D-10 orally, preferably in the morning and at night. Both may be taken in a little water. The treatment will have to be continued for an extended period of time.

The patient should not expose himself to cold and should wear warm clothing. His *diet* should be of a vegetarian foundation. Persistent care will bring a measure of relief if the above directions are followed and much future discomfort may be spared.

INFECTIOUS LIVER
AND GALL BLADDER DISEASES

There are *liver* and *gall bladder* troubles that can come about through infection. The patient feels ill and brings up bile; he feels sick all over and has *diarrhea* and in some cases develops a slight attack of *jaundice*. When such symptoms appear, great care should be taken and the first thing to be given to drink is clay water. Either white or yellow clay will do – a teaspoon of clay to a small wine glass of warm water, to which has been added several drops of Lachesis 12x or 10x. This is a superior remedy that will act as an antidote. The patient needs to fast completely for two or three days, drinking nothing but clay water. If at the end of this time he feels like eating, he can try a peeled and finely grated apple which should be well chewed. This can be followed by a drink of *whey-concentrate* in the proportion of one teaspoon to one half pint of water or fruit juice such as orange, blackberry, raspberry, grape or pineapple. The mixture should be sipped slowly.

In very delicate cases the person may not be able to drink anything but freshly pressed *carrot juice*. Solid food should be

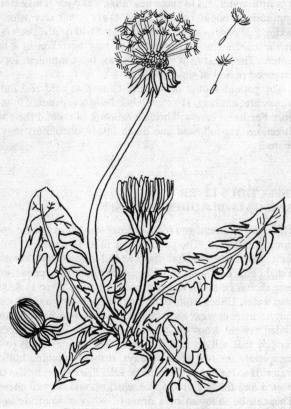

Dandelion (Taraxacum officinalis)

avoided at this stage, because the trouble will be cleared up much faster if the patient fasts. Regeneration will only be delayed by burdening the digestive system with food. In case the patient vomits bile, be sure to give him liquids afterwards. *Horsetail* or *Dandelion* tea will be excellent and for the latter you can use leaves, roots and all.

An extract (which is more potent) of Dandelion called Taraxacum will be found to be wonderfully effective in such cases. Cereal gruels should be avoided because they always contain some fat and in the digestive process the liver will be irritated.

Taking solid food can serve no useful purpose and, again, the value of fasting during the first few days cannot be over-emphasized. Once the grated apple and any of the various fruit juices can be digested and the patient feels hungry again, try Bircher-muesli for breakfast and supper. At midday a little salad may be taken, taking care that the dressing has little or no oil to start with – just lemon and whey concentrate. For several days after recovery fried foods of any kind should be avoided, for a certain amount of sensitivity remains. Even slightly heated oil or animal fat will soon cause the congested feeling in the back of the head or in the forehead to return. A peculiar feeling of nausea may manifest itself, also. Until all germs have been eliminated, normal feeding should be postponed.

Solidago, as usual, should be taken to stimulate the *kidneys*. Or take Horsetail for this too. If the patient runs a temperature, and it is not unusual for it to reach 100° F, then Ferr. phos, 12x, diluted Holly infusion, Aconitum 4x or any other good fever remedy should be taken. One or two tablets or Podophyllum 3x and, according to circumstances, three to four drops of Chelidonium 2x or the combination remedy Chelicynara should be taken. Condensed *carrot juice* is also advantageous. No *liver* complaint should be treated lightly and armed with these remedies you may rest assured that the best possible treatment is being given.

JAUNDICE

Jaundice is much more dangerous than is usually assumed. People who have suffered from it assert over and over again that ever since they had it, they have not felt the same again. They have also observed that fried foods and sweet things no longer agree with them.

There are two kinds of *jaundice*. One is due to congestion or blockage in the gall duct and the other, a result of infection. Both can be serious. As part of the treatment abstain from fats, fried foods and sweets. The bowels must be thoroughly cleansed and the bile must be liquified by taking the following remedies: Chelidonium 2x or Chelicynara, Podophyllum 3x and condensed *carrot juice*. Plenty of fresh carrot juice should be drunk daily, at ¼ pint to a cup. Warm water treatments will help considerably and should always be given, either by putting a hot herbal compress on the liver or covering the liver area with a hot bag – either water or electric. Also, *cabbage leaf* compresses alternating daily with *clay* poultices will provide relief. At the same time the kidneys should be stimulated by drinking kidney tea or Solidago. Other suitable herbs are Horsetail, Birch leaves or Rosehips, the last one being a very mildly acting remedy.

Even when the doctor affirms that the patient is quite well again, on no account should the treatment be stopped. The special diet should be continued for some time as well as the use of compresses and warm water treatments.

An important detail of treatment of jaundice is the care given to the bowels. On no account must this be neglected and if regular bowel action is lacking, an herb enema should be given. The bile must be removed from the circulatory system as quickly as possible, for the longer it remains in the blood and the more concentrated it is, the greater the harm that will result.

Beware of patent medicines in the treatment of *jaundice*. They invariably mask and suppress symptoms only and serious complications can result from the taking of them. It is much wiser to let the illness take its normal course and assist the body in various functions with natural remedies, rather than try to bring about a cure with "over-the-counter" drugs. The healing process cannot be unduly hurried as it must run its course. Most cases under supervision of an allopathic doctor will take 6–8 weeks at least. But, if you employ the aforementioned treatment with its various measures, satisfactory results can be achieved in two weeks. However, it must not be considered complete unless the after-treatment is carried out as well.

Anyone who has had *jaundice* should, especially in the spring, eat plenty of Dandelion salad as that is when it is at its best. Artichokes, chicory, and all bitter herbs, salad vegetables and radishes in small quantities are also excellent for the liver. Bitter salad herbs should be taken moderately as too much can do more harm than good. The repeatedly mentioned *carrot juice* should of course never be forgotten. If this advice is followed and special attention to the after-treatment is given, then the jaundice problem will be completely overcome with the least unpleasant and harmful consequences.

KIDNEY STONE COLIC

There are many people who have *kidney stones* without being aware of it. The same goes for *gall stones*. Their presence is only brought to notice when the stones enter the ureter, or in the case of gall stones, the bileduct. When they get stuck and can neither move forward or backward a renal colic is experienced with excruciating pain. So intense is the pain that it is not unusual for the patient to lose all control knocking into things around him or even rolling on the floor in agony causing great concern to those around him. The pain can last for hours and there is great danger if the proper treatment is not given.

The patient must be placed in a hot bath and with light careful massage, the stone must be made to move from the ureter into the bladder. As soon as the patient is in the water he will feel somewhat better. If the heart begins to give trouble or if he suffers from a thyroid problem (Basedow's disease) he must be assisted with cold water treatment. The best way to do this is to take a cold towel, place ice cubes in it and roll it up lengthwise to form a tube. Wrap this around the body so it passes over the heart area and this cooling effect will bring relief. If necessary place cold compresses on the wrists and forehead, renewing them frequently to keep them cold. The patient should remain in the hot bath for at least one half-hour.

Internal treatment should begin immediately. Magnesium phos. 6x and Atropinum 3x should be taken. If he cannot keep down the medication, then an enema should be given. If, in spite of everything, the patient loses consciouness, there is no need to panic as the unconsciousness will pass off harmlessly and prevent a perforation.

After the bath, which should have been kept as hot as possible, herbal enemas should be given frequently and hot packs applied. If blood comes instead of urine, this means the stone is stuck fast in the ureter and undoubtedly has damaged it. At this stage, it would be a good thing to give *Solidago* by way of the bowel in order to stimulate the kidneys, for, as a rule, the patient will be unable to retain anything given by mouth, if he has an attack. Continue packs and enemas for another half hour and then follow up with another hot bath, compresses and massage. Thus the treatment continues until the stone begins to move toward the bladder. The pain will diminish altogether as the stone enters the bladder. It may take several hours to accomplish, but once achieved, the patient should lie quietly and rest. If he is thirsty, give him diluted *whey-concentrate* to drink as this reduces the internal heat and replaces the liquids lost by perspiration. It will also help to rid the body of toxins which have been forced into the circulatory system by the various treatments. Give him plenty of *Plantain Tea* because this too has resolving properties.

After a slight rest, a busy after-treatment, including hip-baths and massage must follow, as the stone must not be allowed to remain in the bladder, where it could give rise to irritation and bleeding. By these methods, a ureter blockage with its serious consequences or an operation can be avoided. Should the size of the stone prevent removal through natural, physical measures, then, of course an operation would be necessary.

PROSTATE TROUBLE

It is not always possible to cure *Prostate* problems. There are cases, especially cancer of the Prostate, where treatment is difficult and sometimes in vain. Nevertheless, operating is not always the answer either, and if it can be prevented, all the better. For some types of prostate problems there are three remedies: Sabal, Staphisagria 3x and Populus 2x have, in combination with herbal steam baths, led to many cures. However, if trouble-free urination has been re-established, do not take it for granted that no further trouble will ensue. Diseases of the *Prostate* are seldom so well cured that they do not, sooner or later, recur. Help can be given nevertheless but, one should remember, that one does not grow younger, but older.

If the distended Prostate can be softened and reduced to its normal size, the water will once more flow freely, but it is likely that a certain degree of distension will remain. A cool glass of beer, or anything in the nature of a temporary disturbance, can cause the trouble to flare up again. Once more you may take recourse to steam baths and the remedies mentioned. To avoid disappointment, you must know that, although they will probably bring you relief, they may not be able to eliminate your disposition for this particular condition. If you continue taking these remedies after the last attack has subsided – reducing the number of drops or pills and the frequency of the doses – you may be able to influence the gland favorably and keep it from flaring up. This is a condition brought on by the aging of the body and it must be remembered there is no simple solution to this problem.

ECZEMA

Before treating eczema it is of primary importance to discover the cause of the disease. It is usually to be found in faulty metabolism or wrong diet and very often a complete change of diet may be necessary. Without question, the bowels and kidneys should be stimulated to function well; and then we must find out if a chronic or acute skin eruption is involved.

External irritation, such as is occasioned by certain occupations, can play a part in the development of these skin diseases, but many times, heredity may be responsible.

From the point of view of external treatment, some of the best results have been obtained from *whey-concentrate*. Whey is a natural sour milk product which destroys bacteria, helps the circulation and by virtue of the minerals and enzymes it contains, regenerates the skin. As a rule, however, whey-concentrate alone is not sufficient, especially in the treatment of *psoriasis*. It is then usually necessary to powder the skin with a biological calcium preparation such as Calcium Complex with Urtica (Urticalcin) in powder form. The third healing factor is a lanolin cream. The entire external treatment for eczemateous skin diseases would then be as follows:

In the morning the affected parts should be swabbed with undiluted *whey-concentrate*. If this is too strong and the sore places smart or burn excessively, dilute with boiled or distilled water. After this, powder the affected parts with the calcium powder. Make sure that the powder gets well into the fissures. In the evening, dab the area once more with *whey-concentrate*, but instead of using the powder, rub the affected parts lightly with lanolin cream or St. John's wort oil. This procedure should be repeated daily.

Any skin eruption, especially a dry, scaly eruption, needs internal as well as external treatment. It is important to take into consideration the condition of the blood and the lymph. First of all take solidago, a kidney remedy, then concentrated carrots which serve both as a liver and vitamin preparation. As specific treatment include the "Formic Acid Therapy" which has to be employed in the form of injections, because the acid is not stable and will be partially transformed into carbonic acid as soon as it is brought into contact with the gastric secretions. For this reason it should not be given by mouth. The best results are obtained by hypodermic injections in the 6th and 12th decimal potency. During the first two weeks an injection should be given every third day for a week and then once every 14 days, till the cure is complete. Even the most difficult case will yield to this treatment, providing the diet is maintained and very little salt and protein is being taken. Salt, as far as skin diseases are concerned, is an absolute poison, while the metabolic toxins resulting from an excess intake of animal protein have a very adverse effect upon these diseases in general and upon psoriasis in particular.

If there is a discharge of pus from the eruption, Hepar sulph. 3x should be taken. If the trouble is connected with an acid condition of the body or if there is an oozing, burning, blistering rash with painful itching, then Rhus tox. 4x or 6x will be the best remedy. Both dry and oozing eruptions, which burn and irritate at night especially, will be cured by Arsenicum alb. 4x to 6x. In cases of chronic eruptions, both Sulphur 6x and Sulphur iodine 4x to 6x have proven their worth, especially if the eruption is based upon a scrofulous condition. If the disease is the result of a rheumatic or gouty disposition, then Calcium carb. 4x alternated with Lycopodium 6x would be indicated. In all circumstances, a good calcium preparation which incorporates Nettles, i.e. Calcium-complex with Urtica and Viola tricolor (an extract from the pansy) are excellent remedies to combat this disease.

PSORIASIS

There are certain skin diseases like *Psoriasis* which are extremely difficult to heal. A direct method which has been found quite successful is Formic Acid 30x coupled with an external application of Graphite powder. Though the orthodox doctor considers *Psoriasis* incurable, naturopathic treatment as well as Homeopathy can claim a considerable number of cures. Anyone who has suffered from this scaly eruption knows what a terrible strain it is on the nerves. Once the frightening irritation starts up, very few patients can bear it without scratching themselves until they bleed. It was thus with a girl who was suffering from one of the worst attacks I have ever seen. Often by morning, she had scratched herself to such an extent that the whole area was bleeding freely. After three months of intensive treatment the disease disappeared, although two further post treatments were necessary to cope with a few minor relapses.

Although she had several previous treatments, the skin had not been too badly damaged that it could not be healed. For some who have undergone an extensive tar and sulphur treatment and have used eventually grey quick-silver ointment, the treatment is very much more difficult. Also the chances of healing the disease are very poor if there has been previous X-ray treatment. For this reason, I would warn patients never to have this particular treatment. If you impose too great a strain on the body by using irritants such as terpene, turpentine, turpentine wax or other strong turpentine products, a relapse later is very possible.

Psoriasis is not contagious, therefore it cannot be easily spread from one to another. It is, however, possible to pass it on to one's children. Women who suffer from it should make every effort to rid themselves of it before marrying. If you are already married and have children, then they must be given special care. Make sure that they have plenty of calcium and vitamins in their diet and take proper care of their skin.

PSORIASIS CURE
THROUGH RAW FOOD DIET

An interesting proof of the regenerative power of raw food is given in the following letter from a patient who suffered from *Psoriasis*:

"Just now I am in B. where I have had a complete raw food diet. For 23 years I have suffered from psoriasis and have had completed cures of all sorts; until now, all have been without success. Having arrived here, I fasted for seven days, then I took fruit juice, then fruits, nuts and maize bread. For several weeks I have been eating raw salads and potatoes for lunch and fruit morning and evening. I feel quite well and I am glad to say that the eruption has gone. Now and again the sun brings an occasional blemish to the surface, but it never gets bigger, and disappears within one or two days. This does show me, however, that I am not yet completely healed and that I must continue this cure. This does not worry me for I enjoy my fruits and salads. I can't quite put into words what it means to me to know that I shall be quite well again and that I shall have the strength to work and be useful. I only know that I shall be everlastingly grateful."

The reply was as follows: "I am truly glad to be able to rejoice with you, knowing that with a simple, raw food diet you were able to overcome Psoriasis. Now we must achieve a complete cure and you must be patient for a little while longer. The raw food diet has stimulated the various body functions, including that of the kidneys, and has given the body sufficient vitamins and healthgiving salts. This shows that the diet is influencing the functions of the various organs. *Psoriasis* is usually treated externally and in various clinics, this treatment is considered the most important. In this respect, orthodox medicine is in error. *Psoriasis* is one of the worst skin diseases and is not an outward manifestation only and local external treatment should therefore be of secondary consideration. It is important, of course, to keep the skin clean, supply it with sufficient oil and disinfect it properly so that further difficulties do not arise, but the internal treatment is far more important, and your letter is proof of this. If you wish to improve your health further, then let me recommend kidney tea as well as Solidago and sufficient calcium. These you will find will do you a lot of good."

THE ELIMINATION OF FOOT SWEAT

Is it reasonable to get rid of foot sweat? Is foot sweat not a completely natural contrivance for the body to dispose of poisons which it could not otherwise get rid of? This theory seems to be correct, otherwise so many unpleasant consequences could not have resulted from people who have tried to suppress perspiration of the foot. Just recently I had a letter from a woman in Zurich telling me that while her husband was on military service, his foot sweat was suppressed and as a result he developed a skin disease. Skin problems inevitably follow these so-called cures. One should therefore never try to thwart nature in her attempts to dispose of toxins, for the disadvantages will be outnumbered by the advantages gained from pursuing such a course. If you want to get rid of the troubles incurred you will once again have to try to induce foot sweat but sometimes this is easier said than done. A Berlin doctor recommends powdered Carbid which should be shaken into the insoles of the shoe. The slightest moisture exuding from the feet generates heat through contact with the Carbid and draws out more moisture. In this simple way foot sweat can be induced artificially. This doctor used this method to cure several cases which had previously failed to respond to any other treatment.

In any case, it is fundamentally wrong to try to suppress foot sweat. If the odor becomes too unpleasant, wash the feet frequently with a herbal infusion, afterwards oiling them with a good, aromatic, easily absorbed skin oil. Change socks often. The natural functions of the body should never be suppressed because through them the organism is able to protect itself.

THE SPECTOR OF CANCER

Cancer can develop as a consequence of faulty nutrition and a disturbed metabolism. It has been proven that it is not only the inherited disposition that counts, but also excessive protein intake which leads to constant irritation of the cells and thus encourage abnormal cell growth. This, of course, is no reason to go about prophesying that everyone who eats too much protein food and suffers from metabolic disturbance will develop cancer. It would be irresponsible to implant the fear of cancer in this way, for the faults mentioned can very well lead to some other problem in no way related to cancer.

High blood pressure, diabetes or gout can all develop from the same cause and the same cause can produce different effects. The latter depends to a great extent on the disposition of the person. An acid system, for example, will rarely favor cancer growth. He who suffers from gastric acidity can rest assured that cancer is unlikely to choose him for a victim. Much worse is the symptom of lack of acidity. Pain too speaks against cancer for it is only in its advanced stage that cancer becomes painful. There are, of course, exceptions but normally, it is an ulcer rather than cancer that produces gastric pains. To arrive at a correct diagnosis one has to consider, therefore, every factor associated with the particular condition. This is not being mentioned to allay the fear-ridden patient, but to give information to the reader which is likely to prove useful at some future time.

According to observations, I have found that if the three following factors exist simultaneously, cancer should be considered:

1. A disposition to the disease which has been inherited or acquired. I should like to make it understood, however, that it

is the disposition or the tendency that is inherited and not the disease.

2. A diet containing too much protein, and especially animal protein, can also lead to cancer.

3. Irritation of the cells, whether it is chemical such as produced from nicotine and tar substances or an irritation caused by excessive eating, drugs or constipation, etc. The point is that constant mechanical irritation of one sort or another can contribute to the development of cancer.

Every so often an assertion is made that a cure for cancer has been found, but such assertions usually lead to inevitable disappointment. Either the cure does not work or the disease proves to be other than cancer. One should beware of such charlatan claims. However, this does not mean one should sit idly by while the dread disease takes its course. Natural healing has produced some astounding results.

For example, there was the patient of one of our most famous surgeons, who was operated on for abdominal cancer. No sooner had the operation begun when it was found that the growth had spread to such an extent that its removal was impossible. As far as the doctor was concerned the case was irreversible and the patient had just a short time to live. She came to our clinic for help and even in this evidently hopeless case she was not given up. All natural healing methods and remedies were called into use and to the great surprise of the orthodox doctors, the patient began to gain weight and feel better. After a considerable time, when she had forgotten the necessity of continuing to take the utmost care, she unfortunately ate some fruit that had been sprayed. This was a most regrettable mistake, for in her case the slightest poison could have a disastrous effect. Indeed the success achieved over a period of months of careful treatment was lost in a few days. The patient worsened from one hour to the next. This is a dire warning to all who suffer from cancer or have a disposition for it. The importance of diet cannot be exaggerated. It should be rich in vitamins and minerals and extremely restricted in proteins.

Cancer statistics tell a lot about how and why the disease occurs, especially in the so-called highly civilized countries of the world. I can vouch for this for, in my world-wide travels undertaken for purposes of research, I have noticed that, the more primitive people were seldom if ever ill from cancer. This is also true of the North American Indians and Mexicans, uncontaminated by large urban centers and their pollution. On the other hand, I heard from a doctor friend of mine that 40 to 50 years ago it was difficult to find a case of lung cancer for demonstration to medical students but now the cases are abundant. During more than 60 years as a practitioner I have had occasion to witness the increase of cancer in Switzerland where only a few years ago it was practically unheard of.

What conclusions can you draw from these sobering facts? If you want to make sure this dreadful disease does not touch you, return to a simple, natural diet. Avoid the temptations of manufactured foods and take care to shun all chemically contaminated goodies. Unfortunately the chemical industry is much too ingenious in the field of food adulteration, with its dyes, flavors, preservation methods, fertilizing, spraying, bleaching, etc.

As soon as a certain practice becomes illegal, the chemist discovers ten other loopholes in the law and the steady stream of poisons continue to pour from the factories. By the time medicine is able to prove that these things are dangerous to health and may increase the chances of one's getting cancer, millions of people have already saturated their systems with the chemicals in question.

Apart from manufactured foods there are many other causes of ill health. Consider tobacco. This is a case of slow poisoning self-inflicted by the smoker. It is quite possible that today's tobacco is more harmful than it used to be because methods of cultivation and fermentation have changed and additions of a suspicious nature are common, to say nothing of the paper in which the cigarette tobacco is wrapped. How otherwise can the increase in lung cancer be accounted for? It may, of course, be that the decline in general health and powers of resistance is partially responsible too. From the point of view of survival, living conditions have become increasingly unfavorable making it necessary for those who love life to live as close to nature as possible.

You will act in the best interest of your body, if you consume pure foods that have not been tampered with in any way and anything that has been "improved" upon by man. Nature know the needs of your body best. I have had best results with raw foods and "fruit juice days" in cases of cancer. It is important, however, that only organically grown produce is used. Sprayed fruit and vegetables grown with artificial fertilizers are taboo.

As regards medicinal treatment from the plant kingdom there is the Mistletoe, the greater Celandine and Petasites which are very effective remedies. The fresh plant extract prepared from them should always be used.

As yet, the chapter on cancer is not completed. We do not know whether a cure will emerge from the retort of the chemical laboratory or if it will spring from the womb of nature and free us of this terrible scourge. It may well be that the Creator himself has plans to release us in his own good time. Whatever happens, one thing is certain, if we want a better, healthful life we must put a stop to the unnatural tendencies and developments of our age and return to the simple ways of living and eating.

More detailed information on appropriate nutrition in cancer cases and their treatment with biological remedies has appeared in the monthly "Health News" magazine and will be further discussed in a special publication.

ARTHRITIS – GOUT

Four to seven per cent of mankind are afflicted by this dreadful, painful scourge. Two to three hundred thousand Swiss have fallen victim to it and about seven million Americans can speak of *Arthritis* as a personal experience, and many may have suffered from it for decades. No wonder that life holds no pleasures for them. To help as many as possible is the purpose of the following article.

Arthritis often has its origin in a chronically suppurating focus somewhere in the system. It may be the tonsils, a dental granuloma (abscess) or some other purulent trouble which discharges minute quantities of toxins and poisonous end products of protein metabolism into the bloodstream. This has the effect of damaging, besides the joints, the internal organs such as the heart, kidneys, etc. But apart from that, Arthritis is definitely a disease of modern civilization, the outcome of eating the wrong kind of foods. In many cases we have also inherited a disposition for it. An old saying has it: "The fathers have eaten sour grapes and the children's teeth are set on edge." A disturbance of the mineral metabolism makes it mandatory that we change from an acid producing diet to one yielding an alkaline surplus. In the first place meat, especially pork sausages, bolognas, cold cuts, beef soups, foods cooked with eggs and cheese should, if possible, be avoided. If you feel you cannot give up meat entirely, at least confine yourself to freshly prepared natural meat and avoid completely all kinds of preserved meats and pork sausage. Secondly, avoid all processed foods, white sugar, white flour products, canned foods, in other words everything that has been taken out of its original form. The *diet* should consist of potatoes, cereals, unpolished rice, fresh fruits and vegetables or naturally dried fruit (unsulphured) and vegetables containing no chemicals or preservatives. The simpler and more natural the diet, the greater will be its contribution to our everyday health, well-being and long life. The most important remedy for *Arthritis* is *potato juice.* It is not only its basic and known constituents that contribute to the cure of arthritis but possibly, as yet other unknown factors. *Potato juice* should be taken daily and in severe cases the amount should be slowly increased. The potato should be grated and the juice squeezed out and taken first thing in the morning before breakfast. It can be also taken

229

in warm water or added to soup if you wish to dilute it. This most important and excellent remedy is at everyone's disposal all over the world and is easily obtainable. Other healing juices which may be taken daily in small amounts are *kale* and *carrot* juices in conjunction with the potato juice. The best way to take them is undiluted. Sip slowly so that they can be salivated before swallowing.

Externally, apply pulped Comfrey roots to the painful parts and you will find that the pain will gradually disappear. Tincture of comfrey is excellent also. Butterbur (Petasites hybrid) is a good supporting remedy. For teas which you can drink, there is a wide selection: Birch leaves, Masterwort (Imperatoria Ostruthium), Rest Harrow (Ononis spinosa), Anise (Pimpinella anisum), Goldenrod (Solidago virgaurea), Dandelion and Meadowsweet (Spiraea Ulmaria). Fresh plant extract of the herbs are also an excellent help. Of recommended value are Juniper berries, Barberry (Berberies vulg.) and Nettles and in addition, attenuated doses of Colchicum and the radio-active salts of a volcanic spring. These remedies brought together should be taken as follows: 5 drops in potato juice three times daily before meals. Add an extra drop every day until you reach 25 drops if there is no sign of a strong reaction. Then reverse the procedure and decrease gradually to 5 drops and increase again to 30 drops. The dose must be adjusted to individual requirements even if it means reducing it to two drops. This remedy can be used externally also, by taking a few drops in the hand and rubbing gently into the affected part. If a septic focus is the cause of the trouble it must be either healed or in some other way made harmless.

TOMATOES – RELATIONSHIP TO CANCER AND ARTHRITIS

Very often one hears that eating *tomatoes* encourages cancer. Doctors too often voice this opinion which is based on various mistaken conclusions of certain scientists. Many have asked:

"What about tomatoes? Can I eat them?" Cancer mortality has absolutely nothing to do with eating tomatoes. Research carried out by careful investigators has shown that cancer mortality is greatest in those countries where the intake of protein, especially animal protein, is excessive. Ellis Barker gives many interesting statistics in his book on this subject.

A diet in which protein predominates can ultimately lead to cancer development, especially if one has a disposition for it, which can either have been inherited or acquired by faulty feeding. Another factor is the constant irritation of cells through medicinal or mechanical action. Ailments which have become chronic, such as constipation, can easily lead to degenerative changes in the system, which may sooner or later become malignant, if the afore mentioned factors are present.

Many women report that after having received a blow or similar injury to their breasts, it has led to an induration of the tissues involved, which has been diagnosed as cancer. Needless to say that not every blow results in the same consequences. If the disposition for malignancy is absent, the immediate results of such an injury will naturally disappear without leaving any ill effects. Of course this has nothing to do with *tomatoes!* If they were responsible for the disease, we should find the greatest cancer casualty, for instance, in Naples, Southern Italy, where people consume immense quantities of them. But I have come across few cancer patients in this district and, indeed, mortality from this disease is very low there because great emphasis is put on fruit, vegetables and carbohydrates and very little protein, mostly fish. This diet is a contributory factor to the low incidence of cancer in this area.

Sufferers from *arthritis* are often frightened with the same unreasonable argument. It has been propagated by scientists whose experiments have been confined to research laboratories and whose procedures have been far removed from actuality. It is true that green or unripe *tomatoes* are certainly detrimental to health for they contain substances in the nature of toxins which are only dispersed and rendered harmless by the process of ripening. To condemn the *tomato* in general because it is unwholesome in its unripened state is unfair. In reality, ripe *tomatoes* are healthful and contain at least five different vitamins which are a necessity for our bodies.

TREATMENT OF PSYCHOSOMATIC ILLNESSES

If we are to understand the meaning of "Psyche" or "Soul" we shall have to turn to the Book of Books, the Bible, and meditate upon the simple story of creation: "And the Lord formed man of the dust of the ground"; one might say of the elements of the earth. It goes on to say: "He breathed into his nostrils the breath of life and man became a living soul"; or as another translation describes it, "a living creature". In other places we read: "He poured out his soul unto death," and yet again, "The soul of man is in his blood," and "The soul that sinneth, it shall die."

If we pause to think about these scriptures, we must come to the conclusion that the "soul" or "psyche" of man is represented by his emotion-life in his sensitivity complex. With every pint of blood he loses, in a way, he loses part of his soul, his sensitiveness. If too much blood is lost, as in an accident, sensitiveness or feeling becomes less and less until it ceases altogether. First God created in the lifeless body a conglomeration of cells; then he charged the body with the breath of life, the spirit which began to permeate the hitherto lifeless form. And life entered it and man became conscious of himself, began to breathe and feel, and his existence as a living soul thus began. The unity of the body and the breath of life is, according to biblical statements, the living, sentient soul, which must always be considered a Whole. Therapeutically too, we must treat man as a whole if such treatment is to be successful and help him maintain mental and physical health.

RECIPROCAL EFFECTS

Mental disturbances lead to reactions in the physical body as well. Knowing of the reciprocal action of mind and body on each other, it is only reasonable that both components should be treated. It is well known that physical afflictions leave their mark on the mind of the patient which, in turn, reacts by imposing further restrictions upon the body. Every psychotherapist will confirm that mental conditions can be responsible for physical ailments, while the latter can react so severely upon the mind of the patient that he becomes mentally unbalanced. In women, disfunction of the ovaries frequently give rise to mental disturbances, which will disappear when that disfunction has been corrected.

Generally speaking, the whole field of psychosomatic medicine is, as yet, little explored and it is impossible to establish generally valid doctrines and principles. Experience and observation, however, have clearly shown that therapeutic one-sidedness frequently fails to achieve results in the treatment of a particular problem while constitutional treatment – the treatment of the patient as an entity or a whole – succeeds.

NATURAL TREATMENT

Although not natural, the electric and insulin shock could be a step in the right direction. Even if these treatments fall somewhat short of what we understand by natural methods, they are based on a fundamental theory – that shock effects brought on by accidents, fright and other emotional experiences can bring a person back to reason. A change of climate, environment, strenuous walking and breathing exercises, physical training, singing, etc. all are means of inducing favorable changes in the patient's mental outlook. Physical treatments

233

such as showers, hip-baths, underwater message and walking barefoot in the early morning dew are further sources of help which can be employed according to the doctor's suggestions with the necessary understanding in mind of the individual needs. The patient's every reaction to these physical shock therapeutic measures should be noted and anything contributing to the establishment of a happy atmosphere should be encouraged, as these measures alone quite often will work small miracles.

FROM THE REALMS OF EXPERIENCE

I had a very interesting experience some years ago. One of my friends had a daughter who suffered from hysteria, which caused her to bury her head in a pillow and cry for hours. My friend asked me to prescribe treatment for the young lady. The doctor's diagnosis was schizophrenia. The patient's sister who was also a doctor seemed helpless in what seemed to her as a hopeless situation. I took over the patient and my first action was to ensure the functioning of the ovaries by giving the Exanthematic treatment (called the Baunscheidt treatment) to stimulate the menstrual periods which were irregular and insufficient. The first reactions were of a very unruly nature, but as soon as the elimination of the Leucocytes started, a most extraordinary change took place. The girl, now completely in her right mind, said herself that it was just as though a veil had been removed from in front of her face. One single treatment sufficed to bring about a complete cure and even later, after a successful marriage, there were no relapses.

Another instance of such an illness was, where the patient was not having any periods at all. I prescribed Mustard hip-baths and Ovasan 3x to be taken internally. The periods soon reestablished themselves and the emotional crisis completely disappeared.

NEW WAYS

The problem of mental and emotional difficulties is not always so easy to solve, but there are instances where the solution could be quite simple. However, we must apply ourselves to finding the right method of approach. Every improvement in the function of the body, even if it is only the relief from constipation, can perhaps lead to a cure. The use of physical therapy in its many forms can open up new avenues in the treatment of such patients. As usual, diet plays an important part, for we know pure, natural foods keep the healthy person fit for daily work and helps maintain general balance. It is even more reasonable to suppose that this necessity becomes greater for the sick person. All adulterated foods should be avoided. We will want to make sure that the value of the food has not been lessened or destroyed by refining processes and that the fruits and vegetables have not been spoiled by chemical sprays or fertilizers. This careful attention to diet will provide real help for both body and mind. Take care of your circulation and make sure to take Calcium-complex regularly.

CORRECT NURSING TREATMENT

It often happens that the immediate family treat the patient either too gently or else too harshly. Even qualified nurses do not always find it easy to adopt the right method in dealing with psychosomatic illnesses. The patient can be very sensitive and easily upset due to a lack of nervous force, not being able to bear any form of opposition or constant reprimands. Therefore, one should try to help the patient skillfully overcome any shortcomings or deficiencies. Even when the patient has done something wrong, it serves no purpose to require a confession of guilt, for that would have the effect of causing the patient to retreat even further and become more stubborn than before. On the other hand the patient is quite likely to abuse our kindness, so it is best to be firm but kind at all times. This kind of approach will create a stability between patient and nurse or family member in charge. A reproof should not be given in a manner that antagonizes the patient but should consist in a quiet tone of voice so that he will recognize the direction is given in the guise of a helping hand and faithful support. The patient usually will accept such treatment gratefully but if he is antagonized, he will retreat back into himself once more.

AN EXAMPLE OF A DAILY PROGRAM

As recommended by Kneipp, the patient starts the morning by walking barefoot on the dewy grass. This draws the blood down to the feet and draws the energy obtained from the earth up into the body. If the weather is not favorable for this, water stamping followed by physical exercises in the open. In the course of the exercises, rhythmic movements, the singing and vocal breathing gymnastics will disperse any congestions and free the inner self.

Breakfast should consist of pure, natural foods, various fruits, Muesli, whole wheat bread, butter and honey. Avoid the usual breakfast of milky coffee, white bread, etc. and concentrate on those natural foods which are essential to body-building.

After breakfast a period of occupational therapy should follow. The purpose is to capture the patient's interest and concentration and divert the thoughts to something realistic. This is an absolute requisite of the treatment, for he must not be left alone and to his own thoughts which have a tendency to become more depressing as he broods. If one can divert the attention to every day realities, depressing thoughts and feelings will have fewer chances to assert their influence on his mind.

In the world of emotion, it is similar to the working of two transmission wheels; while the belt drives one, no power is transmitted to the other. Applied to the patient, this means that we must see that he occupies himself instinctively, either mentally, spiritually or physically with the realities of life. If we succeed in this, he will gradually be lifted out of his morbid sensitivity, imaginations, phantasies and dreams and return once more to normality.

Artistic occupations for those who have a natural inclination and ability are especially indicated as they divert and satisfy the patient without the need for constant encouragement. They constitute a bridge between a world of phantasy and reality.

The midday meal should consist of raw vegetables, steamed or baked potatoes, natural rice or some other whole cereal. All irritating foods must be scrupulously avoided. A further period of occupational therapy should follow the meal even if it is only washing the dishes or helping in the kitchen. During the afternoon some form of physical treatment should be given. This may consist of a hot bath with sweat inducing packs. Such a bath may be given several times during the week, depending upon the degree of benefit derived from it. If it warrants it, depending upon the patient, alternating hot and cold showers, starting with the hot shower may be given instead of the hot bath. In case of menstrual difficulties, a hip-bath lasting about a half hour at 100° F with herbal extracts added, can do a lot of good. After any one of these treatments there ought to be some form of relaxation such as a walk in the fresh air, which stimulates and gives an optimistic turn to the patient's thoughts. If time is left before the evening meal, it should be employed with further occupational therapy.

Supper should be eaten about 6 p. m. and should consist of a light, easily digestible meal that will not disturb the patient's sleep. Recommended high on the list is Muesli with fruit or a fruit salad with whole wheat bread, butter and honey.

As the day began with the first ray of sunshine, it should end with the fading light and the patient should get ready for bed as it begins to get dark. If he has trouble getting to *sleep* a mixture of Avena sativa, Passiflora and Aconitum will help soothe the nerves. In more serious cases, a combination of Rauwolfia and Avena sativa and Loranthus (a variety of

Mistletoe that grows on the oaktree). Use these natural remedies and arrange your patient's daily program according to individual needs and in this way you will be helping him towards both mental and bodily health.

The diet should be planned on a natural basis and should be rich in vitamins and mineral content. A juice diet or a short fast could, if the patients condition allows it, be tentatively tried out. It is important to have his understanding and cooperation, for such measures demand a certain effort on his part, which often proves too much even for those in good health. Never lose sight of the necessity of helping both mind and spirit. Physical ills need to be cared for, but not be given undue importance. Sympathy, firmness and understanding will help him gradually to think simply, consecutively and logically. Stubbornness will give way, little by little, but in order to achieve success, be careful not to irritate him into being contrary for this will once more throw him back into inward confusion and there will be unpleasant reactions which will have both physical and mental repercussions.

Strong nerves are needed to deal with psychosomatic cases and your own weakness and occasional helplessness must be carefully hidden. Patients must have confidence in the one caring for them as they are exceedingly sensitive and react to unfavorable circumstances very quickly. If you become annoyed because the patient has done something wrong, or if you are unhappy because his progress is not moving ahead rapidly enough, this does not spur him on to improve but rather throws him right back again. One needs tremendous self-control and self-confidence, also a certain calm and reserve of strength, in order to help rather than hurt a neurasthenic or mental problem. If the patient is conscious of a strong hand supporting and guiding him he will come through the wilderness of his distraught feelings with confidence in himself and his future. He will then cooperate with his helper and begin to think, feel and behave quite normally again. For those who are so gifted and feel they have the vocational abilities, the treatment of patients with nervous disorders is not only a very skilled, but also a most rewarding work. It brings peace of mind to these unfortunates by providing a bridge over which they can cross from confusion to the reality and confidence of their own free will and ultimate happiness.

THE HEART, AN INDEFATIGABLE ORGAN

Even before man becomes conscious of his existence, the *heart* begins to beat and continues to do so day and night until the day he closes his eyes in death. How grateful are we to this organ that serves us faithfully during our span of life which reaches 60 years for many and even 80 or 90 years for the more fortunate ones.

MATCHLESS ACTIVITY

Where could we ever find a machine that would work as efficiently as our heart? When we begin to study the structure of the myocardium we cannot help but be overcome by the immensity of divine creation. Every muscle fiber consists of a bundle, the fibrils, which in turn are divided by cross walls, surrounding every single cell with a protective cover. The outer walls of the heart consist of thousands of these elastic cables, through which a network of blood vessels provide nourishment and a network of nerves register the stimuli. We must admit that this living miracle deserves more consideration than we give it. Young people and athletes tend to treat the heart in an irresponsible and careless manner. The heart can be harmed in two ways; physical exertion can overtax it and worries may be just as harmful. The sympathicus serves to stimulate the heart while the vagus nerve slows it down. Both of these impulse conductors work in a rhythmic fashion according to demand, which translated means the heart beats either slower or faster. Between every beat the heart stands still for about $1/6$th of a second, the only rest it ever indulges in, which of course does not make up for all the activity we expect of it throughout our lifetime. This organ with all its capabilities and unerring service to man is truly an astonishing work of art.

In this twentieth century it is not all surprising to learn that about 50% of all people today show some sort of abnormality in their heart function. Modern man seems always to be under pressure and hurries even when he doesn't have to, although he may be careless about attending to his other responsibilities. This imbalance certainly does not provide for peace of mind as we find it among those who enjoy their work, and not view it as a necessary evil in modern society. "Haste makes waste" so the saying goes, but a steady pace is much to be preferred.

The endocrine glands, especially the thyroid, influence the operation of the heart which is noticeable in Basedow's disease. If we regard the heart rhythm, the pulsation, on paper by means of an electrocardiagraph, any malfunction of the heart can be observed. If the recording shows two entwined curves this indicates two hearts beating simultaneously. How is that possible? The answer is simple if you are a pregnant woman. If, however, three curves become visible, the happy mother-to-be will know that she may expect twins.

COMPLICATIONS DESERVING ATTENTION

It is interesting to note that the heart may continue to beat even after death. On the other hand it is also possible for the heart to have ceased to beat, although death has not yet occurred, as in the case of asphyxia. A strong electrical shock, for example, causes a spasm in the heart which may temporarily suspend its function but death itself does not occur until later, when the oxygen supply is cut off and carbon dioxide accumulates. Vesal, the father of modern anatomy, wanting to determine the cause of death of a nobleman he had treated, performed an autopsy during which he noticed, to his horror, that the heart was still beating. Witnesses who were present accused him of having performed a post-mortem examination on a living person and he was sentenced to death. This illustrates that life does not necessarily coincide with the activity of the heart. It has been observed in criminals who were sentenced to death in the electric chair that the heart stopped beating minutes before the actual occurrence of death.

A physician being aware of this fact was permitted to give an injection to a "dead" person in order to relax this spasm, because the doctor in his diagnosis had attributed the sudden recession of the heart beat to such a spasm. His assumption proved to be correct; the person who appeared to be dead, came back to life and had to be subjected a second time to this dismal kind of punishment. Every day new, astonishing facts connected with the functions of the heart are being discovered either accidentally or as a result of research, and certainly many more interesting and puzzling cases could be cited here.

INTERESTING AIDS

The discovery of the so-called heart hormones is the result of such an accidental discovery, made by a Hungarian professor who injected into an old sheep over a long period of time an extract from the heart of a young lamb. Due to this, the vitality of the old sheep increased markedly, its heart rhythm gained in strength and it was once again able to climb around on the hills. When this sheep was killed, the assumption of an actual rejuvenation having taken placed, was proved correct by the presence of young heart cells in the process of dividing. They were similar to those found in young sheep at the time of growing up. A heart of a young growing animal, therefore, must, for some reason, have the property that causes divisions of the nucleus of the heart cells, thus promoting the formation of new cells. This process no longer exists after the animal has grown up and reached maturity. The cause for the rejuvenation, which is called heart hormone, is still unknown, even until this day. Since we are dealing with a perfectly harmless substance, the experiment was also used on humans and the results were quite satisfactory, especially when given as a treatment for dilation of the heart, and in cases of a worn out or exhausted heart. Knowing of this excellent effect should not lead us to believe that if we abuse the heart and cause damage to the muscles, that there is a recourse to heart hormones which can easily correct it. This is not the case. The most sensible way to assure proper heart function must not be overlooked and that is normal care and consideration of it. Only in case of real need should heart hormones, homeopathic treatment or other remedies be considered. In case of need, the following plant remedies are available to us: tincture of Arnica root, Crataegus, Cactus grandiflorus, Strophantus, Spigelia and the nourishing heart preparation, Avena sativa; also the homeopathic preparation, Calcium Carbonicum and refined, diluted gold. A heart tonic made up of these substances may help to lessen many problems. In certain cases, individuals benefit from a tea prepared from the woody material found inside a nut, separating the two halves, such as a walnut.

If we make sure not to overstrain our hearts when we are young by engaging in very strenuous sports and we take reasonable care of our heart, we can last a long time without suffering any ill consequences.

LYCOPUS EUROPAEUS, A REMEDY AGAINST PALPITATION OF THE HEART

Lycopus Europaeus, commonly known as "Wolfstrapp" can be found in Switzerland in areas of up to 1,000 meters (3,280 ft) and in the valleys of Tessin and Puschlav. The European Lycopus is very similar in content and effect as that found in Virginia.

242

Lycopus produces excellent results in the treatment of *over-active thyroid* conditions and its accompanying heart palpitation. Even in cases of very strong pulsation, a dose of 5 to 10 drops has a very tranquilizing effect. If a *hyperthyroid* condition has existed for a long time Calcium-complex is recommended, since people who suffer from heart palpitation usually show a calcium deficiency. Many times, excellent results have been achieved with people who thought they suffered from a severe heart ailment by simply giving them Lycopus and calcium. It is interesting to note that a somewhat increased metabolism can be normalized with Lycopus and a calcium therapy, if at the same time a homeopathic marine plant preparation such as *Kelp D-4* is taken. However, it is important that no iodized salt be used at the same time. A combination of Lycopus and Calcium-complex is also very helpful in cases of over excitement of the heart. Even though a calming effect can be felt almost immediately, the preparation should be taken for several days. It is important that the person find out what is an appropriate dose and this will depend on individual sensitivity. For extremely sensitive people, 5 drops of Lycopus taken 3 times daily will suffice. Since the preparation is harmless the dose may be increased, if need be, to 20 or even 30 drops at a time.

CONTEMPORARY HEART POISONS – PACE AND HASTE

The ever increasing pace so characteristic of our modern world is one of the worse poisons for our heart. Even though productivity has not increased simultaneously, it has become the custom to cram many activities, especially those connected with our job, into a short time span. Related to this of course, is the shortened work week which has become more and more popular today. The increased free time is hardly ever used in a wholesome way such as pursuing a hobby, working on an art project, or acquiring more knowledge through a study course.

Instead, we continue at the same rate and pace we use for work and seem to find enjoyment on weekends in the midst of the mad world of freeways and expressways. The result is a state of complete exhaustion instead of recuperation from the week's work. Driving at high speed creates anxiety and inner tension and acts detrimentally towards the heart – like a poison. It is not only the fast pace and haste which are so harmful, but the effect it has on the heart and blood vessels caused by air pollution from exhaust gases emitted from heavy traffic, especially traffic jams. Especially bad for the blood vessels is the lead contained in the gasoline.

Contrast this with the benefits to be derived from taking a short ride over traffic-free back roads to a near-by forest or mountain. Have you ever experienced the pleasure of exploring on foot, in a leisurely manner, the paths that lead one back to nature? Try it sometime with your family. It will be a real enjoyable experience for the body, the heart and the mind.

This relaxing exercise in a clean environment would then permit us to go back to work on Monday morning, refreshed and relaxed instead of tense and irritable as is the case so often today, when we misuse our leisure. We must mention here also, the tendency to allow too little time to get to our work. This is an exploitation of our strength. We should always leave the house early enough so that it will not be necessary to rush for the bus or tram. Even a short run with a brief case can be taxing on the heart. Obese people should especially be careful about this, remembering the proverb, "Haste makes waste". It has become a habit to hurry at all times as if one was going to a fire, even if the gained time is wasted later on in an idle telephone conversation or an unimportant chat with a neighbor. Even babies come into the world in a hurry as the obstetrician induces labor to bring about birth prematurely so that his leisure plans will not be interrupted. This certainly is not wise, for the heart is not a machine that can be driven at maximum speed, ignoring its normal function, without suffering some kind of damage. Even young people who participate in over-strenuous sports activities can experience a case of dilation of the heart or other related diseases. Modern athletic competition no longer gives importance to purity and beauty of style, but requires the athlete to give his all, no matter how damaging the result may be. The idea is to win at all costs, a philosophy that shapes the thinking of coaches as well as participants in athletic events. Establishing new records and beating old ones governs the spirit of today's competition.

SMOKING – A POISON FOR THE HEART

That smoking is harmful to the heart is an acknowledged fact, and a fact to be considered especially by women. The question of why women smoke, if it is so harmful, has many answers. One may be found in the assumption that it helps to strengthen their self-image; or it may be the need to imitate whatever is popular at a given time, for no one wants to be out of step with the prevailing trend. Another is the mistaken idea that smoking calms the nerves in this fast pace of life, and it helps one to get a grip on oneself. It is a fact that 50 years ago hardly a woman smoked. The new trend we may attribute to the general change in life style that we have recently undergone. Abundant proof exists that nicotine is harmful as it constricts the coronary arteries and really has the same effect as a slow acting poison. The unfortunate consequences do not become evident until 20 or 30 years later, which makes it all the more difficult to convince people to stop smoking. There is no question that nicotine is harmful to men, but more so to women whose bodies are much more sensitive to its effects. According to statistics more men today are smoking pipes, which are not as bad as cigarettes since the toxicity is lessened due to a filtering system and a different preparation of the tobacco. Nevertheless, there are plenty of good, valid reasons to make us realize how much easier and more sensible it would be to refrain from punishing the heart while there is still time.

ONLY ONE HEART

Despite the unsuccessful efforts to transplant that most important organ in our body we must not forget that we have only one heart from which we expect faithful service during our entire lifetime. It is a miracle in itself that it is capable of rendering this service to us without interruption. How should we show our appreciation? By properly caring for it. It is a lack of appreciation to hasten its deterioration by careless overexertion and willfully feeding it with poisons we know to be harmful to it. Thus a shortened life can be charged up to either ignorance or a disregard for the principles of healthful living. There are no supermen. All of us pay the penalty for abuse of our bodies and belated regret, realization and life style changes, after the damage is done, will do no good. It will be too late to do anything about it.

If we are willing to make the effort to break our bad habits early enough, we can bring about a restoration and strengthening of the heart with the help of natural medication. For example, the heart is greatly strengthened by Crataegus, an extract from Hawthorn, which serves to strengthen the nerves of the heart. A tranquilizing effect on the heart is obtained from a harmless plant, native to Virginia, Lycopus, which is also grown in Switzerland. If wheat germ oil is taken simultaneously, the result will be truly astonishing. But, no matter how good the remedy, the effect will not be lasting, unless we cease to subject the heart to harmful external influences.

BEWARE! HEART ATTACK!

An elderly physician once said, to my amazement, that he hardly ever came across a case of heart attack among his patients during his early years of practice. And this, despite the fact that country people had to work much harder physically because modern machinery was not available to them. Why then, we might ask, is heart attack one of the most frequent causes of death today? It cannot obviously be linked to physical exertion from everyday labor, because technological advancements have diminished the need to work so hard. So the labor-saving devices, while making life easier, have not contributed to a life without heart attacks. Why wouldn't less demanding physical exertion result in better health conditions and less heart problems?

This reminds me of my stay in Vermont, U.S.A., when Professor Raab, the famous research scientist on blood circulation, talked about the "loafer's heart" of our generation. He did not mean that the loafer's heart resulted from loafing around, which certainly is not the case in today's busy world, but rather, the point he wanted to make was that "loafer's heart" is a result of one-sided activity and a lack of healthy activity outdoors.

The normal balance between work and relaxation is disproportionate. Not only in the United States, but here in Switzerland as well, we have all developed the bad habit of using the car for every little errand instead of walking. It is very unusual for a person who owns a car to take regular walks, not even when it is just a short walk to the corner store. Everyone hops in the car, nobody ever walks. Thus we are a generation spoiled by the many technological inventions that make life easier all the time and make muscles suffer from lack of proper exercise. Many are not aware of the danger that results from this way of life. Our blood circulation suffers and may even cause a deterioration of the entire vascular system as well as of the heart. One-sided mental activity may lead to tensions, circulatory constrictions, spasms, high blood pressure and many other infirmities, which are all potential causes for heart attacks especially in people in their 40's and 50's.

THE HAPPY MEDIUM

Many times of late I have received obituary notices of dear friends and relatives whose busy and productive lives have been suddenly interrupted by *heart attacks*. An analysis revealed that, in all cases, these people had long ago ceased to engage in any regular program of physical activity. Because they were too busy with the material things in life, they didn't have time to hike or take long walks in the forest or along country lanes for leisure activity. In the years prior to their death they no longer participated in the activities of, for example, the Sierra Club or found time to do a little gardening. Neither did they have time to participate in a sports activity that they may have liked in their youth. They never became aware of the fact that their life-span was being shortened considerably even though they may have had plenty of vitality. This may sound contradictory, but it is a fact that one-sided abuse of energy under pressure and haste puts great strain on the body. Limiting one's responsibilities and duties and avoiding today's fast wearing pace would assure a much longer service of the heart. Thus, we can conclude that most heart attacks are self-inflicted. Everything that is not regularly utilized or exercised in the body, degenerates and the organism tends to atrophy if all activity is taken away.

There is a happy medium between the over-taxed heart of a professional athlete and the under-taxed heart of a loafer. To achieve this medium should be the goal for everyone who does not want to put an end to his life prematurely. To avoid a heart attack in the late 50's or early 60's it is advisable not to give up participation in some kind of field sport at least through the 40's. This makes it unnecessary to medicate oneself in the later years. There are times, however, when we are warned ahead of time by certain symptoms. This happened to me a few years ago when I suffered from extreme heart seizures or what are sometimes called cramps. An examination produced negative results. This led me to take a closer look at my life. It revealed that for months I had been working only mentally with little physical activity. During this time my life was filled with problems and worries. This analysis was enough to pursuade me to immediately change my ways and to renew the sport I have cherished so much, hiking in the mountains again. And sure enough, my condition improved rapidly.

Recommended Modifications:

A change of life style will be of benefit to all of those whom we classify as manager types, office business men, functionaries, parliamentarians or those holding sedentary positions. They should all realize that it is much wiser to take some prophylactic action than to be concerned solely with the monetary benefits which their widows and children will inherit due to an untimely death which could have been avoided. Let us not be deceived. Nature has its own iron laws which we can not disobey with impunity, without paying the price. If your assessment or analysis of your life shows you are in danger of having a *heart attack*, wouldn't it be the sensible thing to modify your timetable? A wise man will listen to counsel. So, wouldn't it be wise to buy less gasoline, for example, and use your legs more to assure that your body cells get enough oxygen? As far as diet is concerned, stick to natural foods of high nutritional value. The body will welcome such a change and show its gratitude through increased efficiency and a longer trouble-free operation.

THE SICK PERSON WITHOUT A SICKNESS

If you own a car you may at times hear a noise when you are driving it, a noise that comes and goes. You may take the car in for a check-up, but just at that time, the noise is not there, and naturally the mechanic cannot find anything wrong with it. A few weeks later though, your car stops in the middle of the road because the defect which was not taken care of, developed into a serious problem. Now, you must be the mechanic!

It is even harder to detect a disorder of the human heart, especially if it is not a question of an actual organic disease. At times all possible methods of examination used do not disclose any clue of a malfunction. Thus, it has happened quite often that, after a thorough medical examination, a doctor will pronounce his patient hale and hearty and a short time later the patient dies from a heart attack. This has happened to persons who have just left the doctor's office and are leaving the building. This is not necessarily the doctor's fault because, at times, all possible methods of examinations do not disclose any clue to a certain malfunction. The medical observation is not sufficient in the case where someone feels very ill and the cause of the illness cannot be found. It takes many years of experience to understand what the person is trying to tell you. Sometimes when dealing with women, these complaints are passed off as hysterical or psychosomatic, but by arriving at this conclusion, the root of the problem is never reached and the patient is forced into deeper despair.

HYPERTHYROIDISM

Not long ago I observed a girl who had just returned to the Engadine from a trip to Italy. Her big, shiny, bulging or popping eyes showed signs of an over-active thyroid. She explained that her doctor had practically taken her apart without finding anything wrong although she complained of feeling very ill and extremely weak. She could sleep for 24 hours at a time if no one awakened her. Long sleeping periods can be attributed to the increased iodine content of salt air which seems to affect those who have a thyroid condition. An active thyroid affects a person in either of two ways: They feel an unnatural desire and need for sleep or they become very active, vivacious and nervous. It is essential for such a person to be aware of what the problem is, for it will enable him to adjust to his environment accordingly and begin remedial measures.

Years ago I sent a patient suffering from the same symptoms to her doctor to have him check her metabolism. Since he felt there was nothing wrong with her thyroid, he was reluctant to check her out. She insisted. To his astonishment the test revealed a substantial increase in her metabolism, a condition generally associated with calcium deficiency. Naturally, she immediately went on a high calcium diet to correct the metabolism.

250

A Calcium-complex preparation, in this case, is highly recommended and a homeopathic preparation, preferably Kelp D-6, extracted from the marine plant of the same name. It is a source of great satisfaction to see these symptoms disappear when the body, with the aid of natural medications, resumes its natural functions again.

VEGETATIVE DYSTONIE

Many disorders of the nervous system are purely psychological in nature or they may be caused by a malfunction of the endocrine glands and this disease is called "vegetative dystonie." The term is quite descriptive although it doesn't tell much. The term encompasses all disorders of the sympathetic or vagus nervous system, unless the disorders are of an organic nature. "Vegetative dystonie" therefore is a rather broad and complex concept. All of the following symptoms, not attributed to organic disease, would be classified under this term: vascular spasms, sudden sweating, cramps in the vascular system or gall bladder, spastic stomach aches, intestinal and heart disorders, including organic neurosis.

Since this new all-encompassing term has been coined, there are fewer people around whom we would classify as "sick" people without identifiable illnesses. Thus, if the doctor cannot find an explanation for a certain complaint, he simply attributes it to "vegetative dystonie." This is convenient and of benefit to the doctor as well as to the patient, at least from a psychological viewpoint. To be suffering from an illness without a name is a rather uncomfortable affair. By giving it a name the patient is satisfied if only for the sake of not being called a malingerer (one who pretends to be sick to escape work, etc.). A skilfully handled psycho-therapeutic treatment has always brought forth good results, especially if combined with certain remedies to strengthen the nerves such as a preparation consisting of a trituration of Avena sativa, Calcium gluconicum and other plant extracts and a preparation of

Ginseng with Avena sativa. Depending on the condition of the patient, an anti-spasmodic preparation made from Petasite would be indicated.

VISIBLE AND INVISIBLE GOITER

Many people, and more prominently, women often complain about a palpitation of the heart without being able to explain its cause. For example, when climbing stairs every one becomes aware of a more rapid heart beat. However, if one has a rapid heart beat that manifests itself without physical exertion or emotional upset, it is wise to undergo a thyroid test. A hyper-active *thyroid* has certain characteristics. Besides heart palpitations there is generally a considerable loss of weight and an inner vibration in the chest area also is present. There may be other symptoms such as loss of hair, severe nervousness and diarrhea. The metabolism is increased and the eyes have a distinct bulge. Any combination of these signs leads the physician to suspect an internal enlargement of the *thyroid* or a *goiter*.

Goiter as a result of a hyper as well as a hypo-active thyroid is more frequent in Switzerland, especially in the Alps, than many people think. This is true also of any landlocked country and the middle plains of the U.S.A. Many people get used to this unpleasant symptom and resign themselves to a constant state of nervousness and hyper-sensitivity.

Causes and Cures:

Although iodine deficiency plays a major part in goiter, minerals and trace elements are essential for prevention. Our experience has been that calcium is of equal importance as iodine. It is therefore recommended that the diet should be high in calcium which will enable one to avoid the many problems that goiter brings. Cole slaw or cabbage salad has an abundance of calcium and so does sauerkraut, kohlrabi, turnips, carrots, red beets. The latter two can be taken as a juice. Also, a good calcium-complex preparation is an excellent direct supplement. One has to be careful with commercial products containing iodine. In cases of hypersensitive people, those who suffer from a highly over-active thyroid condition, the use of iodized salt alone will sometimes cause palpitation. A person who is sensitive to even traces of iodine should avoid products containing them. A calcium therapy never causes similar complications, neither does the small amount of iodine that is found in certain vegetables. For example, watercress and all the other kinds of cresses, lettuce und leafy salad greens all contain tolerable amounts of iodine that will not upset the most sensitive person. Marine plants prescribed in homeopathic doses, such as Kelp D-6, D-5 and D-3, are excellent iodine derivatives. For seasoning there is a herbal salt which contains freshly processed cress in addition to trace elements from Kelp that is useful as a prophylactic against goiter. If *goiter* is present, and it is not caused by a hyperthyroid condition, Kelp tablets will produce excellent results since they contain all the minerals found in marine plants. Additionally they help to reduce overweight without any side effects. *Goiter* not only detracts from one's appearance and is physically annoying, but it also places a burden on the mental process because of its effect on the memory and the nervous system.

Surgical removal of the *goiter* can be avoided in many cases if a proper treatment with natural remedies is administered in time. This will insure restoration of normal body functions and lost physical strength, which is not always the case after surgery has been performed.

IODINE

Iodine is a strange substance that still puzzles many scientists. Given in great quantities it is a dangerous poison, but the body cannot exist without it. This element is among those which are needed in small traces but is of such importance that it may be compared to a push button that has the power to start and stop a sophisticated piece of machinery. The human body contains approximately 1/20th of a gram of iodine, half of which is found in the muscular system, 1/10th in the skin and a large portion in the endocrine glands, especially the thyroid. Here we find iodine attached to an amino acid, a compound called Thyroxin.

It is interesting to note that the so-called iodine level, that is the amount of iodine contained in the blood, is the same level for all people all over the earth, no matter where they live, in the mountains, at the seashore, in the polar regions or at the equator.

Where can it be found?:

Iodine is present in the rocks from which it is released in the process of weathering when rocks decompose. It dissolves in rain water and is carried to the oceans by the rivers. This is one of the reasons the ocean is so rich in iodine and other minerals. While various salts remain in the sea, iodine evaporates and is returned to the soil by means of rainfall, dew, fog and snow. Every year hundreds of tons of iodine are returned to replenish the soil. In valleys between mountains an iodine deficiency is often encountered. This can be explained by the fact that the water, being flushed too rapidly, carries with it large amounts of dissolved iodine instead of restoring it to the soil.

The consequences of iodine deficiency:

It is possible for a person to become mentally retarded due to a deficiency of iodine. If the thyroid fails to produce enough hormones, myxedema in severe cases could result. This deficiency may cause physical as well as mental difficulties. It can kill all emotional activity and may result in extreme disinterest in regards to work or job related activities and it may increase the desire to eat. The entire metabolism is affected, normal heart activity is slowed down considerably, with low blood pressure following. When sexual potency is low or lacking, this will very much affect the temperament adversely. It is not infrequent to observe a miraculous change in such a person if he is given iodine in the form of marine plant tablets containing *Kelp* and if his diet is changed to a natural basis.

Goiter is in almost all cases a result of an imbalance of the iodine content in the blood. It was interesting for me to observe that goiter connected with hypo-thyroidism favorably reacts to a treatment with iodine of potassium. On the other hand, the so-called *Basedow goiter,* caused by a hyper-active thyroid, responds best to a treatment of iodine combined with calcium therapy. Iodine in this case may be given in only minute doses, that is, in homeopathic amounts. When a marine plant preparation is prescribed it is best to begin with a Kelp preparation D-6, then after a few months change to D-5 and continue reduction, until after about two years the patient reacts favorably to the Kelp pills in uncontrolled strength. When this is the case, the person may be regarded as cured. At this time it is also advisable to continue to maintain a diet rich in calcium and to supplement it with a Calcium-complex intake.

OBESITY

It may be surprising to you to learn that *obesity* is related indirectly to iodine. The thyroid and gonad glands work together and if an obese person is given iodine in plant form, such als *Kelp* pills, the thyroid begins to secrete more hormones which, in turn, activates the entire metabolism. The gonads become more active and the body fat decreases. Iodine is more important than we think, because this mysterious element is responsible for operating the "gears" of our body according to the proverb: "Minute cause, immense effects." Watercress, even though it cannot be compared in effect to that of marine plants, nevertheless, contains a modest amount of iodine which can be of good service to our thyroid.

PROBLEMS CONNECTED WITH MENSTRUATION

Excessive as well as insufficient blood flow may create a great deal of discomfort for a woman. If the menstrual flow is too heavy it means an unnecessary loss of blood, which may lead to a slight case of anemia. Women who suffer from this condition should make sure that they do not engage in any strenuous physical activity beginning a few days before the period.

A preparation made from Tormentilla has proven to be a simple, reliable, natural remedy. It is a combination of fresh blood-wort with the juice of green blooming oat plant. It additionally has a soothing effect on the nerves. Too light a flow of blood causes an imbalance of emotions for many girls and women. The marine plant *Kelp,* from the Pacific Ocean, is very beneficial in cases of this sort because its iodine-potassium content is of greatest value. Generally, two or three Kelp pills suffice to normalize the flow. Women who have been suffering for a long time from the discomforts of insufficient menstrual flow should take a preparation that stimulates blood circulation. For total eradication of the disorder another preparation Ovaria D-3 influences the function of the ovaries and thus brings on a regular rhythmic period. This should be taken simultaneously with the former.

In addition to the above mentioned botanic medicines it is also recommended to take sitzbaths with thyme and camomille added to the water. Since a cure of menstrual malfunction goes hand in hand with the relief of emotional depression, every woman suffering from a similar condition will be glad to follow this advice. I should add here that women suffering from hyperthyroidism must take Kelp in homeopathic doses.

Ups and downs during menopause:

During the time of change of life practically every woman suffers to a certain degree from ebullition. At times a woman may be affected so strongly that her nerves and emotions are totally upset. It is important to take good care of the body during menopause. Excellent results are obtained by exercising regularly out-of-doors; activities such as hiking and the practice of taking deep breaths of fresh air are very beneficial.

Certain physical applications may also contribute to improving the condition, namely, daily brush massages of stomach, back and legs and bi-weekly hip-baths with hay flower added to the water. Extreme emotional depression may be relieved through Kuhne-baths. Physical exertion as well as occupational strain should be avoided at all costs. In addition one must learn to get along without coffee, tea and alcoholic drinks.

These precautionary measures make it easier to sleep at night and help to improve the overall condition. The following preparations will be of benefit in affecting a necessary relief of unpleassant symptoms: Salvia, Ovaria D-3, Ignatia plus Sepia D-6 and Aconitum D-10. They all help to assure a sounder and more restful sleep, which in turn favorably influences the emotions bringing about a balance that relieves depression.

The fact that this unpleasant condition can be relieved in such simple ways is certainly good to know. Thus, being acquainted with the various aids available, there is no reason to suffer all the inconveniences that accompany change of life.

KIDNEYS

If we compare our body to a modern chemical plant, the air conditioning unit responsible for getting rid of poisonous exhaust fumes would correspond to our lungs. In case of a prolonged break-down of this unit, the workers would die from gas poisons released into the air. The result would be just as drastic if our lungs stopped functioning. In order to assure a continuous well-being of the workers it is of utmost importance to get rid of the poisonous solid waste materials. In the case of our body, this is accomplished by the kidneys with some help from the liver. If the kidneys stopped operating for only two days uremia would set in. The non-excreted kidney toxins would cause metabolic poisoning. This can be observed in cases of enlarged prostate, the so-called prostata-hypertrophy. If the *prostate* swells and blocks the ureter completely, it must be corrected within 48 hours. This can be accomplished with the help of herbal steam baths or by means of a catheter. If immediate attention is not given, uremic poison may set in and this could be a threat to one's life. *Kidney stones* may bring about the same condition. In this case, prolonged hot baths are very beneficial. They should be accompanied by a light massage of the kidney and bladder area. To prevent the formation of kidney stones Safflower wort has proven to be very beneficial.

Noteworthy characteristics of the kidney structure

The structure of the kidneys are a true miracle. All constructive problems are solved so efficiently that the ancient anatomists called the kidney a "viscus elegantissimum" meaning elegant organ. The kidney consists of about a million bell or goblet shaped filters. Each of these filters is surrounded by a two-walled capsule and is separated by conducting tubelets which supply blood and filter out the urine simultaneously.

About two liters or not quite four percent of this liquid is being transported to the bladder by way of the ureter and then excreted. The remainder is reabsorbed by the bloodstream so that the entire filtering activity in one day amounts to about 60 liters (63.4 quarts) of fluid.

The kidneys look like a pair of peabean or peanut shaped organs. The filtering units are located on the outside. Towards the inside of the passages which become broader we find the large vessels and the beginning of the urether.

Harmful influences:

Aside from the heart and the liver, no other organ suffers more from the consequences of our modern way of life and its "civilized" diet. In may practice I have been able to observe the extent of the damage refined white sugar has done to the kidneys. Often a patient was relieved of all pain if he totally abstained from all food items containing sugar. This was proven by the fact that pain returned without fail when sugar was given to the patient again. This holds true for any kind of manufactured, refined sugar. However, natural sugars extracted from dried grapes, figs, bananas and other fruits never cause any such complications. The kidneys can also be rendered a great service if the intake of salt is minimized. Bacterial poisons likewise have a detrimental effect on the kidneys. That is why infections such as measles, scarlet fever, diphtheria, and angina affect the kidneys adversely. Permanent damage to the kidneys can be prevented if proper care is taken in curing such diseases fully and in making sure that normal kidney functions are properly supported and stimulated during and after any illness. For kidney stimulation, excellent benefits can be derived from the fresh plant extract Solidago, a remedy that should be on everyone's medicine shelf.

Very dangerous for the kidneys are metallic poisons such as lead. This is why painters and lithographers may invariably be faced with some kidney problems unless proper methods of precaution are taken.

The kidneys will function better if we also protect them from dampness and cold influences. For example, during warm or hot weather, we should make it a practice to take cold drinks in small sips only. If we bathe in cold water or feel cold after having gotten wet we should immediately restore the proper balance in our body by applying warm water packs.

Helpful hints for detecting certain disorders:

The kidneys should be given a little more care and attention than usual because many times problems with the kidneys do not evidence any pain at the beginning and thus may pass unnoticed. If the amount of urine excreted is less than normal over an extended period, we should have an examination right away; this holds true if the color of the urine changes. If blood is present or if the urine is cloudy, or we notice any other residue in the urine it should be a cause of great concern to us.

When little crystals are found in the deposit, this indicates that there is a likely tendency for kidney stones or kidney gravel to develop. Don't wait for pain. Seek treatment immediately.

If we examine the *urine* deposits under the microscope, the urinalysis will disclose interesting pictures that we cannot help but be amazed at the diversity of the crystaline formations. All sorts of prismatic forms and entire bundles of needle crystals can be seen. This is the result of uric acid, sulphuric acid and benzoic acid crystallizing. The amino acid Leucin crystallizes in an especially interesting way, forming a crystal more compact than a snowflake.

Such observations turn an examination of the uric sediments into an interesting study. Indeed, the scholarly expert can draw valuable conclusions from the images that the microscope discloses to him during an examination of the urine deposits. The fact of whether or not the patient adhered to a certain prescribed diet can even be ascertained. If the urine contains lots of sulphuric crystals it is evident that the patient ate foods containing sulphur, i.e. eggs, beans, peas, lentils, and radishes even though he was instructed not to do so. If the examination shows any oxalic acid crystals, this proves that the patient ate spinach, rhubarb, salad or sauerkraut. If lots of creatinine crystals are evident, the patient obvioulsy did not abstain from eating meat.

An examination of the urine thus can be very informative, more so than is often thought, even among professionals. We may learn something about metabolic disorders or certain organic diseases or any other kind of functional disorders through urinalysis.

Knowing how important the proper functioning of the *kidneys* are, we should not consider it a luxury to have a thorough, comprehensive examination at least once a year. Diabetes, for example, is another disorder that can be detected by *urinalysis*.

In view of today's demands on our health resulting from the ever increasing pace of life, it is of paramount importance to keep up the care of our body at least to a degree we would take care of an automobile. We all know that it is more economical to take care of a car problem when it first begins and thus avoid a major repair through neglect. We should give our body the same consideration, for as a heavily burdened organ like the kidney, many pains and much discomfort could be avoided later on if prompt attention and care are given it.

RUBIASAN TREATMENT

The excellent effect of *Rubia* in cases of *kidney* colic is well known. This famous root of the Madder has the property of dissolving *kidney stones*. The patient must, at all costs, avoid the possibilities of colds and exhaustion. During the treatment, as well as thereafter, he should be placed on a special diet to assure success. The patient must avoid all artificially flavored or refined food items containing white, bleached flour and of course, refined sugar. Furthermore, he should not eat spinach, asparagus, rhubarb, brussel sprouts and especially pork, lunch meats and cold cuts. Vitamin A is very necessary to overcome the deficiency that promotes the formation of *kidney stones* and kidney gravel. Eat plenty of carrot salad and drink carrot juice to counteract this problem. If bleeding is present, no animal protein should be eaten, the only protein allowable being curds. Better results can be obtained if the patient adheres to a diet of wild rice, vegetables and salads.

Physical applications are beneficial also. At night a warm, moist compress made with hay flowers and camomile should be applied to the kidney area for about a half an hour. Hot hip-baths will also help. If the stones should cause any bleeding, the patient should take Millefolium (Yarrow), Hamamelis virg., Echinacea extract, Tormentilla and Cantharis D-6.

Careful execution of these recommendations make up what is called the Rubiasan treatment. One should drink less liquids when taking this treatment. After finishing taking the box of pills, a week should elapse before taking any more and during this recess drink as much liquids as possible to provide for a thorough flushing of the kidneys. This will prevent the formation of new gravel stones. Then begin another week of treatment with a limited intake of a Solidago preparation and weak kidney tea. Follow this up with no medication for another week but taking plenty of fluids. The treatment is completed after a third week on medication and a fourth week where, again, plenty of liquids are consumed.

Even though the stones will have disappeared after this treatment it would be wise to repeat it in a shortened form every three months, just to be on the safe side. Diet must be continually observed. If available, a tea prepared from the plant Chanca pietra found in the tropical jungles of Peru will enhance the effectiveness of the Rubiasan treatment.

THE URINARY BLADDER

The urinary *bladder* is a hollow organ made up of muscle fibers, the inside of which are lined with a mucous membrane. Under normal circumstances the bladder has the capacity to hold about ¾ of a liter (almost a quart) of fluids. Since the fiber cells have a rubber-like elasticity the bladder is able to expand greatly without suffering any damage. According to the amount of fluid present, pressure is exerted on the walls of the bladder. When the pressure mounts this triggers the feeling of having to pass water. The amount of fluid present in the bladder is not the only force causing the urge for elimination but external influences such as exposure to cold contributes to it. Cold feet or stepping on to a cold tile or cement floor causes a strong need to pass water, even if the bladder is only partially filled.

When suffering from a *bladder* infection the urge to pass water may also be present, but often it is not possible to do so. This creates a painful condition because the bladder is one of the most sensitive organs which reacts to emotional as well as physical stimuli.

BLADDER INFECTION – CYSTITIS

Generally a *bladder* infection is a result of a cold. An old saying has it: "Whatever results from a cold can only be taken away through heat." This ancient law of natural therapy can also be applied to the bladder. That is why hot herbal packs, compresses and hip-baths are very successful aids in treating this infection. The water used to prepare the compresses should be as hot as the hands can bear it when wringing out the cloth. The hip-baths should have a water temperature of 37–38 degrees C. or 98–99 degrees F. in order not to cause any congestion. This should be carefully observed, especially if the patient suffers from high blood pressure or a weak heart. The hip-baths should be continued for ½ hour, adding hot water from time to time to maintain constant temperature.

Certain bacteria such as Staphylococcus, Streptococcus and Colibacillus also are responsible for bladder infections. In rare cases the *bladder* may be affected by tuberculosis, a condition more likely to occur if the patient already has a kidney tuberculosis, which permits the bacillus to enter the bladder through the kidney and manifest itself at the slightest irritation of the bladder. The cause for this Cystitis must be searched for especially in chronic cases which need special treatment to be fully eradicated.

The symptoms of *Cystitis* are stinging and burning sensations in the ureter when passing urine. Due to the irritation a strong urge persists to pass water. The urine generally contains some red and white blood cells, is cloudy and appears white and slimy.

Supplementary treatment

The treatment with the above mentioned warm wet packs can be greatly augmented through the use of several botanical remedies. One of the best medicines, counteracting any kind of inflammation is a preparation made from extract of Echinacea. Doses of 5 to 10 drops should be taken every hour.

Also, a preparation made from Solidago and several other plant extracts speeds up the cure and at the same time stimulates the kidneys. Cantharis D-4 takes away the unpleasant feeling when passing *urine*. And a preparation made from Usnea containing natural antibiotic substances, fights off all harmful bacteria. Meanwhile, it is best to stay in bed as long as the infection has not completely subsided.

In the case of a constricted urethra, the duct through which the urine passes, an enlargement of the prostate or bladder stones, the treatment must be adapted accordingly and thus expanded. In cases where urination can no longer be controlled due to a muscle weakness, some bladder medication should be taken. The same kind of medication has proven excellent in the treatment of enuresis in children. The plant Galeopsis is also very beneficial and should be mentioned here too.

BED WETTING (ENURESIS)

Bed wetting is a difficult problem that affects mother and child alike. Even though it may be the result of some emotional disorder, certain remedies, physical applications and a non-irritating diet may greatly support the organism on overcoming these emotional problems.

If an intelligent child suffers from *enuresis*, provided he does not have a cold or any other physical condition or weakness, this can generally be attributed to an emotional conflict. It can be an unpleasant home atmosphere or the child simply may have been spoiled by indulgent parents. The first step, if it is the former reason, should be to create a happy home environment free from anxiety and a "hurry-up" pace of life. It should not be difficult to find the cause for the emotional problem. Skillful empathy on the part of both mother and father will help reveal it. There may be a variety of reasons such as fear, jealousy, ambition, over-exertion due to anxiety, or provoking television programs that children should not be permitted to see.

To be a bed-wetter has great disadvantages for the healthy, intelligent child as well as for the handicapped one. This problem should be attacked with all energy at once.

All available natural remedies to strengthen the bladder and kidneys should be considered. Furthermore, a sufficient amount of biological calcium and salicylic acid should be prescribed. In order to cure the various afflictions stemming from enuresis, the following remedies can be recommended: kidney tea, bladder drops, Galeopsis, Usnea preparation and a herbal preparation of Silica and other plants. The treatment must be supported by an appropriate diet, free of salt and fat. The diet should consist of wild rice and millet combined with fresh vegetables and salads. At the same time a glass of *carrot juice* should be taken daily. As with all types of liquids, it should be taken in small sips and be well salivated. It is important to train a child to salivate and masticate food well at all times for the sake of good digestion. No fluids should be given the child after 4 p. m.

Great improvement can be brought about through physical applications. A warm, moist hayflower compress placed on the lower abdomen daily stimulates the blood circulation of the urinary organs. From time to time the child should be given a hip-bath with hayflowers added to the water. It is important that the child does not get cold, but rather his whole body should be warmed thoroughly by keeping the tub covered with a large towel or heating the bathroom. Cold feet should be prevented. Make sure the child has adequate foot-wear, warm socks and adequate clothing to protect his body when going to and from school. Make sure that the child gets plenty of exercise out-of-doors. This will stimulate the circulation and give the child a feeling of warmth throughout his entire body. Take hikes or walks through the forest with him and have him breathe deeply. It will do you good to do the same! In the evening try to cultivate an atmosphere of soothing relaxation. Encourage a joyful and happy outlook as this is the one thing that contributes to a speedy recovery. It brings with it emotional balance, and helps overcome the emotions that have been a basic part of the problem. Engrossed as we sometimes are in our daily routine, we tend to forget how important it is to our health and the health of the child to preserve a feeling of being wanted, a wholesome interest between parents and children. This will help eliminate the emotional stumbling blocks to the child's problem.

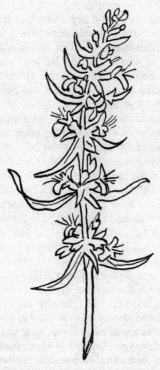

Ysop (Hyssopus officinalis)

ORCHITIS

Orchitis is an inflammation of the *testicles*. It is a rather frequently occuring disease and its treatment tends to be neglected by men reluctant to see a doctor. Because of this, I would like to talk about the causes and subsequent treatment of this inflammation at length. By overlooking the condition and not properly caring for it you may invite later infertility which can result in serious emotional problems, especially for younger men.

Orchitis is generally caused by germs that are carried in the bloodstream and they need not be of the venereal type either. Tuberculosis of another organ, for example, could be responsible for Orchitis. Mumps, or other infectious diseases may be the cause. In any case, treatment of the basic underlying cause should never be neglected.

The plant extract from Echinacea along with other extracts has proven successful in cases like this. Take 10 to 20 drops every hour during the day. During the night, apply a mud pack to the inflamed area. In order to increase the healing power and to keep the paste from drying out, add a tablespoon of St. John's wort oil to the paste. An alternative is to use a compress made from squeezed cabbage leaves. If this causes a strong reaction one should stop using it immediately, and stick to the mud packs. These always have a soothing effect. It is important to keep the bowels open and induce regular movement. These suggestions will work if you follow them conscientiously.

OVERCOMING SUSCEPTIBILITY TO ECZEMA AND SCABIES

Cases of *scabies* (Milchschorf) in children are often the consequences of genetic predisposition toward dermatitis in one or the other marriage partner, passed on over generations from parents or grandparents. If scabies is improperly treated the child may become every receptive to any infection due to lowered resistance. For example, let us consider for a moment a child suffering from whooping cough which was suppressed or improperly treated. The bacterial toxins were not completely eliminated. It is likely that the child will suffer consequently some damage to his heart or develop asthma, two conditions that are very difficult to improve or correct.

Any kind of *eczema* as well as scabies must therefore be treated correctly from the outset in order to totally eradicate them. I am trying to direct attention in my writings to fighting this disease by means of an appropriate liver treatment. The first step in this direction is a salt-free diet of the kind described in my book entitled: "The Liver, a Regulator of our Health."

IMPORTANT RULES FOR DIET AND OTHER RELIABLE REMEDIES

If we are careful in our choice of protein we can count on rapid success. Lactic protein, such as curds, buttermilk, and sour milk to which freshly grated horseradish has been added, have proven excellent in cases of eczemas. A person suffering from eczema often cannot drink any whole milk and he should abstain from it. Nut protein in the form of almond milk or soy bean milk are both very helpful. One should stay away from eggs, especially boiled eggs which cause strong reactions in persons suffering from eczema. The same holds true for all kinds of cheeses with the exception of curds, cottage cheese and most white cheeses, which cause no complications.

The *diet* consists basically of wild rice or, if unavailable, brown rice and products rich in calcium. Cabbage, sauerkraut and kohlrabi leaves are among these vegetables. A biological Calcium-complex preparation makes the assimilation of calcium from food much easier and ensures against a deficiency. Medical advisers sometimes recommend calcium injections which may be theoretically and logically correct but, I do not recommend it, since I believe it to be more wholesome to supply the body with sufficient amounts of calcium obtained from food sources or to take the complex by mouth.

It is very important when suffering from *eczema* to stay away from sweets of any kind. This includes candy, ice cream, cakes and pastries. White sugar has harmful effects and it may even create a condition of allergic sensitivity in certain people. White flour, although not quite as drastic in its effect, should definitely be avoided. It is recommended for therapeutic reasons to confine one's diet to whole grain products.

From experience we have learned that the most effective natural remedy in treating eczema and psoriasis is Viola tricolor, an extract from the pansy. Calcium-complex preparations should be included too. These may be used externally as a powder to dab the affected areas. A whey concentrate and Usnea extract have the same soothing effect and should definitely be incorporated in the treatment, not only externally but also taken by mouth. *Eczema* is generally accompanied by hypo-active sebaceous glands which make it necessary to supply the skin with sufficient oil. St. John's wort oil or a good lanolin preparation will accomplish this purpose.

Other important advantages:

As with most diseases it is important to deal with psychological challenges as they may subsequently be the cause of the illness worsening. That is why I have devoted a chapter to "Get well through joy." A lot of attention was given to the same question in my book about the liver since this organ is notably sensitive to emotional influences.

Knowing how to deal with one's illness is a step forward in the right direction, for mental balance is the sane approach to all problems. One must gear oneself to undergo and accept treatment through natural therapy instead of chemical. If one adheres strictly to a natural diet he can be sure he is pursuing the right course. It is absolutely necessary to carry out the treatment for six months to a year. The treatment is not expensive since it is mainly a question of correcting one's dietary habits. Reactions and side effects are minor and usually do not occur at all, if skillfully approached.

In summary it should be stressed that in case of eczematous skin eruptions, the liver needs special attention and care. The same goes for the kidneys which should by all means be protected from exposure to dampness and cold. Furthermore, we must take care that the skin does not come in contact with strong detergents, floor waxes or other household products containing turpentine. With the kidneys and liver functioning properly the skin is freed from excessive work and thus the unpleasant itching will subside and, with it, the eczema symptoms will disappear.

For those who follow the above suggestions conscientiously, success will unfailingly appear but those who think that drugs and chemicals alone will suffice may go for years without ever getting better. The more stubborn the case of eczema, the more patience is needed to obtain satisfactory results.

NETTLE RASH

Nettle rash is a peculiar condition that is very unpleasant for the one afflicted. It is also known as Urticaria and the question as to what causes it is asked over and over again. The itching variety of Urticaria is accompanied by little red dots on the skin. It is thought to be due to certain sensitivities to agents or foods. It is actually a question of hypersensitivity, generally referred to as an allergy. Where a tendency of this kind exists, certain foods such as strawberries, fish, cheese, sea food, pork, salami, etc. may be the cause of an allergic reaction such as Nettles. It is not unlikely that a reaction will occur to certain medicines even if these are biological preparations such as arnica, to cite one.

To deal with this unfavorable predisposition, the first thing to do is to avoid every agent that could be a possible cause for Urticaria. A prolonged observation may be necessary to determine the exact cause of the allergy. Sometimes the sensitivity may have its origin in a hereditary disposition, which makes it all the more difficult to overcome. It is possible to train the body to get use to those agents that have caused problems and thus eventually eliminate the annoying symptoms. This can be accomplished by exposing the body to very minute quantities of the causative agent at a time. The sensitivity may be also successfully treated by raising the calcium level and by taking sufficient amounts of a preparation made with different plant extracts to form a Calcium-complex.

WHAT IS AN ALLERGY?

The question is easily answered if we think of an *allergy* as a hypersensitivity to a certain kind of variety of different agents. This hypersensitivity may have such drastic reactions as comparable to poisons. I am acquainted with the son of a druggist who literally becomes ill if even the tiniest amount of egg is in his food. A late friend of mine in New York reacted in a similar way to wheat. Whenever he ate a piece of bread or pastry made with wheat flour he became deadly sick. Professor Abderhalden once told me of one of his assistants whose head swells every time he eats white beans. Often we encounter allergic reactions people have to flowers and fruits. Some cannot eat strawberries, mangoes, rhubarb, blueberries, etc. Certain kinds of flowers and fruits may even cause herpetic skin eruptions when even touched. *Allergy* to animal fur like those of cats, dogs and rats is quite common. Then too, some people are allergic to some animal protein or fats. Others cannot even look at a crab or lobster or any other shellfish without getting violently ill. To be allergic to rye or wheat, however, astonished me somewhat.

How to counteract this condition:

Many people have asked: "What can be done to counteract this condition?" but, until now, I have not been able to give

271

them an answer that would have satisfied me personally. It is possible to undergo a series of tests given by specialists, which I understand is a popular and rather standard practice among Americans. As a rule, it is rather expensive and requires an additional sum of money in cases where immunization with antibodies becomes necessary. However, the effectiveness of this kind of treatment can never be guaranteed.

One of the best ways is to *test* oneself according to the following method: everytime an *allergic reaction* is noted, one should write down everything that was eaten, touched or smelled. In time, a comparison of these notations should reveal the recurrence of a certain material, a food item, a fruit or a flower. This repetition may then serve as a clue as to the cause of the allergic reaction. Then, of course, the most obvious thing to do is to avoid at all cost the responsible agent.

A person suffering from an allergy often shows a calcium deficiency which makes it necessary to eat foods of high calcium content as well as augment the diet with a Calcium-complex preparation that will raise the calcium intake more rapidly. This will help to control if not eliminate the allergy.

SPASMS AND CRAMPS

There is a variety of more or less severe *cramps* that may be caused by a certain nerve or brain disease such as Encephalitis, or may be brought on by an infection such as Tetanus. Severe cramps also may be the result of urine poisoning such as uremia or eclampsia. Every one of these cramps require specialized individual treatment. What we want to deal with here are the simple, frequently occurring muscle *spasms.* Sometimes they are noted as muscle twitching or clonic cramps of rather brief duration, but returning in quick succession, or long lasting muscle contractions known as tonic cramps.

These simple forms of cramps can be successfully controlled through using a hayflower or camomile water pack on the affected area. Otherwise, one may take a hot shower directing the hot spray to the cramp area. Depending upon the particular nature of an individual, physical exertion may cause severe contracting cramps in the rectal region. These cramps may be so severe as to cause the afflicted person to cry out in pain. Obviously, this leads him to believe he is suffering from some severe illness. In reality, however, it is nothing but a quickly passing cramp that can easily be relieved by taking a hot shower for a few minutes. Direct the water onto the afflicted area for fast relief.

Menstrual cramps, which cause great discomfort to women, fall into the area of spasmodic cramps. Many different kinds of headaches also may be brought on by spasms. This is particularly the case with migrain and the much feared "Fohnweh" (discomfort caused by warm, humid winds that pass through the Alpine regions).

It is a relief to know that it is unnecessary to take highly toxic medication to relieve these pains and cramps. Instead, a preparation derived from petasites officinalis has proven very reliable in controlling cramps without causing harmful side effects.

OUR "NASTY" SYMPATHETIC NERVE

A modern telephone certainly can be considered a technical miracle. But what if it breaks down? It is then that we would prefer the simpler older system which can be quickly repaired.

In comparison, our sympathetic nerve system is a miracle of much greater magnitude than a telephone. If ever anything goes wrong with it, it may have tragic consequences, which is the reason we call it our sympathetic nerve.

Never before in my life have I had such bad experiences with my sympathetic nerves as recently, during a period of much stress and worry. It was in such a state that I left St. Gallen to head for the Engadin mountains. Shortly after the onset of the previously mentioned anxiety provoking condition I felt such severe spasmodic pains in the stomach area that I could hardly sit any longer. Unfortunately I did not have any Petasites preparation with me which would have released the cramp. My stomach did not quiet down until I vomited. During the night I suffered from severe pains which felt as though my stomach had contracted into a painful bundle. After my arrival in the Engadin I was able to control the nausea with Nux vomica D-4 and Crataegus which helped to calm my heart. Nevertheless, during the night, I was very uncomfortable, and even though I fasted the entire next day, the cramps did not subside until evening when a prolonged hot shower released the spasm.

It was this experience which helped me understand why one of my friends, who had many worries related to the sale of his business, had to have surgery several weeks later, because of extremely painful stomach ulcers. Doctors are correct in assuming that practically all stomach ulcers can be traced to spasms caused by aggravating circumstances. Constant spasmodic cramping of the stomach muscles unfailingly has resulted in ulcers.

Precautionary measures better than cure:

It is better to conquer difficulty and worry by means of self-discipline than to have problems control us. Often this is a question of experience and practice, for even if we know how to react in difficult situations, old habits often prevail and serve to prevent us from making correct decisions. People of a calm and tranquil nature find it much easier to remain collected and composed when facing unpleasant and distressing surprises than those who are prone to make split-second decisions without giving sufficient thought to the result. The sympathetic nerves unfortunately are not subject to our voluntary control (reason), but rather to our feelings and emotions. It is thus important to be composed so that unpredictable situations may be taken in stride. When the wise Solomon advised us to take better care of our hearts than of anything else he had a good point in mind. Since the heart is the source of life, we should heed his advice. By subjecting our emotions to proper and collected control we are able to harvest many benefits including those pertaining to our health. Of utmost importance though, is the fact that we are rendering a welcome service to our sympathetic nerves.

RELIABLE AND INEXPENSIVE REMEDIES FOR INSOMNIA

It is certainly an aggravation not to be able to go to sleep in spite of being tired. But it is even worse to lie awake for hours because of tensions of the day being transformed into problems at night of insurmountable magnitude. Unpleasant daytime experiences prevent sleep and create a state of depression and the wheels, which are supposed to stand still during the night, turn faster and faster. Suffering from restlessness the individual turns from side to side and finally, in order to put an end to his suffering, he reaches for a sleeping pill to overcome his *insomnia*. This, of course, is the most inappropriate way he could have chosen, for in no time, if he continues this habit, he will have developed a dependence on this crutch. He tends to forget that this destroys the body's ability to react and respond in a natural way and that continued use of sleep-inducing drugs, whether they are habit forming or not, has a destructive effect that can be far reaching. It is far more important and wiser to isolate the cause of the problem that keeps one awake and by resolving it, we will eventually restore our ability to fall asleep.

A variety of aids:

Many have found it possible to put the cares of the day out of mind when going to bed by reading a book, a magazine or some interesting article which, if one reads long enough, will eventually lead to drowsiness and uninterrupted sleep. Reading in bed is the safest kind of self-inducing "drug" that you can take. In cases where the nerves have been overtaxed, it is helpful to massage the aching area of the head with the finger tips. This gentle massage generally relaxes the tension and

275

results in sleep. A warm bath just before going to bed is a wonderful relaxant. Anything that recirculates the blood and drives it back to the external areas helps to induce sleep, since insomnia is often caused by too much blood congestion in the brain. Our busy life today suffers from a lack of balance which accounts for unequal distribution of physical and mental work. Often we overtax our mind and do not provide sufficient exercise for our bodies which consequently diminishes our ability to relax. We cannot rid ourselves of the many problems that haunt us and still subject our already heavily burdened mind to even more stress. Is it any wonder that we cannot fall asleep?

A radical approach to inducing sleep is provided in a letter recently received from Australia from a former patient living in Elwood. She wrote me about how enthusiastic she was over a book written by Kneip. Her enthusiasm led her to provide a cold water treatment for her entire family. Her husband, who had been suffering from insomnia for months, had been relieved by applying cold water packs to the back of the head and neck just before going to bed. This treatment resulted in a deep and wholesome sleep. One of their daughters, also suffering from insomnia tried her father's method, and was able to fall asleep without any trouble. This was a spiritual and emotional relief that was of great benefit to her.

Today, health books have a wide circulation in every country. The thought that my health books, which are available all over the world, translated into several different languages, could be effective even as a sleeping remedy long after I am gone is quite a pleasant thought to me.

More cold water applications:

Sauna baths, once popular in only northern countries, are now accepted in many other areas of the world. In Switzerland and northern European countries it is common for people in the winter to take a sauna bath and then roll in freshly fallen snow. The claim is that the body's power of resistance becomes greatly strengthened by this exercise. *Walking* barefoot in the snow and water stamping are all favorite activities. All of these activities cause the blood to be drawn from the brain, which, when practiced before going to bed, makes restful and wholesome sleep possible. Information on various applications coming in from different countries may benefit us too, since it contributes to the list of already available remedies.

I was greatly surprised to encounter a sauna bath among people living in a Finnish Colony in Brazil, of all places. What purpose is there for a sauna bath in an area where the temperatures reach 40 degrees Centigrade (105 degrees Fahrenheit). The answer is: whatever one is used to, seems to become a necessity, which is true for these Finnish people who built their sauna in a hot foreign land. It helped them to overcome nostalgia for their homeland. Nevertheless, in the tropics the evenings are cool and thus the sauna bath was a welcome addition to a life pattern developed here. After the sauna bath a nearby jungle creek invited us to a cool bath which stimulated the circulation and helped to provide restful sleep. Perspiring in a sauna bath differs from perspiring in the heat of the day in that it brings about a relaxed feeling and enables one to sleep soundly at night.

EPILEPSY – NEW VIEWS
CONCERNING ITS TREATMENT

Epilepsy, also known as "falling" sickness is frequently mentioned in old writings and biblical accounts and although it has been around for thousands of years, the therapy known to us today is still not adequate in attacking the symptoms. Bromine, used in various combinations, Luminal, Cominal and other drugs prescribed to reduce the severity of the attacks, can hardly be called satisfactory to neither the patient nor the physician. If the patient is sensible enough to avoid alcohol, nicotine and other harmful stimulants, he may be able to obtain somewhat more satisfying results than drugs provide.

A dietary treatment consisting of raw foods, rich in vital elements is of definite advantage. Observation shows that attacks appear less frequently and are less violent when the patient adheres to a proper diet. It appears also that a new road to success has been found by positively influencing the mineral metabolism. As a rule, epileptics show a low calcium level and often excrete a lot of calcium, especially that bound to phosphorus with the urine. A calcium therapy is therefore advisable, in connection with a proper diet, and will prove quite advantageous. In addition to eating foods high in calcium, the patient should take a preparation of Calcium-complex, which in addition to being very effective, is free from any harmful side effects. This is an advantage which a bromine treatment cannot claim for itself, since it has a damaging result to the body over a period of time and the emotional and mental health of the patient suffers.

All sorts of evidence:

Recently I received good news from South Africa, from a patient whose attacks formerly occurred on a daily basis and had diminished to only one a month and the monthly attacks were milder than formerly. The success is attributed to the patient's taking of the preparation Calium-complex and another preparation of Vitamin D. Since she was overweight she added *Kelp* pills to her medicinal diet. It is likely that the organic iodine contained in the marine plant pills was responsible for the strong influence upon the endocrine glands. No doubt other minerals found in *Kelp* also helped.

In any case, as various studies showed, *epilepsy* today can be treated with less harmful preparations than bromine. As mentioned before, in addition to a dietary arrangement consisting of non-irritating, alkaline-based foods, a biological calcium preparation should be taken. Vitamin D helps make it easier for the body to absorb the calcium and they should be taken together. The main treatment is *Kelp* and in pill form, it should be taken three times a day. None of these are specific medications but rather nutritional supplements supplying the body with what it needs most. Another product which has proven excellent is the oak mistle, Loranthus emopaens, a plant native to the Balkan area. It is unfortunate that to this day, specific remedies are prescribed without giving due consideration to the possibility to what the body may lack without which the illness cannot actually be improved or cured.

Not everybody needs the same amount of every substance. Depending on the individual's nature, his temperament, and his hereditary disposition, the need for a particular element may be greater than normal so that more vitamins, mineral salts or other substances are needed to reconstitute a proper balance.

A report from an acquaintance in America, who had been suffering from *epilepsy* since her youth, confirms this assumption. She wrote that she was aware of the excellent effects of *Kelp* since she had been taking it for more than ten years. She also mentioned that she thought that a biological calcium preparation had helped her even more than the Kelp. Since her attacks were minor but recurring frequently, it was a source of satisfaction to learn that she was able to overcome them by taking *Kelp* and calcium supplement and by adhering to a diet rich in calcium. Apparently her need was greater for the calcium, in this case. Each one's requirements may differ.

Biologically oriented physicians come to the same conclusion, as the report from one of my friends in New York shows. He related the example of a famous doctor, 80 years old, who is totally nature-oriented. This doctor also emphasizes the excellent effect of calcium on the general state of health, especially when combined with Vitamin D. Although already mentioned, I would like to re-emphasize the importance of a non-irritating diet, low in salts.

TRAGIC HEREDITARY DISPOSITIONS

When young people get married they hardly ever think about the prerequisites of health which they may be transmitting to

279

their offspring. It is understandable that the happiness they have in having found each other is based on emotion rather than reason. The things deliberated on before marriage are generally of material rather than a spiritual nature. Even though the emotions may be ruling it is still of paramount importance to consider the make-up of the two individuals involved, because the health of their children will be very closely related to this question. None of us are perfect and only a few feel so strong and healthy as not to be aware of some weakness of either a physical or mental nature. If any unfavorable, negative genetic factors should be present, it would be better if one partner did not possess the identical weakness, but instead had a positive predisposition to offset the severity of the defect in the other. If the parents of both partners, for example, are emotionally unsuited to maintain a healthy balanced life, minor emotional stress on the children would manifest itself through some mental defect becoming noticeable.

If there is a history of diabetes in both families of the young couple, some basic mistake in their diet will be enough to double the unfavorable predisposition in one or the other descendent so that insulin treatment may become necessary. Susceptibility to TB, ulcers, cancer, arthritis, rheumatism and many other physical conditions may be transmitted genetically. With this in mind it does not appear unreasonable for young people, before they wed, to consider the task of examining their particular genetic predispositions in order to determine whether the founding of a family appears to be advisable from the standpoint of health. If, however, one should elect to take the risk, it is even more important to consider the medical question closely since much harm can be avoided through a reasonable approach and by taking a corresponding action. If, though, after close consideration, there are no possible existing conditions, then it would not be necessary to take any precautionary measures.

Basic prerequisites:

Many young people, even though properly brought up and otherwise responsible, hardly ever think about any necessary medical prerequisites before marriage. Their conversational subject matter is often limited to questions of housing, furnishings, vacations and excursions, leisure activities and hobbies and perhaps questions of whether to have children or not.

As we are all aware, many companies, especially governmental agencies, have prepared long questionaires for job applicants. The exact answers are supposed to determine whether the applicant has all the necessary qualifications. Well, it would be just as informative and certainly appropriate with regards to the founding of a new family, if the prospective parents would fill out such a questionaire. Any good physician or psychologist could easily recognize from this, what kind of medical risks are to be encountered with respect to offspring.

If two people, for example, both suffering from hypothyroidism, were to marry, it is possible for their offspring to be mentally retarded children.

The risks involved in cases of epilepsy are well known and this is the reason why people suffering from *epilepsy* are advised not to have children. Laws prohibiting the marriage between close relatives have been created because the transmission of negative hereditary dispositions becomes stronger in proportion to the closeness of the blood ties between two people. Originally the hereditary taint was not present otherwise Adam's children could not have intermarried in order to fulfill the divine procreation mandate. The same holds true for Noah's descendents who, together with their wives, were the sole survivors of the deluge. They too would not have had the necessary positive genetic predispositions. With respect to disease, since no negative factors were present, intermarriage among close relatives did not create any problems.

Mature people, aware of their responsibilities toward their offspring, will not overlook the above mentioned precautions but rather give them due consideration, for only in this way they may be spared much possible suffering later on. They will be able to found a healthy family, thanks to their reasonable and sound attitude that will be reflected in strong healthy children which are certainly needed in our trying times today.

HARMLESS WEIGHT-REDUCING GUIDELINES

The great number of problems created by overweight are best known to those who are suffering from it. I read in a widely publicized scientific journal that any tendency toward corpulence is attributable to overeating. I, however, do not go along with this particular theory or the assumption of the doctor who wrote the article. It is true that overweight is often caused by improper diet or a diet that is too rich. The unfortunate consequences, in that case, have their origin in a too well developed appetite. But there are people who gain weight despite the fact that they eat very little. Unfortunately, these people cannot reduce their weight by simply cutting down on the amount of food they consume.

Disorders of the endocrine system:

The above mentioned situation is created through improperly functioning endocrine glands. I was able to observe in my office cases where the *gonads* as well as the *pituitary* gland and even the thyroid were accountable for problems of obesity. If such functional abnormalities have been existing since youth, the *gonad glands* are generally undeveloped, or at least inactive with no hormone production. Often, in such cases, fat is deposited on the hips and waist only and never on the extremities. In women the breasts show a considerable fat deposit instead of being made up of well developed milk producing glands. Sagging breasts are often an additional worry of overweight women. This problem could be related to a malfunction of the ovaries.

This type of obesity cannot be dealt with either by means of special diets or any other kind of treatment. It can be overcome only if the causes are being treated. This means a stimulation of the production of the *gonads*, the *thyroid* and the *pituitary*. When choosing remedies we will certainly want to turn to marine plants such as *Kelp* preparations which are of excellent value. *Bee pollen* will be of additional help since it is known to have stimulating effects. In order to take proper advantage of the various things available for our diet, we should drink plenty of *beet, carrot* and *celery* juices. Young stinging nettles or *horseradish* grated, should also be eaten daily. As a supplement to our diet, oysters, shrimp and octopus have great therapeutic value. Extracts from animal glands may be helpful but only if given in appropriate dosages, because they may otherwise do more harm than good. *Exercise, walking, hiking, jogging* and deep breathing, preferably in mountain or ocean air, are excellent for stimulating the glands.

Uncontrolled appetite:

Where the *appetite* is the cause of *obesity* it requires a different kind of attention. People, whose digestive functions work well or, whose body metabolizes food efficiently, have a tendency toward a ferocious appetite. In such cases it is best to apply the old and tested principle to *stop eating when the food tastes best.* A *diet* prescribed for this situation is one low in carbohydrates and fats and high in raw and fresh produce. The raw vegetables may be taken either as salad or as a juice.

For success it is most important to avoid all kinds of sweets and white flour products. Cream soups should be added to this list also. Since beer is one of the worst things an *obese* person can drink, this may be a real stumbling block for some men. If one is serious in his determination to reduce, he will make the effort to abstain from alcoholic beverages of all kinds. As regards meat, it should be limited to lean muscle fiber meat. Every opportunity should be taken to trim off excess fat and dispose of any animal fat that may be in the kitchen. One exception is fresh butter, which may be eaten in limited quantities. All kinds of cress, green leafy salad vegetables, horseradish, peppers (green), yeast extracts and vegetable broths can be eaten since they have a stimulating effect on the endocrine glands and assist the metabolic process.

Medications claiming to melt down fat are very dangerous and should be avoided at all costs, for one's health is more precious than a trim figure. On the other hand, preparations containing algae and cellulose, which expand in volume, may be tolerated for a short period of time. Unflavored gelatin in water, drunk a half hour before meals is said to expand in volume and thus shrink the appetite. These may be all right when the patient is excited about accelerating his weight loss but experience shows that he will grow tired of these remedies over a long period of time and will neglect them. The best weight reducing plan is one that utilizes *marine plants*, since they contain minerals in concentrated form and iodide of potassium. They not only stimulate the activity of the endocrine glands and consequently reduce weight but, what is more important, they positively influence the general state of well-being. People suffering from exophthalmic goiter are usually sensitive to iodine and must, therefore, take this medication only in homeopathic doses.

Kelp is known to be one of the richest of all the marine plants. It will suffice, therefore, if the person takes one or two Kelp preparation pills in the morning and at night, combining this with the diet mentioned previously and a steady reduction of weight will be noticed from month to month. A rapid loss is highly undesirable but a slow steady weight loss along with the supplementary medication will improve a person's sense of well-being and still leave enough energy to have a healthy enthusiasm toward work and everyday obligations. Many patients who have lost weight by taking *Kelp* can testify to this.

THE STOMACH

As with any other organ in our body, the stomach is a miracle of divine creation. The mucous lining of the stomach like all other mucous membranes consists of elastic rubber-like tissues. It has a connective tissue padding, permeated by a network of arteries, veins, lymphatic vessels and nerves. All of these minute vessels and nerve bundles taper off on the inside to very fine, microscopic end loops, surrounding the stomach glands. The inner lining of the stomach is not smooth, but rather rugate, the larger rugas or wrinkles being subdivided into smaller ones, giving the appearance of the structure of an auto radiator or, depending upon the type of modern heating unit you have, it appears in enlarged form of a rib structure. This rugate inner lining of the mucous membrane is covered with about five million tiny stomach glands. They secrete in precise amounts pepsin and the enzyme rennin (the gastric juice that coagulates and curdles milk and from which rennet is made) depending upon the particular requirements of the food that is eaten. A sufficient amount of hydrochloric acid has to be secreted because pepsin requires an acid complement for it to be effective.

HUNGER AND APPETITE

Whenever we are hungry or have a certain desire for a particular food, this natural body reaction stimulates the secretion of stomach juices. If, however, we eat without appetite, forcing ourselves to consume whatever is set before us, we will undoubtedly have problems with digestion, which in turn may lead to other complications. Of the two, natural hunger is more to be desired. This can be provided by working normally, getting plenty of fresh air and by not eating between meals. If your work is not located too far from home, walk instead of riding. If you have a jaded appetite try chewing on bitter herbs such as Centaury or take artichoke tincture.

Our emotional or mental state may stimulate or suppress our appetite. This explains why an emotional state strongly influences the flow of gastric secretions.

An example of how emotions govern gastric juice flow and the desire to eat or not to eat is easily explained. If you come home after a day at the office and learn that the dinner is not what you like, then your hunger will disappear. On the other hand if something has been prepared that is your favorite food, immediately your gastric juices begin to flow and you look with anticipation to sitting down to dinner because you are hungry. The frame of mind is important when eating. Happy people, who are always in a good mood, digest their food much better than those who are worried or upset. The process of digestion is not helped either, by sitting down at the table when plagued by problems or when aggravated by openly discussing and debating them. Meal-times should be a pleasant experience for the whole family and arguments never should be precipitated during the meal. When over-exhausted, it is wise to rest up, unwind, relax and contemplate for a little while before eating. The manner in which the food is prepared tends to make the meal more or less desirable. When prepared with love, a meal tends to taste better. By the same token, a nicely set table which does not show the haste of the daily routine, but which shows care and attentiveness most certainly promotes the desire to eat by stimulating the flow of gastric juices, encouraging digestion and the assimilation of food. It is not hard to understand that the atmosphere at the table likewise contributes to better digestion. Every meal should be a family feast of gratitude, where not only is the food enjoyed and appreciated, but also where stimulating conversation takes place.

Skillful *seasoning* of food is an art and likewise of great importance. This is not accomplished by using salt alone but by striving to get to know how many of the different kinds of *herbs* provide different taste sensations. Most *herbs* serve to stimulate the mucous lining of the stomach to increase its secretion and as a result, aid the digestive process. You will find too that different *herbs* complement different foods and bring out their flavor.

It is too bad that much of the pleasantness of eating is lost due to the hurry-up pace of life, TV-prepared dinners, which are filled with all kinds of imitation flavors, inhibitors, retardants to prevent spoilage, etc. and the individual eating habits of different members of the family who seldom find time to sit down together to a family meal. Is it any wonder that even young people are suffering from gastric ailments, indigestion and ulcers. Gastroenterology is one of the most successful specialty fields in medicine today because it seems as if every other person has a stomach problem!

Additional cause of stomach disorders:

Stomach problems, while not the number one illness, have been moving up the scale of disorders that are giving trouble to many people. In the U.S.A. this is especially the case, where people are in such a hurry all the time that they literally gulp down their meals, often not even taking time to sit down at a table because they do not want to lose time away from the office or their place of business. If one has acquired the habit of eating food too hot or swallowing it too rapidly, it should not come as a surprise when gastric problems surface. It is just as harmful to wind up a hot meal and rapidly cool off by eating ice cream without first letting it warm up in the mouth. Very cold food on top of very hot food is a sure way to stomach problems.

In cases where the mucous membranes are chronically irritated or inflamed, one need not be surprised if this condition eventually develops into *ulcers.* Undue emotional stress, nervousness and worries which lead to spasms are major causes of the formation of ulcers. Often I have watched ulcers disappear as soon as a patient had learned how to remain calm and collected.

Natural remedies made from Bismutin, Magnesium, Kalium phos. and other preparations, contribute greatly to a cure; and do not discount the importance of *raw carrot juice* in this treatment. Naturally, it is better to treat gastritis on time before it reaches the ulcerous stage. For this purpose St. John's wort oil is excellent when taken in the morning and at night, a teaspoonful each time. This simple, natural remedy has proven effective over a long period of years.

GASTRIC ACID

Gastric acid is a peculiar miracle, consisting of diluted hydrochloric acid which in some inexplainable way does not harm the mucous membranes or cells. The hydrochloric acid is formed from the chlorine of the saline solution circulating in the bloodstream. The healthy gastric mucous membranes are saved from self-digesting by anti-enzymes, which to this day have not been identified. If, however, the mucous lining has suffered some damage or a chronic infection gains hold, something drastic happens. The protection from the anti-enzymes is no longer fully effective and the gastric juices begin eating away the mucous lining with the result that *gastric ulcers* develop. When the concentrated acid gets to the ulcerous parts the so-called hunger pains set in.

As soon as some milk is taken or some dry rolled oats are chewed, the acid is neutralized and the pains temporarily subside. Even more effective is wood ash when scalded in boiling water. The filtered caustic solution is able to neutralize the acid because of its alkaline content. Ashes from birch tree have proven to be excellent.

Hydrochloric acid acts like a disinfectant and kills germs which cause fermentation and decay. When there is little hydrochloric acid present, fermentation begins sooner, accompanied by gas formation and bad breath. It is peculiar too that cancer of the stomach generally develops when insufficient amounts of hydrochloric acid are present. The reason for this has not yet been explained to anyone's satisfaction. It is obvious to everyone how difficult it is for man to find answers and explanations for that which we receive from the hands of the Divine Creator. It makes one think of the foolishness of even giving thought to the presumptuous ideas of the evolutionary theory. Since it requires such painstaking efforts to find clues to the disclosures of divine secrets, how then could we possibly believe that all these miraculous creations have come about through their own effort, with no direction from a Superior Being. Only a fool is capable of speaking the words: "There is no God."

It is possible to cure *stomach ulcers* with the help of raw potato or cabbage juices. Advantageous also is carrot juice which is nutritionally very effective and strengthening. Of course there are other useful medications such as Hamamelis, but it is unnecessary to reach for something expensive in the apothecary shop as long as there are products from gardens or supplies from the kitchen.

It is an undisputed fact that more men than women suffer from *gastric* or *duodenal ulcers*. The explanation for this may have its origin in the fact that women are seldom affected by anger and tension to the same degree as men. Emotional stress and anxiety are the main causes for the formation of gastric ulcers. Irritation of the stomach lining, especially when the condition persists or recurs often, may be responsible. Thus, it is important to isolate the causes for the irritation of the mucous membrane for only then can they be avoided. Do not eat exceedingly hot foods nor mix ice water with them. And remember that hot spices, alcoholic drinks and strong medications generally aggravate the condition rather than help it.

It is seldom that *ulcers* form at the entrance to the stomach, since they are much more frequent in the region of the stomach "exit," the "small curve." As mentioned before, the first symptom is that of an irritation of the gastric membrane. This irritation alone may have already caused some pain, but generally, it goes unnoticed and untreated. When hunger pains set in, which are so-called because they characteristically appear when the stomach is empty and disappear when some food is taken, the membrane is already affected and there is a strong possibility of an *ulcer* beginning. The stomach wall, thus no longer protected, is being eroded by the action of the gastric juices and it is this which makes the pain felt. Normally the walls of the stomach are saved from self-digestion by a protective enzyme. If the mucous membrane of the stomach is already damaged so that pain is felt, the patient need only take food and the distress is dramatically relieved because the gastric acid must now act on the food and is simultaneously absorbed by it.

If the pain sets in about one half hour after meals, this indicates that the ulcer is located in the duodenum, generally one half to two inches away from the stomach exit. A neglected ulcer, one that has not been treated, shows a crater-like formation. Even though the lining of the stomach becomes thicker, due to the ulceration, the ulcer may eventually penetrate it, creating a perforation which allows the chyme (a pulpy semi-liquid into which food is changed by action of the stomach) to get into the abdominal cavity. This triggers a very painful *peritonitis,* accompanied by vomiting and an increase in the pulse rate. The abdomen becomes swollen and tightly stretched like a board. The patient's life is in danger and he needs immediate expert medical attention and must be hospitalized without delay. Providing his overall health is good and he is being treated by a skillful surgeon, he may have a good chance to survive.

It is possible for *duodenal ulcers* to grow and eventually affect other organs. This endangers particularly the pancreas and even the liver and the intestines. Simple *gastric ulcers* are generally associated with a high acid content in the stomach, and the person may experience some belching or a sour tasting regurgitation. Improperly treated ulcers may turn into cancer, a condition much more difficult to detect, since it is not normally accompanied by pain and thus not often diagnosed until a later stage appears. Experience shows that a malignant ulcer is almost always associated with a lack of gastric acid, where as a simple ulcer thrives on a hyper-acid condition.

The treatment:

Fasting has proven to be excellent as a treatment for stomach ulcers provided that the body has stored up ample amounts of energy.

Raw *potato juice* can be recommended as a specific remedy and, taken regularly during the day, it has a marvelous curative effect. Raw *cabbage* juice, likewise, is excellent. If it is found difficult to drink these raw juices by themselves, they may be added to a minestrone or oatmeal soup. The soup should be cooked and allowed to cool a little before adding the juice.

Condensed *bilberry* and *licorice* juices have also been proven to be excellent. The thickened juices should be taken daily in doses of one-half to three-quarters of an ounce. Before swallowing they should be kept in the mouth for a minute or two to insure proper salivation which will hasten the curative effect.

The diet should exclude any spicy ingredients and any kind of roughage in order to prevent further irritation. Provided the overall condition is excellent, one or two days *fasting* per week will assure good results. The *diet* should be made up largely of milk, cottage cheese, cooked porridge and cereal soups. Even when a complete cure has been effected, and when the pains have totally subsided, it will be necessary to refrain from alcohol, nicotine, pork, luncheon meats, animal fats and strong spices for a long time. As a matter of fact, it would not be a bad idea to eliminate these items altogether from the diet. Doing this would certainly be a step in the right direction to the practicing of preventative care and, considering that there are many other palatable foods which are not harmful to the body, the sacrifice involved seems not too great.

Gastric ulcers are often the result of nervous tension. It is advisable, if good results are desired, to free oneself from worries und anxieties as quickly as possible. It is no longer a great big problem to get rid of *stomach ulcers* if the methods outlined above are carefully followed. Still, the best way to keep from getting ulcers is to avoid foods that may cause them and to train oneself to stop fretting and avoid worrying about things that may never happen or that are beyond one's control.

APPENDICITIS

Many people have a misconception with respect to the appendix, which refers to the first part of the large intestine, where the small intestine merges with it. It is the vermiform appendix which usually gets inflamed and requires surgical removal. The vermiform appendix is located exactly in the center between the navel and the right iliac bone, the most protruded structure of the pelvic bone. If we imagine for a moment, the face of a clock, with the navel forming the center, the appendix would be in the same position as the small hand when it is on eight o'clock.

Occasionally, an infection of the ovaries is mistaken for an attack of appendicitis. When the area of the appendix is depressed by the hand and suddenly released, the sensation of pain is radiated to the right, where in the case of ovarian inflammation, the pain would be local and of a dull nature. The inflammation may also be diagnosed through the rectum. *Appendicitis* generally makes itself known through severe, sudden pains in the lower right side of the abdomen, appearing without warning and usually being accompanied by nausea and vomiting. As a rule the tongue is coated and the patient runs a slight temperature. In case of doubt the physician may take a blood-test to determine whether the number of white blood cells has increased. Often the usual number of 6,000 to 9,000 has jumped to 15,000 and the pulse rate also climbs above 100.

Years ago the surgical removal of the vermiform appendix was considered hazardous, but today, with highly developed surgical technique it is a simple matter, free from complications. If difficulties are encountered this normally has nothing to do with the operation itself but may be caused by other existing circumstances. The risk of thrombosis or embolism is naturally higher in people who have varicose veins or who show tendencies toward venal congestions. This condition may be greatly reduced or even eliminated with help from simple, natural remedies. Echinacea extract preparation, taken before and after surgery decreases the susceptibility to infection and also supports and speeds up the healing process.

Danger of infection is much greater in tropical areas and if one intends to visit the tropics and is suffering from a chronically inflamed appendix, it should be removed before departure, a necessary precaution that will make the trip safer and more enjoyable.

A conservative treatment:

A conservative treatment of *appendicitis* stresses foremost, a liquid juice diet and bed rest. *Carrot, beet, bilberry* and *grape juices* are particularly recommended. The juice should be diluted with spring water by one to two parts. Sip the liquids slowly, allowing them to be well salivated before swallowing. Add to one tenth quart of the juice 10 to 20 drops of Echinacea extract preparation. The burning sensation can be relieved by using cold milk packs and nausea can be controlled with Nux vomica, taking 5 drops to a glass of water, also in small sips.

From the beginning it is very important to empty the bowels completely. This can be accomplished by taking a harmless laxative tea or herbal laxative. If the bowels fail to react quickly an enema is in order. Either camomile, savory or sanicle tea can be used, preferably with 20 drops of Echinacea purpurea added.

Although the appendix, as has been discovered recently, serves an important function and is not just an unnecessary appendage, yet generally speaking it is better to have it removed when inflammation occurs then to run the risk of a perforation and a resultant peritonitis. Surgeons who routinely remove an otherwise healthy appendix when performing an abdominal operation, however, are from nature's standpoint guilty of incomprehensible action. The body's every scar carries with it the possibility of later irritations and disturbances. Anyone who lives sensibly, keeps his bowels working well, and who makes sure that infectious diseases are well cured, will generally be able to keep his appendix throughout life without any danger of inflammation. It has been discovered that once the appendix has been removed the bowels are somewhat more sensitive. This indicates that an operation should be resorted to only when actually necessary. Even then a person should proceed with caution, looking for a competent and conscientious surgeon to be sure that the operation will be performed with utmost care. Second operations have at times been necessary when an instrument or a piece of gauze was left inside the patient. Such examples of carelessness can only occur when persons have not yet mastered their profession.

IS DIARRHEA HARMFUL?

About 50% of the population suffer to some degree from diarrhea, and this is especially true of women rather than men. We hear again and again that it is harmful to allow constipation to exist for any length of time and there are ample remedies available for its treatment. In comparison to this, only a few people suffer from diarrhea. We do not mean a quickly passing diarrhea, but rather a condition that prevents normal evacuation for long periods of time. Not much has been written about it, even though diarrhea of this kind is more harmful than constipation. In these modern times, where tour "packages" abound and more and more people travel to different parts of the earth, diarrhea has become more common. It appears that the main culprit is drinking water. Thus, the common tourist ailment in different countries is called by different names, as in Mexico, where it has been aptly named "Montezuma's revenge".

It can be harmful and oftentimes quite serious because it causes dehydration through loss of body fluids. Minerals that the body needs as well as the nutrients provided by food are washed away and replacements have little chance of remaining in the body until the condition is corrected. Most people are taken completely by surprise when diarrhea occurs and momentarily are caught off balance as to what remedy to pursue. Once it strikes, a *whey* dilution should be taken since germs or bacteria have difficulty surviving in an acid condition, which is what whey supplies. If diluted *whey* is not effective, decrease the dilution or try it without dilution. The main thing is to stop the action and *whey* is as good a remedy as any other medication.

The salivary glands:

If we are to understand diarrhea, we must familiarize ourselves with the secretion process of saliva and the functions and the duties of salivary glands. *Saliva* is a fluid that the salivary glands secrete or empty into the mouth to keep it moist, as an aid to chewing and to start the digestive process. The secretion is made up of enzymes and a variety of minerals, determined by the type of food eaten. Few people are aware of the fact that the different glands namely the salivary glands, the mucous membranes of the stomach, the glands of the liver and the pancreas, secrete several quarts of *saliva* per day. It is the function of the *saliva* to partially metabolize and start the digestion of the food so that the body is able to absorb it more readily. When they have completed their task, the large intestines take over, reabsorbing the valuable materials, making them again part of the body fluids.

In cases of diarrhea the valuable fluids are lost. The body is depleted of important minerals which cannot be replaced quickly enough through food intake. As a consequence the body is weakened and the equilibrium of the mineral metabolism becomes highly disturbed. A temporary attack of diarrhea does not mean a great amount of valuable fluid will be lost, but if the condition is allowed to exist for several months it could have dangerous consequences. For prolonged attacks, a liquid made from *potter's clay* will help to destroy the bacteria and toxins produced by this illness. *Yogurt* has also been established as a good counteracting agent and should be taken at the first sign of diarrhea.

Actually the correction of this condition depends foremost on a change of *diet*. Avoid all fruit, raw vegetables, sweets, cooked cabbage, and every other food that may cause fermentation and gas formation. Milk is recommended, unprocessed, if possible. The *diet* may include cottage cheese, any of the mild cheeses such as Emmental (Swiss) cheese, rolled oats, rye crisps, zwieback, potatoes boiled in their jackets and natural rice. Not everything is forbidden in fruits; apples, bananas and blueberries or bilberries have a constipating or healing effect. It is very important not to eat fruit and vegetables at the same meal, a precautionary measure, because it prevents fermentation. Make sure to chew well everything you eat, and salivate the food adequately before swallowing. A short fast is beneficial too because it gives the digestive tract a rest during which time the bacterial flora can be restored and regenerated.

One of the most important remedies, besides the ones that have already been considered, is a tincture prepared from the fresh plant tormentilla or blood-wort. It is most effective when taken in conjunction with the nerve-relaxing oat juice, Avena sativa, a combination referred to as Tormentavena. This combination can control even the most stubborn case of *diarrhea* within one or two days by taking 5 drops in a little water every hour and if possible, refrain from eating. This is a simple and completely harmless plant remedy and can be given even to infants. Other temporary relief may be obtained from raw oats, when these are well chewed without anything else added to them. Wood ashes or charcoal from lime wood have a beneficial therapeutic effect.

296

When diarrhea has been brought under control and even when it can be considered completely overcome, one should try to fortify the result. To complete the healing process a new bacterial flora of the intestine should be created. There are three remedies that will help bring this about: Acidophilus in powder form and two lactic acid preparations, a *whey* and biofermentation process. It generally takes a long time for the intestinal flora to be sufficiently strengthened so that the intestine may once again function normally without assistance. Careful attention and patience are the key to licking this problem.

CONSTIPATION

"Death resides in the intestines" says an old proverb, the warning and meaning of which we should carefully consider. It is an undisputed fact that constipation is the cause of many ailments. People who have been complaining about *headaches* for years never think that their discomfort could be caused by a transfer of accumulated metabolic poisons from the intestines to the bloodstream. *Stomach*, *liver* and *kidney* disorders may also stem from constipation or irregular intestinal activity. The same holds true for *skin eruptions*, *pimples* and various kinds of *eczema*. It may be even a case of where certain diseases or disorders do not respond to any kind of natural remedy until constipation, which again leads to renewed poisoning, is completely eradicated.

If the condition is allowed to go untreated, it may give rise to grave consequences. Malignant growth leading to intestinal obstruction may be the result of constipation that has been existing for as many as 20 or 30 years. An artificial exit of the colon is certainly not a desirable answer to the problem. Often we do not recognize the automatic devices that our body possesses until it is too late, at the moment when all these natural prerequisites fail to function properly. They should never be neglected and every consideration must be given to the natural law and its requirements. Even the most skillful surgical act is nothing but a makeshift solution, compared to the previously natural condition. Only someone who has had to put up with the burden of an artificial rectal opening is able to appreciate and comprehend the marvelous working of our sphincter (ring-like muscle that surround the opening and closing of the anus). Let us not take these things for granted and let them go so far as to neglect proper intestinal activity.

There are women who complain about having spent a small fortune for *laxatives*. This is not surprising when we consider the many overpriced chemical remedies sold over-the-counter, which at most offer temporary help. It takes more to fully cure the condition than just making it disappear for a few days. Just as a tree needs proper fertilizing and pruning in order to grow strong, the natural function of the human body needs to be supported instead of suppressed inadvertently. Man has the tendency to become too dependent on modern scientific research instead of heeding the advice of nature.

Many people on the face of the earth would not want to take any of the best artificial laxatives, even when offered to them free. Neither the Berber tribes in the Atlas mountains, nor the Incas in the Cordilleras, nor the Weden of northeast Ceylon as well as many other tribes would have any use for them. Why? Because their diet is usually high in fibrous material, which provides mechanical roughage for the intestine. They do not eat white bread and pastries made from bleached flours and refined sugar which all contribute to constipation.

To accurately judge the excellent working condition of the organs we must take into consideration how these people live close to nature and practicing a way of life that would never lead to ulcers. They actually practice nature's principles. On the other hand, we have come to accept our way of life, rushing here and there as the norm, and have come to feel that this is appropriate for this modern day. However, this is a misconception because the restlessness, anxiety, vexation, and continual rushing, is reflected in a contraction of our sympathetic nerves and as a result, it brings on spasmodic *constipation.* On top of that, if we take strong laxatives we are only "adding insult to injury" to our now oversensitive intestines.

We can profit from the experience of a farmer, who knows what to do when his livestock shows signs of improper intestinal activity. From linseed he will prepare a potion and feed it to the animals. This causes a mucilage formation in the intestines, which in turn relieves the problem. The same linseed, biologically prepared, can have the same effect on humans. Another very effective remedy is psyllium seeds or powder that can be taken in water as is. They do not have to be boiled as linseed does and are more palatable. If one does take linseed, it should be ground fresh each time as it goes rancid rather quickly. However, there are prepared linseed products on the market which are available if one does not want to bother preparing his own. The linseed preparation serves as an excellent stimulation to increase intestinal activity when it is taken together with Bircher Muesli and nuts. Most nuts, as a matter of fact, do help intestinal activity. One reason for this is that, many times, *constipation* is caused by malfunction of the liver which in turn influences the intestine. Even in severe cases of *constipation,* good results have been obtained by treatment with various liver preparations i.e. Rhizoma preparation, Chelidonium D-2, Concentrated Carrots, and the bile-liquifying Podophyllum D-3, D-4. Where constipation is caused by a malfunction of the liver, the above remedies will provide relief.

While nervous tension can cause *constipation,* diet is really more important. The farmer knows that he cannot keep his animals in the stable all the time; they need exercise and a change of diet from time to time. We can take a lesson from this and make sure we get enough exercise and pay attention to our choice of food and its variation. Avoid chocolate and sweets which can cause intestinal problems. Likewise, cheese,

cheese products, eggs and anything prepared with eggs, like cake, etc. should be avoided. Instead, eat plenty of carrots, raw sauerkraut, cole slaw and bitter salads such as dandelion greens, chickory and endive. To vary the diet eat soaked prunes and nuts together with a slice of whole wheat kernel bread. Add Bircher Muesli and ground linseed for an appetizing breakfast. During the berry season add fruits to the Muesli and top it off with *Yogurt* for a tasty and healthy dish. Carbohydrate producing foods and dough products made with bleached flour must be avoided. Natural brown rice on the other hand causes no complications. Potatoes constipate, so leave them off the menu. Observe proper eating habits, not gulping down your food, but masticating it well before swallowing. It is better to refrain from eating when in an aggravated state as this is a sure way to invite *constipation* and a badly upset stomach. Eat slowly and relax at the dinner table and you will enjoy a leisurely meal that leads to good digestion.

Hayflower hip-baths taken in the evening just before retiring will relax and act as a natural sedative. Relief may also be obtained from a special juice diet. This has a stimulating effect on the metabolism and thus increases the productivity of the kidneys, liver, intestine and pancreas. Hundreds of people have been able to overcome their constipation with help from a Rhizoma preparation which acts as a cleansing agent, regenerating the body fluids. Aside from the many excellent natural remedies available today, lasting results can still be obtained when the many mistakes in diet and the tension ridden way of life are avoided. If you get to the root of the problem and make those necessary changes you can lick the problem.

Starchy diet and constipation:

Many people suffering from *constipation* claim that a *diet* high in carbohydrates makes their condition worse. Looking at this argument closely, we are inclined to agree, for in such cases the pancreas produces an inadequate amount of starch-decomposing enzymes. Thus, it is positively true that starchy foods indeed lead to *constipation*. Potato starch is particularly bad; the eating of potatoes should therefore be restricted or eliminated altogether until the pancreas is functioning properly. Too many make the mistake of not paying enough attention to those foods which are known to cause problems. They have the mistaken belief that there must be some kind of miracle remedy that will do the job without any sacrifice on their part. But wouldn't it be wiser on our part to avoid all foods that could be responsible for the disorder instead of waiting until we have the problem and then depend on a remedy to overcome it?

In addition to potato starch, grain starch may also produce or further constipation. Bran content of whole cereal or bran by itself neutralizes the constipating effect. Rice starch is least constipating of all and it is easily digested and therefore recommended for children and infants. Since the usual kinds of white rice, long and short grain, are very low in mineral content, only unprocessed natural brown rice should be included in the diet. It can be very palatable when well prepared. Do not overcook or soak rice for long periods of time. It is best when still firm and in that form is most beneficial for digestion. Naturally, the cooking time will depend upon the type of rice. Some white rice is "precooked" and requires 8–10 minutes of simmering. On the other hand, natural *brown rice* requires cooking up to one hour before it is ready to serve. Rice gains good flavor when garlic, onions, chopped parsley and vegetable or chicken bouillon is used instead of water. In tropical countries coconut water is used instead of tap water and this produces a very nice flavor. Rice may also be prepared in the oven and sprinkled with grated cheese to which sliced tomatoes have been placed on top. When well prepared, natural rice is so palatable that even those who formerly did not like rice will find it an excellent dish. And it is very nourishing. Since we eat with our eyes, if one has been accustomed to eating the white, fluffy kind of rice, it will take a little adjustment to become accustomed to the darker colored natural brown rice, but you will be glad you changed after a very short time.

Important points to be considered:

Another advantage of *brown rice* is its therapeutic effect on the body. It is so nourishing that it can sustain one over a long period of time. It is filling too, so that even a small quantity is satisfying. This is good for the pancreas, an organ often weakened by eating too large quantities of food. If one sticks to a natural diet, chews well, eats slowly and salivates the food before swallowing, the pancreas is being paid a service, and excellent intestinal activity is assured. Often small mistakes in eating habits can rob us of the vital elements so necessary for good digestion. Thus, by limiting starchy foods we can supplement the diet with vegetables and salads and sesame seeds. Proper caution and selection of diet pay off.

DYSBACTERIA

Much is being written about the principles of proper modern nutrition today. Whole grain products, wild or brown rice, wheat germ, natural honey, buttermilk, yogurt, curds, cottage cheese and vegetable oils, high in polyunsaturated fats, are being recommended as nutritionally sound food, and rightly so.

But it is of interest to note that in a family of five, all eating the same healthy natural food products, not every member benefits to the same degree. One member of the family may be strong, healthy and in good physical shape whereas another may be skinny and weak, and a third member could be anemic and pale. This leads us to the conclusion that not always can sound nutritional principles be equated with the intake of good food of high mineral and vitamin value. But the important thing is: is the body absorbing and assimilating these vital elements?

Dysbacteria is one of the modern illnesses responsible for loss of energy in thousands of people. Some degenerate totally without knowing what is the matter with them. The main cause for this illness is drug medication. Two modern groups, sulfonamides and antibiotics are responsible. To counteract this it is suggested that the patient be given a preparation made from Cynaram polygonum and Boldo and other plant extracts which liquify the bile. To successfully combat dysbacteria he must take *whey* concentrate as well.

Another preparation made from lactic acid, *yogurt* and *acidophilus* bacteria has proven to be one of the most effective and harmless remedies against dysbacteria. Taken in conjunction with whey concentrate its effectiveness has been greatly increased. A few days after taking it, normal appetite will return and the intestine will begin to function properly again. The patient too feels a lot better and notices a definite improvement in his body due to returning energy and strength.

As soon as the intestinal bacteria have recovered, assimilation of food improves and in turn, causes the terrible fatigue to disappear. The body is once again being properly nourished. To add to the energy, the person will profit by a juice diet extending over two or three days. Carrot, beet, celery and tomato juices can be recommended. There are some on the market that are made by the process of lactic acid fermentation and these are excellent. For the duration of the fast the juices should be diluted with water or mildly carbonated mineral water. To avoid hunger pains, a little rye crisp can be eaten.

I have often recommended a weekly "juice-day" because of its excellent effect on the general health. This provides an opportunity for the digestive organs to rest, which results in a better absorption of food. Thus, the amount of food eaten is not important; what is important is that it is well assimilated and fully utilized.

INTESTINAL PARASITES

When grandmother in olden times took a look at her grand-children and concluded from the symptoms she saw that they were suffering from *worms*, she was usually right. There would be shadows under the eyes, itching of the nose, nervous behavior, lack of interest in playthings and restless turning back and forth in bed at night. She used to give them tansy or wormwood tea. When the small thread-like worms became visible in their stool, then grandmother would make the children drink milk to which crushed garlic had been added. Even though the children hated to take this concoction, it was usually effective and if the results were not totally satisfying, the garlic milk was also used as an enema. Thanks to their close attention, under close supervision the children were rid of their worms in short order, and it was a good thing too because these worms can damage a child's organism severely.

The same precaution grandmother used should be followed today. These tried and effective remedies have never been replaced by drugs, and garlic is still one of the most effective means of removing *worms*. Any child who is pale, tired all the time, and moody should be carefully examined. A neglected condition can have serious consequences on the normal growth as well as the emotions of the child and prompt attention is needed to restore the body to a natural healthy condition.

OXYURIA VERMICULARIS AND ASCARIS LUMBRICOIDES

Worms should never be considered harmless or their existence accepted as a necessary evil. Although in most cases we are dealing only with pin or round worms, these *intestinal parasites* can be quite harmful to our health. Oxyuria, the little pinworms, are often the cause of much discomfort. Both these as well as ascaris, the round worms, secrete poisonous metabolic substances which are absorbed by the body. This causes a change in the blood picture and the overall feeling of the person is negatively influenced. Unfortunately children with calcium deficiency are especially prone to helminthiasis (infestation), which constitutes a double burden for them since their power of resistance is already lowered and the damage is thus magnified.

The ascaris lumbricoides, the earthworm-like round worm, attaining a length of 10 to 17 inches has, in addition to its poisonous metabolic secretions, other detrimental effects. The eggs which are transmitted from vegetables that have been fertilized with cesspool manure, develop into small larvae, which penetrate the intestinal wall and are carried into the lungs where they settle and develop further. The patient may appear to be suffering from an obstinate case of bronchitis. From the lungs the worms work their tract, from which their eggs emerge in about 70 to 75 days after the initial infection takes place.

But the journey of these worms has not yet ended. When fully developed, not only are they found in the intestines, but sometimes in the nose and mouth, much to the horror of the victim. At other times they may bore their way into the bile ducts, causing jaundice. Or they may bore through the intestinal wall, which can precipitate peritonitis. Their number may rise to several hundreds and they actually are capable of blocking the intestinal canal, which could be fatal. I could go on enumerating the many dangers to which worms can expose us, but perhaps this will suffice to convince us that worms are not a harmless matter, but worthy of attention.

The eradication of oxyuria vermicularis and ascaris lumbricoides can be greatly facilitated with help from *papaya* preparations. They are made in granules, derived from the most effective parts of the tropical bush plant Carica-papaya, and actually digest the worms in the intestine. The *papaya* plant is a tree-like bush with large leaves similar to the fig tree, but much larger. The fruit is the size of a melon and it contains enzymes. But it is from other parts of the plant that the preparation is made that destroys the worms.

Although ordinary worms treatments can sometimes have ill effects, the papaya preparation treatment is quite different. While it is completely effective it is quite harmless to the body. Whereas other modern worm medicines kill the worms by poisoning them, leaving the body to dispose of them, papaya is based on a different principle. It does not poison, but the simple enzyme it contains, a protein decomposing substance, attacks the worms and digests them in the intestine.

It is important to maintain a diet low in proteins while undergoing the *papaya* treatment, otherwise the proteins from meat and eggs use the worm killing enzyme for their own digestion and it will no longer be available for its intended purpose.

Sometimes it is felt that worm remedies are ineffective, because after a short time, the little parasites may be noticed again. This does not mean that the remedy is necessarily at fault, because it is possible that a new infection has been contracted through negligence. This happens during the night, when the little worms leave the body in the warmth of the bed and desposit their eggs in the minute skin folds near the anus. This causes itching and naturally one begins to scratch and thus the eggs get under the finger nails. Since children have the habit of putting their fingers in their mouth, these eggs are transferred back again into the digestive tract. It is also possible that the microscopic eggs are shaken from the sheets when the bed is made, dispersing the eggs into the air, from which they are inhaled together with the dust from the room.

Cleanliness cannot be overemphasized. The room should be dusted daily with a damp cloth. It is also indispensable to change the linens frequently. Tight fitting panties should be worn under the night gown or pajamas to avoid involuntary scratching. Fortunately not everyone succumbs to this infection because the natural resistance of the body and good digestion do not permit them to develop in the first place.

THE TAPEWORM

Tapeworms are more dangerous than the small ones that were just discussed. The tapeworm is extremely stubborn and difficult to get rid of because of the barbed hooks on its head by which it attaches itself to the intestinal wall. When small pieces one quarter to one third of an inch wide and four to eight inches long are found in the stool, this does not mean the body is getting rid of it. Rather, these are egg containing reproductive parts, cast off by the full grown worm. Even though the tapeworm casts off parts from the end of its body, it does not get any shorter because it continues to grow at the other end where the individual body parts begin. Such a tapeworm can produce hundreds of thousands of eggs which eventually find their way into the cesspool. This is why it is so dangerous to fertilize the vegetable garden with cesspool manure. The worms may be spattered up from the ground onto the vegetables in a heavy rain and thus provide a source for a new infection. The same goes for fertilizing the pasture where sheep and cows graze as they stand a good chance of becoming contaminated.

There are various kinds of tapeworms. When eating meat that has been inadequately cooked, it is possible to become infected with the so-called bladder worm of either the beef, pork or fish type. These bladder worms then develop into tapeworms in the human body.

Even more dangerous than the cattle or fish worm is the dog tapeworm or tenia echinococcus. It is only about one quarter of an inch long but the size has no relationship to its hazardness, for this little worm is capable of causing greater damage than the larger cattle worm. Although known as the dog tapeworm, sheep, goats, pigs and even cattle have been known to become infested with it. When this happens, blisters the size of a walnut form in the lungs of cattle, and in the case of swine, these formations are found in the liver.

As reported to the Swiss Information Service to Physicians in 1963, 508 cattle and 62 swine were infested with the tapeworm, and this was a potential danger because it can spread. As far as domestic animals are concerned, extreme precautions need to be taken especially with dogs and cats. Adults who are generally meticulously clean, often are offended when reminded to take precautions when handling domestic animals. Often they think nothing of patting their animals while eating. Also, many think it is a show of affection when a dog or cat licks the hand or the face, but there is a danger attached to it. Young animals should be trained with this danger in mind. To minimize risk it is better to abstain from feeding raw lungs or liver to dogs.

Since field mice can be infected from the feces of dogs, it can then be transmitted to people from the cat that catches the mice. The larvae of the dog tapeworm can cause small blister-like swelling in the human liver which can be quite dangerous since worm medication is only effective in the intestines and not in the liver.

A further danger lies in the fact that the eggs can develop into minute grubs in the intestines, bore through the intestinal wall and then be carried by the bloodstream to various parts of the body, where they form cysts varying in size. This can be fatal. Thus, when playing with domestic animals, exercise due precaution because the pleasure of fondling them may turn to regret later on. If you must play with them, be sure to wash your hands thoroughly before eating anything.

Because international travel has become a way of life today another danger presents itself. In our travels we come into contact with many strange people and their animals. This is an area in which there is always a possibility of risking infection through the transmission of eggs and parasites. This danger, always present, should make us more aware of the need for meticulous cleanliness and hygiene.

Instructions for the *diet* and recommended treatment are as follows: A meatless diet, plenty of vegetables, raw carrots and fruits. No potatoes, no bread, and nothing made of flour. For lunch: Lentils, carrots, onion and garlic, all cooked together in one pot and seasoned with fresh horseradish. Twice a day a small dish of raw sauerkraut and in the morning, a handful of peeled pumpkin seeds and two tablespoons of unsweetened cranberries, chewed well. Follow this up an hour later with 1–2 cups of tapeworm tea without sugar. During the day sip a glass of garlic milk.

Recipe for tapeworm tea: $1/6$ oz. powdered Aloes, $2/3$ oz. Black Adler bark, $2/3$ oz. Senna leaves, 1 oz. Valerian root and slightly more than 1 oz. of Peppermint leaves. Mix them altogether and make an infusion. Use 1 tablespoon for every cup of boiling water. Do not cook. Another more radical method that can be used as a treatment is Kamala powder. It is to be used only in stubborn cases. Use one teaspoonful 3 times a day.

While taking the treatment it is important to maintain a normal bowel elimination without using a laxative. Concentrated carrot juice is very effective as is also the papaya preparation. When examining the stool make sure that the body as well as the head of the worm is expelled. If the head remains, the treatment will have to be repeated within two or three weeks' time. The first day of treatment should produce results but if not, continue for another day.

In case there is no response to any kind of treatment, there is a remedy that has been successfully used in Africa. This is the root of the pomegranate tree. One teaspoon of this root in pulverized form should be taken every morning and evening; or a tea can be made by boiling the root and two cups should be taken daily.

DANGERS OF THE TROPICS

For many people who visit the tropics, wild game seems to be the only thing that should be feared. However, there are other threats even more perilous and these stem from a variety of minute living creatures. The microscopic creatures constitute a far greater danger to health than all the creatures of the forests and rivers of the tropics. One of the most dreaded of all tropical diseases for travelers or tourists is amoebic dysentery, a persistent and sometimes fatal disease which resists all but the most energetic treatment. Not only is this disease contracted in the tropics but is an ever present danger in the subtropics as well. Thus Italy, Greece, the Middle East, Mexico and many of the sub-tropical islands of the earth are fertile fields for this disease. Ever present is also the danger of *elephantiasis*, a disease in which parts of the body, particularly the legs, become greatly enlarged due to parasitic worms that block the flow of the lymph. Other fatal diseases are spread through mosquitoes, the most well-known being *malaria*, characterized by chills followed by sweating and fever. No doubt one of the most dreaded tropical diseases is *sleeping sickness*, spread by the bite of the tsetse fly. In addition to those mentioned, add *psittacosis*, a contagious disease of parrots and other birds which is spread to humans and is characterized by diarrhea and high fever. It is highly communicable.

Precautionary measures:

Below are several points that everyone should bear in mind when traveling in the tropics:

1. Raw meat should never be eaten. Meat roasted on the outside but still rare on the inside must also be avoided. The same applies to raw fish of any kind. In the Far East raw fish prepared by a process of fermentation results in a very palatable dish and is prized by many as a delicacy. Nevertheless, for the tourist it can be very dangerous and should not be consumed.

2. Vegetables should never be eaten raw. Salads of any kind must be totally eliminated from the menu when traveling in the tropics. If they are grown in the garden of a friend where one can be sure the vegetables were raised under sanitary conditions, possibly one can take a chance, but to be on the safe side, it is inadvisable. Vegetables may be washed in a solution of potassium permanganate, but this does not provide 100% protection either.

3. Fruits, which cannot be peeled, must not be eaten. It may be difficult to resist the temptation to eat luscious strawberries or cherries in January in certain tropical regions south of the equator, but it is not worth taking the risk of exposing one's self to the great danger of possible infection. Even though some fruit may be peeled, there is always the chance that your hands may transfer the bacteria from the skin of the fruit to its fleshy part which would have the same effect of eating it with the skin on.

4. All drinking water must be boiled before drinking it. Drinking water in a restaurant is unsafe as is also any bottled soft drink to which ice has been added. However, it is possible to drink coconut water which is healthy and delicious, drunk directly from the coconut itself. Palm water, which is contained in the marrow of the palm tree in the jungle, is also pure and safe. Even for those who refrain from alcoholic drinks, it would be better to quench the thirst with beer rather than run the risk of drinking contaminated water which could lead to one of the dangerous tropical diseases. Be cautious at all times, and when in doubt, don't take a chance. It can take a long time to cure any of the tropical diseases because some can be fatal.

5. Walking barefoot, although a pleasant and happy habit in temperate zones, is very dangerous in the tropics. Avoid it. Various parasitic larvae may penetrate the skin of the foot and travel via the lymphatics and the bloodstream to various parts of the body where great harm can be done. If you are a nature lover, who cannot resist the impulse of walking barefoot, make sure you do so only on beaches where the sand has been cleansed by the ocean tides. Even the sand dunes further back from the ocean and, which are not in direct contact with sea water are an ever present danger and should be avoided. In tropical and subtropical regions the sand further back is often contaminated with excrement from birds, releasing hundreds of thousands of parasites that can be easily transferred to the foot while walking on the dunes.

6. Shaking hands as a form of greeting is not recommended in these areas either. A simple bow or nodding of the head is much safer, since it excludes any possible transmission of parasites. There is no guarantee that the native shaking your hand did not scratch himself five minutes before, and is sheltering several thousand parasites under his fingernails. If you must shake hands, wash them thoroughly as soon as possible afterwards.

7. If you are on a safari or just hiking overnight it is advisable to take along a mosquito net at all times in hot, humid, tropical regions. A net is an excellent protection and prevention from insect bites that could result in malaria, sleeping sickness, elephantiasis, and many other tropical diseases.

Many an enthusiastic traveler may find the joys and expectations that he is looking forward to dampened, if not spoiled, by so many precautionary measures. However, it is better to take a sensible and precautionary approach and, thus being forewarned, one can guard against any perilous circumstances. Among my closest friends I can count many who have had to pay dearly for their inexperience and ignorance of the hidden dangers encountered when traveling in the tropics. Some, who have lived in the tropics for extended periods, have returned home with grave diseases that have permanently damaged their health or have resulted in their premature death.

The precautionary measures mentioned previously are not meant to spoil one's expectations and joys of traveling, but rather they should serve as warnings and guidelines to help a person undertake a trip by being adequately prepared. Preparation does not mean heavy and cumbersome equipment added to the weight of your already heavy baggage. No, it is only a question of some valuable advice which should be stored in your memory so that you can draw upon it, should the need ever arise. The old adage "an ounce of prevention is worth a pound of cure" is more simple to follow than being compelled to search for remedial measures after a disease has caught up with you.

THE LIVER –
CAUSES AND SYMPTOMS OF DISORDER

It should become more and more apparent that the liver is one of our most important organs and needs to be kept functioning properly. Since the liver does not send out an alarm until a disorder has made considerable progress, it is to our advantage to be especially aware of certain symptoms which can serve as early warnings. If we recognize the symptom in its early stages, we will be in a good position to take precautionary measures to overcome the problem long before it reaches serious proportions.

A pure unadulterated diet of natural foods contributes to maintaining a healthy liver. Where this diet has been substituted for modern prepared foods, the liver suffers. Almost fifty percent of the people living in Switzerland are ill, because they are overfed with rich foods that they crave to satisfy their palate. Overindulgence is largely responsible for these disorders in our "civilized" society, whereas the opposite is true in the Far East where malnutrition is the cause of liver ailments. It is astonishing to find that even in countries where rice is grown and is the staple food, only white rice appears on the market. The only exceptions are in rural areas where the farmers prepare their own natural rice.

Most people are totally ignorant of the nutrional value of rice and of the many benefits which it offers in its natural state.

If certain existing eating habits in Japan, Korea and China were not adhered to, the resulting deficiency of elements would be disastrous. One habit contributing to good health is the eating in abundance of the marine plant known as sea weed or *kelp* as part of their daily meals. This plant is so rich in many minerals the body requires that it counterbalances whatever existing deficiency might exist. The only elements not storeable are calcium and fluoride. A deficiency of the two minerals particularly affects the teeth and this accounts for the widespread tooth decay among so many people. It is usually in rural or primitive areas that natives retain their teeth throughout a lifetime. Among the isolated islands, the natives of the Fiji Islands still have the most beautiful and remarkable teeth.

Sometimes the liver actually goes on strike even though we are applying the basic principles of nutrition or observing an occasional day of fasting. This can happen if we are subjected to constant worries, despair and annoyances. Living in tension and fear aggravates the problem too. In this case, a sensible approach to nutrition pays off only if we have a proper emotional disposition to go with it. Granted, it is not always easy to remain calm and collected in our modern, confused times, where so many things seem to go wrong. Thus we have to stop every once in a while and take stock of ourselves and contemplate on the best avenues open to us. Keeping cool emotionally may be the best service we could offer to our liver. Thus we have to couple a sensible diet with emotional control, a philosophy that governs sound health principles, if we want to keep our bodies and minds at their peak.

The question of fat:

Without question the enemy of the liver is *fat,* especially animal fat. However, one cannot avoid totally all fat since the liver needs some unsaturated fatty acids to function properly. It is therefore important not to use any fat in which the unsaturated fatty acids have been destroyed. Heated fat should be avoided. This automatically would eliminate fried foods.

These few basic rules make up a liver *diet.* Abstain from butter, onions and meats prepared by frying in fat, as well as French fried potatoes. As a matter of fact, any kind of processing requiring frying or baking in fat must be eliminated. Natural oils such as sunflower, sesame, linseed or any other cold pressed oils may be used in limited quantities in the preparation of salads, because, strangely enough, a moderate amount of these natural unadulterated oil is actually beneficial

314

for the liver. This does not mean that a healthy person must be more careful than a sick one, but it certainly would do no harm to heed the advice on oils. A little less fat would mean a lesser burden for our bodies, although this fact may be disputed by some cooks who adhere to the old idea that it takes a large amount of fat to keep a person healthy. This idea is untrue because the body benefits more from a limited intake of fat, since it is able to produce its own fat. People, who become obese despite the fact that they consume very little fat, confirm the above assumption. However, drinking too much beer will have a tendency to increase weight. The malt supplies the carbohydrates which in turn produce unwanted fat deposits. The majority of well-fed or over-fed people actually need much less fat than they consume. They could reduce their fat consumption by half and still be well nourished. This action would not constitute a deficiency of any kind nor would it lead to ill health. On the contrary, it would increase the chances of maintaining good health; it is an excessive amount of fat that is responsible for ill health.

The protein problem:

Once we have learned how to handle the fat problem, we should take a closer look at the question of *proteins* for the simple reason that our liver needs a good protein supply for maximum efficiency. Legumes, that is peas, beans and lentils, as well as milk, are excellent suppliers of protein. Not only the liver but the whole person benefits from natural protein, and a special source we might look to is sour milk, curds, cottage cheese and *yogurt*.

If a patient suffering from liver problems desires a meat protein, the meat should be broiled, never fried. Avoid fatty meats. Very lean, muscular meat, preferably beef or veal, is best for those who cannot do without it. Since pork is the most harmful of all meats, it should be eliminated from the diet. Among the Judaic laws of the Old Testament was one which forbade the Jews to eat pork of any kind and, as it so happened, this abstinence proved to be in the interest of their health. Neither was the Jew allowed to breed pigs, which is still the case today. But a few are clever enough to get around it by paying the Arabs to raise the pigs for them. But word of these hypocritical and secret methods get around, otherwise we would not have heard about it on our last trip to Israel. It is amazing how easy it is for a man to deceive himself, and it is certainly a misconception to believe that the circumvention of the law is accomplished with less difficulties when done secretly than if it were done publicly.

Fish protein is a food that should not be overlooked. It is important that only fresh fish is used and its preparation requires the utmost care. If fish is slightly tainted the danger of poisoning is very high, and if not carefully cleaned, there is the additional danger of poisoning. The eating of fish always presents certain risks especially with scavenger type fish that consume anything they come upon. *Fish* should be either broiled or boiled in water to which a little vinegar has been added.

The *egg* also is a good source of protein and many people make use of this valuable source. Hardboiled eggs, omelets and egg salads should be avoided by anyone with a liver problem; indeed, in this case, meat would be a better substitute for eggs. It is important to make sure that the eggs which we consume come from healthy chickens raised on natural feed. When eaten raw, or soft boiled (2–3 minutes), in its liquid stage an egg is considered a valuable source of nutrients. Eggs are harmful though, for anyone suffering from rheumatism or arthritis and should not be eaten in any form. In this case one can eat legumes or other high protein vegetables.

It is a good thing that there are other, more advantageous protein sources than eggs. The soybean, for example, is an excellent supplier of vegetable protein. In certain areas of China soybean protein is the single most important protein available to its inhabitants. The lack of milk protein and fish protein in many tropical regions is very critical. The need for protein presents a particular problem for the Chinese. Since meat is not produced in sufficient quantity to supply over 800 million people, it became necessary to find a substitute for meat and the soybean was selected because it is an excellent source of protein, and has taken the place of animal as the prime supplier. In many parts of the world today the Chinese custom to germinate the soybean has been followed and the resulting product bean sprouts has become a very palatable vegetable dish when mixed in a salad or cooked in a mixture of other vegetables.

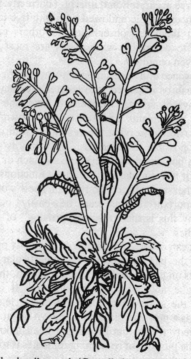

Shepherd's pouch (Capsella bursa pastoris)

A SELECTION
FROM THE PLANT KINGDOM

An assessment of therapeutic effects

Only a limited number of herbs are considered in the following pages since the extensive domain of the plant world demands far greater attention than can be given in this limited space.

To establish the actions or effects of a plant or any other natural medicine, one must first of all possess the gift of being able to observe accurately and interpret correctly. In every age there have been people endowed with intuitive insight which has enabled them, by observation of others and personal experience, to determine what plants are most suitable for healing a given condition.

For observance and experimental work, the effect of various substances can be observed with greater accuracy after a two or three days of fasting. Needless to say, one would only experiment with plants and substances known to be non-poisonous. After observing the reactions from one or more plants, it is possible to judge its relative merits – how it has affected the bowels, the kidneys, the stomach or the appetite or whether it has stimulated the various functions of the body in some other way. If the body is in good working order, certain important effects can be easily perceived. In Homeopathy this is the so-called "proving" of remedies on healthy bodies.

A doctor can observe the effects of a remedy on the patient himself. If the patient reports that a particular remedy has other effects on him than those already known, the doctor will naturally take note of such observations. If other people experience the same effect, then the doctor learns that this medicine has a new and hitherto unknown effect. In this way, a new remedy which, until then had been unknown, is discovered. The purpose of combining remedies is to enhance the effect of one through the addition of another.

Combinations:

If there is a calcium deficiency to be overcome, it is necessary to make sure there is not an underlying Silica deficiency at the same time. Or suppose you want to get rid of night sweating and at the same time dispose of a bad *cough*; for the first, Sage (Salvia off.) would be considered and for the second, either pine bud or plantain (Plantago lanc.) extract would be the accepted remedy.

In order to cure different illnesses, the doctor can choose from a suitable combination of remedies. He must, however, be careful that the remedies are complimentary to each other, for there are some that vitalize the body while there are others that debilitate it or have the opposite effect. In former times, when physicians were not so well informed as they are today, they discovered remedies by accurate observation and careful comparison of their findings. However, usually a knowledge of pharmacology is required to be able to choose and combine remedies correctly. Some combined remedies produced excellent results and their use was continued. However, if it was found that the combined remedies did not complement or harmonize one another, and the effect produced was negative, then this was noted and the remedy discarded. The importance of combining different substances is illustrated in the case of vitamins. Research has shown that some combinations are essential if they are to produce results. For example, an easily assimilated *calcium* preparation is not necessarily absorbed into the system, if there is a deficiency of *Vitamin D*, while the latter cannot benefit one if there is a deficiency of calcium. Thus, one complements the other and together in combination they are beneficial and accomplish their work.

In the body we find the same interdependence of functions. The hydrochloric acid and the digestive ferment, pepsin, work in close association with each other in the stomach. *Pepsin* can break down the food proteins only if the gastric environment is kept acid through the presence of hydrochloric acid. There are many associations like these and if we are to find and produce remedies to fulfill their purpose, we must know of them.

It is, therefore, by no means permissible to combine any kind of herb or extract with another in the happy expectation that eventually one may be lucky and come upon something outstanding. There are herbs and other natural remedies, the components of which, when combined, can deteriorate rather than benefit the system. To ascertain the overall effects and to be able to combine them correctly requires not only very accurate observation but also a certain amount of intuition that comes from experience and training. One cannot always go by the material components, for there are many substances and factors which are yet unknown and undiscovered but nevertheless play a part in the total effect. Thus, it is necessary to reckon with unknown as well as known factors.

There are combinations of remedies that have come down to us from the Middle Ages. Some of them are used as effectively today as they were then, and this is undoubtedly because of their wealth of vitamins and certain ferments. Even though in the beginning, knowledge of such factors did not exist at the time these remedies were originated, nevertheless the skilled observers of that time became aware of their effects and a new remedy was born and employed regularly afterwards. Practical experience in such circumstances is just as valuable, if not more so, than chemical knowledge.

Unknown factors:

Very often a certain substance, such as an alkaloid, is held responsible for the effect produced by a plant. If you extract this alkaloid and administer it, the symptomatic effects will be the same, but the aftereffects will probably be different. The chemist is unable to explain this, because his analytical procedures are not refined to the point where he can pin-point those substances which are commonly termed "unknown" factors and which are responsible for the total effect produced by the plant. It is therefore necessary that all natural remedies be taken as an organic whole, in the same form as nature produces them. To consider in a herbal preparation merely the so-called "active principle" shows a superficial understanding of the subject. For example, if we extract arnicin from Arnica plant, it will never have the same effect on the heart and blood vessels as the extract that has been obtained from the whole Arnica root. The same applies to carrot juice. By using just the pure carotin as a vitamin, the same effect cannot be obtained as it would be by using the ordinary juice of the carrot.

The lactic acid of the Sauerkraut also differs in its action from the pure product, because the former is associated with other substances in the Sauerkraut which possess their own curative properties. Unsophisticated nature is, as all examples prove, the most sophisticated source of our remedies. Nature is and will remain the best and most reliable pharmacy to fill our prescriptional requirements. Any researcher gifted with an awareness of her pattern will not be disappointed in his search for truth. All he has to do is unlock her doors and the answer will be promptly found.

Wild Leek (Allium ursinum)

This outstanding herb has been wrongfully neglected for a long time and in quite a few herbal remedies it has not even been mentioned. *Wild leek* has also been called Wild Garlic on account of its similar smell. The leaves, which look like Lily of the Valley, are used medicinally and as both plants grow in the shade of the forest, one is often mistaken for the other.

The *wild leek* usually grows on damp but, nevertheless, healthy ground and it grows so plentifully along the sides of streams and brooks that it could be actually scythed. The considerable sulphur content of this plant acts on the skin, the bones and the bronchial tubes, especially when there is an abundant secretion of mucus from the latter.

Intestinal *flatulence*, with a burning sensation in the abdomen and an irritation of the bladder, with a strong urge to urinate, will considerably benefit from wild leek. So too, will repeatedly occurring intestinal catarrhs, when the mucous membranes of the stomach and intestines have become very sensitive.

Best of all, however, is the effect that *wild leek* has on hardening of the arteries and in this respect it can lengthen considerably the lives of older people. Wild leek juice or wild leek wine can act to prevent a stroke, and if a person has had one, this simple plant can restore him to health better than some of the most expensive drug medicines. Elderly people, who have *high blood pressure* and are in danger of a stroke, can ward it off with four plant remedies:

1. *Wild Leek* (Allium ursinum)
2. *Mistletoe* (Viscum album)
3. *Hawthorn* (Crataegus oxyacantha)
4. *Arnica* (Arnica montana)

Why risk the danger of paralysis when there are such simple natural remedies which will prevent a stroke and at the same time, strengthen the heart and the system of blood vessels and give new life to the body.

Wild leek may be eaten fresh and uncooked as a salad or in a salad with other vegetables with excellent results. Steamed, it becomes a spinach-like vegetable and, although not as good as the raw vegetable, it is still better than ordinary vegetables. Taken as a wine or extract in the form of drops, it has more often than not proved its worth. If you do not wish to gather it yourself, you can make good use of the extract in which the full goodness of the plant is preserved.

NETTLES (Urtica urens)

When the snow has completely gone and the warm spring wind once more thaws the ground, life once more begins to stir in Mother Nature's womb. On sunny slopes, steep paths and even on rubbish heaps, the green, finely serrated leaves of the nettle appear. Hardly anyone notices it, but quietly it grows while using its juices to prepare a medicine that can bring health to many, and indeed, save lives of those who know about it. Many a sufferer of *tuberculosis* would not have died had he but gone out of his way a little to gather nettles and avail himself of their help. By means of its healing properties, how many children might have had their lymph glands restored to normalcy. Much hard earned money would not clink, all to no purpose, into the pharmacist's till, if young nettles were used as a restorative. No other plant can equal the nettle in cases of *Anemia, Chlorosis, Rickets, Scrofula, respiratory diseases* and especially *lymphatic problems.*

It is most appropriate that nature has given this plant the protection of a stinging exterior. Without it, we would probably never have the opportunity to avail ourselves of its healing power. Animals, with their instinctive knowledge of what is beneficial for them, would not leave any for us were it not for the plant's protective sting.

The *stinging nettle* contains an abundance of calcium, phosphorus, iron and many other important minerals. It also belongs to those rare plants that contain Vitamin D. We already know that this vitamin is important in the development of the bones as well as for the assimilation of calcium. Eating raw nettles, either as a juice or pulped, has a quick and reliable effect on *rickets.*

Many years ago I gave a lecture in Winterthur and mentioned that the *stinging nettle* was a wonderful help to those suffering from *tuberculosis.* A year later, I again gave a lecture in that same hall and a man from the audience announced that he had heard me describe the wonderful healing powers of the stinging nettle. His wife was ill at home with tuberculosis of the lungs. Since the doctor could hold out no real hope of a cure, he began giving his wife food that was rich in calcium. Every day he gave her the juice of raw nettles, finely chopped and added to her soup. In a year's time, to the astonishment of the doctor, this man's wife had completely gained her health. I myself was just as surprised as the 300 members of my audience. He admitted that the daily nettle hunt and the trouble of putting them through the mincer to extract the juice had been well worthwhile.

Young nettles can be finely chopped and sprinkled on soup as a garnish or on salads. Since the juice is not very tasty it is better to mix it in with whichever soup you prefer: vegetable, potato or oatmeal. A tablespoon per day for an adult and a half to one teaspoonful for a child has sufficient medicinal properties to take effect. For an infant, 5–10 drops of the extract a day in different dishes of mashed foods should suffice. If you want to profit from at least part of this healthy remedy and at the same time enjoy a pleasant dish, steam the young nettles in oil with a little onion. This will give you a green spinach-like dish and it goes well with mashed potatoes.

Perhaps some of my readers feel that they have no time to find and prepare these plants and would prefer to buy the juice already extracted. Of course they can do this; but no prepared medicine can have as good an effect as the extracted juice from a plant freshly gathered, and nothing is so inexpensive either.

Calcium-complex contains urtica, which is the Latin name for stinging nettle. As the name implies it is a calcium preparation with the addition of raw nettles. How Homeopathy makes use of the nettles will be explained in the section "Homeopathy" under the subheading "Urtica".

MUGWORT (Artemisia vulgaris)

It is said that Roman soldiers put *Mugwort* in their sandals in order to ease their march into Helvetia. Whether that is true or not, the medicinal properties of a *Mugwort* foot bath for taking away tiredness from aching feet and legs has been proven time and time again.

Those who have spent their holidays in the Canton of Tessin, Switzerland, must know *Mugwort* well, for it is one of the toughest weeds in that district and grows to a height of five to six feet. Anyone not well acquainted with the various members of the Artemisia family might mistake it for Wormwood, as it not only produces similar effects but also resembles it in taste and smell. Apart from an etheric oil and bitter substances, the Mugwort also contains insulin, which is a substance resembling carbohydrate, that can be utilized by diabetics, without the need to engage the pancreas (the Islets of Langerhans) in its digestion. Diabetics should pay attention to this plant. The finely chopped leaves can be used in salads as an additional flavoring and it was also well known in former days as an ingredient in stuffing geese or fowl.

In cases of chronic diarrhea, stomach or intestinal catarrh and now the widespread worm problem, Mugwort is an ideal remedy.

In cases of *Hystero-Epilepsy* – a form of falling sickness which appears to be connected with ovarian disfunction – the fresh plant extract of *Mugwort* is one of the few effective remedies. It is a diuretic and encourages the menstrual flow when it has for some reason become retarded. Five drops of the fresh plant extract in a glass of water, sipped throughout the day, will suffice.

PIMPERNEL ROOT (Pimpinella saxifraga)

In the Middle Ages, women must have often sat talking together as they do today and exchanged advice on all sorts of subjects. The medical practitioner often lived miles away from a hamlet or township and there were no telephones to summon him. Sometimes it might have happened that some noble lady was unable to give her new-born son sufficient milk and, often within her own walls, some wise old woman could be found to give advice. Later, a young girl would be hustled through the gates with orders to find some pimpernel roots. Having been well washed these roots would be placed in the noble lady's bosom and within six to eight hours there would be so much milk that the pimpernel roots would have to be quickly thrown away.

Thus the ancient stories and sagas tell us of the wonderful effect produced by the little pimpernel. Today we have other remedies that may be easier to apply (Lactobono, Rizinus communis 3x) but wherever the pimpernel may be found, it will prove as great a help as it did in ancient times. Women might try it to see if its effect is just as good as these legends say it is. Today, pimpernel's main attribute is the wonderful effect it has on the *vocal cords* in cases of *catarrh* and *sore throat*. Pimpernel roots, chewed all day, will have a much better effect than the expensive patent medicines with all their promising advertising and labels, and in addition they are far from palatable. In the wintertime when catarrh is so prevalent, one can appreciate how well pimpernel serves. If *hoarseness* is allied to the catarrh, the chewing of pimpernel roots should be alternated with rowan berries; the latter can usually be bought in a dried state at the pharmacy. In real bad cases, raw fir bud syrup is another excellent aid.

Formerly, pimpernel root was recommended in cases of skin eruption or calculus. A protection against contagious diseases, pimpernel, was to our forefathers on a par with Butterbur (Petasites hybrid.) and Masterwort (Imperatoria). Hence the old proverb:

> To be healthy, eat garlic and pimpernel
> and live to a ripe old age as well!

ANGELICA

When the black death, the plague, raged in the Middles Ages, terrified humans swept through the woods and forests seeking help. They dug up *angelica* by the running streams and damp clearings for they felt certain that this plant would help them. Next to a plant called the "plague root", angelica was considered the most important remedy for the plague; and in the contemporary descriptions of these dreadful times, one can read the most remarkable stories of the reliable help these remedies gave. They affirm that anyone who kept a piece of angelica root in his mouth all through the day would be preserved from the plague. Be that as it may, nevertheless the strong taste of this root is due to an etheric oil and Valerian, Malic and Angelic acids it contains.

The fresh plant extract has a marvelous effect on the digestion, on *loss of appetite*, on irritation of the gastric mucous membrane and also on *stomach cramps*. Moreover, it has an excellent effect on *bronchial* and impacted *catarrhs*, if a few drops are taken with a little honey once an hour. For the stomach, take ten drops in a glass of water three times a day, half an hour before meals.

The seeds of Angelica may also be used. And now I will tell you how the genuine Angelica liqueur "Vespetro" is made. The recipe follows:

Angelica seeds or chopped Angelica root	2 ozs.
Fennel seeds	¼ oz.
Anise seeds	¼ oz.
Coriander seeds	⅕ oz.

Grind all the seeds together in a mortar or some kind of a suitable mill and then add 8 fluid ounces of pure alcohol to it. After 8 days strain this mixture through muslin or cotton wool and mix it with a solution of 2½ pints of water to which 1 1b. of sugar (preferably grape sugar) has been added. And there you have it!

There is no better or more pleasant remedy for *digestive problems* or *flatulence*. Let us imagine a monastery in the Middle Ages – there the monks enjoy a glass of the golden drink before appearing for duty in the morning; and late in the evening a guest arriving chilled would be given a glass of "Vespetro", and just a small sip would have a quicker and better effect than the chemical liquor or tablet of today.

LADY'S MANTLE (Alchemilla vulgaris)

Is this little plant so called because its leaves are shaped like a cloak, or because it can ward off women's illnesses in particular, and so protect them from harm? Perhaps both attributes have influenced the choice of this name. Let us take a closer look at this plant. To do so we must leave the flat countryside and climb up into the hills. We don't have to climb too high, for Lady's Mantle grows at about 2,000 feet in the alpine meadows of Switzerland. Close by it grows Silver Mantle, a plant which is richer in appeal, but modest from a point of view of nourishment. Lady's Mantle favors rich soil and it can be found growing alongside the proud Aconite in places where the earth contains the humus and nitrogen in which these two plants delight. But you can come across it near a shepherd's hut, in companionship with the giant Dock; it grows very large in this area because of the rich soil.

Its healing potential is of particular benefit to women. In any womb problem or in cases of leucorrhoea, it is a wonderful remedy when mixed with white clover and white dead-nettle. Lady's Mantle is also a simple, reliable help for weak ligaments which could lead to a prolapse of the womb. It has also proved its worth in cases where there is unsufficient strength in the connecting tissues, causing a predisposition to hernia. Where such constitutional problems are concerned, an infusion made from the plant should be taken regularly for at least a year.

The freshly pulped leaves of the Lady's Mantle are very good for healing wounds quickly when applied externally. If one sustains a scratch or a cut while walking or hiking in the mountains, there are plenty of effective remedies all around; a few St. John's wort flowers rubbed on the cut, or pulped Arnica, or Lady's Mantle will make an inexpensive, but healing dressing.

A good ointment can be made from the fresh plant and root which, when dressed over a wound, is very effective; also for less serious ruptures. Children's diarrhea can be stopped with the use of Lady's Mantle without any side effects.

OATS (Avena Sativa)

It is a well-known fact that horses derive their health and strength largely from eating oats. For humans too, it is a strengthening food, but that is not all. It is also a wonderful remedy. Whenever our *stomachs* are *upset*, we should make it a rule to take *oatmeal* gruel or porridge, for this will be sure to right the trouble.

Even in its earliest stages, when it is just tall grass, it has remarkable healing powers. Few people realize that when the ears are just beginning to form, when it is juicy and breaking into flower, this green grass is at its richest in Avenin, which is unsurpassed as a nutrient for the cells of the nervous system. A perfect nerve nutrient can be prepared at home simply by putting the flowering oats through a mincer. Cover the green mash with warm water and let stand for about two hours. Then strain and sweeten with honey, grape concentrate or unrefined sugar. The oats can also be put through the mincer together with raisins or currants, covered with water and strained as before. In this way they are sweetened during preparation. This oat drink is a wonderful *tonic* for everybody in these nerve-racking modern times and, if taken regularly over a period of time, will calm and regenerate the nervous system to a surprising extent.

Even after the oats have been harvested the straw can be used as an infusion, although it is not as effective or as potent as the juice from the green, flowering oats. It will be found however quite effective in cases of *catarrhs, coughs* and *fever* conditions. It is especially good for children whose skin function needs stimulating and the infusion can be added to their bath water.

The possible uses of the oat are not yet exhausted, for the oat grain together with its husk, makes an excellent tea. Sweetened and taken when the mucous membranes of the stomach or intestines are inflamed, it makes an excellent therapeutic.

Homeopathy employs the juice from the green oats for its wonderful *nerve remedy* "Avena Sativa" – which is the Latin name for the oat plant.

LILY OF THE VALLEY (Convallaria)

This woodland plant with sword-shaped leaves and delicate white bells not only brings joy to our hearts in the spring but also strengthens and stimulates this organ. As long ago as the Middle Ages, Lily of the Valley was esteemed and well-known as a heart medicine. Later, when the more potent but less safe plant, Digitalis (Foxglove) was discovered, Lily of the Valley fell into disuse and was practically forgotten. An English doctor, by the name of Withering, discovered Digitalis in the tea mixture of an old woman, who used it to cure *dropsy*. This happened in the year 1785 and Digitalis has been used ever since. However, in recent times, we are beginning to realize that we have wrongfully neglected Lily of the Valley and have now realized that the plant having the most drastic effect is not necessarily the best one. The use of Foxglove as a heart medicine over many years has confirmed this suspicion. Although it is reliable enough as far as action is concerned, it is at the same time an unsafe remedy on account of its cumulative effects. Prolonged treatment with it may damage the heart muscle seriously. This danger does not exist in the case of Lily of the Valley, for within four hours the glycosid, which is the effective substance, is broken down by the body, although its favorable action continues much longer.

Convallaria is best used in the form of a standardized fresh plant extract. It strengthens the *heart muscles* and extends its favorable effect to the blood vessels as well. The same dose as Digitalis acts more gently than the latter and produces no side effects such as are engendered by cumulation. Digitalis sometimes proves ineffective in cases of weak hearts after influenza, pneumonia or other lung and infectious diseases, while Lily of the Valley invariably does the job more effectively. It can and should be used as a pre-operative heart tonic and it will have a salutary effect on the heart if used post-operatively. Those who engage in competitive sports, where a strain is often placed on the heart, will find this plant an excellent conditioner.

I have had excellent results with it in heart complications which occurred during or after kidney diseases and have found it very reliable in the treatment of arteriosclerotic conditions, i.e. high blood pressure and symptoms characteristic of degenerative and *premature aging processes*. It is also eminently suitable for the Climacterium, the period known as the *change of life*. The unpleasant heart symptoms brought on by *hyperthyroidism* will be alleviated by Lily of the Valley while Digitalis would hardly produce the desired results.

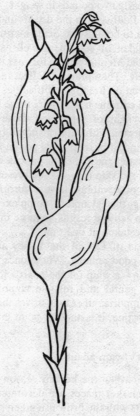

Lily of the valley (Convallaria majalis)

SQUILL (Scilla maritima)

Along the shores of the Mediterranean an extraordinary plant is found. It shoots up out of the dry ground on a stem more than three feet high and is crowned with white blossoms. It has no leaves and if you dig down for its root, you will come upon a large bulb which on the average is about six inches in diameter and nearly two pounds in weight. This is the genuine squill plant that flourishes in the dry ground and the aromatic air and is known to botanists as Scilla maritima. It contains an esteric oil, scillidan or scillain as well as other interesting substances and old Mediterranean folk use it both internally as well as externally. They praise its effect in different kinds of heart troubles and on breathing difficulties. It also aids those who suffer from extreme cold, whose urine is pale and watery, whose pulse is light or rapid and those whose upper air passages are affected with catarrh. It will be found especially helpful in the kind of heart trouble accompanied by difficulty in dispersing water and expelling mucus caused by catarrh, while itching of the skin may also be present.

More recent observations have confirmed the efficacy of Squill in curing this symptom complex. Large doses are unnecessary. To achieve results no more than five drops of 3x potency need be taken at one time.

A combination of Lily of the Valley and Squill together produce a very good remedy. Where once it was necessary to give Strophantin – a whip for the *heart* – it is now possible to help with the gentle and reliable combination mentioned above, which supports rather than drives the *heart*. Because its action is long-lasting, it is another point in favor of using it.

MISTLETOE (Viscum album)

Each December when the holiday season rolls around, shop windows and market places are decorated with the famous Mistletoe, plants with the brownish green stems and the white berries. How many people realize that these plants contain within them the most wonderful of healing powers? Mistletoe is not only used in the observance of an ancient custom but it is also important in the treatment of prematurely aged *arteries*. The fresh extract of the Mistletoe is one of the most wonderful cures for the loss of elasticity in the *arteries*, a hardening of the arteries accompanied by high blood pressure. Combined with wild leek and hawthorn, it will safely arrest the progress of this tragic accompaniment of old age. Mistletoe, combined with the Indian drug Rauwolfia serpentina, becomes a high blood pressure remedy par excellence. They work together to release the discomfort of high blood pressure and provide a measure of relief that calms and soothes the person afflicted. For the treatment to be effective it is important that salt and too much protein in the diet be avoided. The importance of Mistletoe as a remedy can be illustrated by the amount used in Germany alone: 180–190 tons.

Mistletoe extract is also indicated in *headaches* which are accompanied by *dizziness*, in spells of vertigo where there is a tendency to fall backwards, in people whose gait is wavering, those who get attacks of "pins and needles" in the limbs and who suffer from chronic *cold feet*. The extract, used in conjunction with *Rauwolfia*, is beneficial in sudden attacks of *palpitations* which are coupled with *vascular spasms,* difficult breathing and nightly attacks of *asthma*. For treatment take five drops, three to five times daily.

In search of an effective herbal remedy for cancer, Mistletoe should not be ignored. The fresh plant extract as well as homeopathic injections have proven invaluable in this respect. It is a matter of record that people who have suffered for years from pains in the joints because of chronic *arthritis* were completely relieved by homeopathic Mistletoe injections.

BUTTERBUR (Petasites hybridus)

Petasites has proven itself during the past few years as a valuable remedy, especially in cancerous growths. Since it produces severe aggravation of the symptoms (which in itself is a favorable sign, as it proves that the remedy is indicated and improvement, if not complete cure, can be anticipated), the mother tincture is usually not tolerated by the average patient and it has to be potentized to 1x oder 2x or even higher. To find the individual potency tolerance it will be necessary to ignore the usual directions and begin with a potency of 1x. If this has an unpleasantly strong reaction, 2x or 3x should be tried, as the higher the potency, the weaker the reaction will become. This does not indicate that the curative action of the remedy becomes correspondingly less. It is merely a question of the tolerance of the individual.

Alternatively, one drop of the tincture can be put into a glass of water and frequent sips can be taken during the day. After a week or so, the body will have gotten used to that particular strength and will be able to tolerate a somewhat higher concentration. Increase the dose to two drops of the tincture in a glass of water, and later on you may be able to increase it to three drops.

It affects *tumors* and all other pathological cell changes very forcibly, but is nevertheless quite harmless. Thus, strong reactions need not be any cause for alarm. Recently, I spoke to a professor of medicine with whom I had left samples of the tincture for experimental purposes, and he confirmed that *Petasites* is a "strong" remedy. He said one drop doses gave rise to severe reactions in sensitive patients and especially those with diseases of the respiratory tract, must take it highly diluted. Doctors complain that our natural remedies are not potent enough to produce satisfactory therapeutic reaction, yet there are fresh plant extracts as spectacular in effects as many chemotherapeutic drugs, with the added advantage of being harmless and non-toxic. Although poisonous plants are used as remedies, unlike our orthodox colleagues, we use only the whole plant and in those instances, only in attenuated dilutions.

Petasites is the best natural remedy available for *cell degeneration.* It is best given in combination with Mistletoe; where drugs have failed, this treatment has been successful.

RUDBECKIA (Echinacea purpurea)

When I was in Mexico, an Indian told me about the fatal result of an injury. Apparently a machete, an instrument used for cutting down undergrowth in the jungle, had glanced off a hard root giving the barefoot Indian wielding it a deep cut. He washed the wound in the river and without bandaging it, continued with the group of other Indians who worked all day in the jungle as woodcutters. They used horses and mules and it is very possible that their manure lay on the paths. The wounded man must have stepped on some because in a few hours he had cramps and soon got so stiff he couldn't walk. His companions took him back to the base camp, but the next morning he was dead. It was quite obvious that the cause of his death was due to *tetanus* bacillus. Not all Indians are so negligent about treating accidents. There are those who let the wound bleed profusely and bandage it with a cloth without washing. If there are no antiseptics on hand, the best cleansing agent is the blood flowing from the wound and the congealed blood will, for the time being, prove to be the best protection against infection. The bandage also hinders the intrusion of dangerous bacilli to a certain extent. Indian, who have a good knowledge of plants, usually know which medicinal herbs to bind over their wounds. They know which herbs stop bleeding and which heal.

During my stay in Mexico, I noted many things which were a useful addition to my knowledge of plants and their properties. There is one special plant that is much used in Mexico and is well known to the natives, and this is *Echinacea*. It prevents *infection* and *inflammation* in a most remarkable way. It has many friends among those who practice healing according to the biological method, and it is for this reason that Echinacea has received much attention in Europe and in many other countries. Echinacea has also been recognized as an *antidote* to the unpleasant secondary effects of Penicillin and also in cases where a resistance to Penicillin exists.

My own experience with echinacea:

A short time ago I had an interesting experience in the treatment of *wounds*. While scything early one morning, I slipped on the steep part of our meadow heavy with dew and cut my foot quite badly. Evidently I had cut a small artery as the wound bled profusely. Usually I would wash a cut with undiluted *whey* extract because this lactic acid preparation is a wonderful antiseptic. Now however, I wanted to try an experiment with Echinacea. I placed a pad of cotton flannel that had been soaked in the Echinacea tincture on the bleeding cut. Then I gathered more Echinacea leaves from the garden and bound them around the wound as the Indians do. I could now finish my work outdoors. When the wound stopped bleeding I tied a handkerchief around everything, making it easier for me to get around. That night I left well enough alone but expected my foot to be painful. By comparison to other times, I hardly felt any pain at all and the throbbing which usually accompanies such a cut, was just not there.

I was both pleased and surprised that such a simple plant should have such a remarkable effect. On the third day I unwound the bandage without disturbing the 2½ inch cut. Except for about one third of the upper edge, the ball of the foot behind the big toe was cut through. But the treatment it had received enabled it to graft itself on again. I dressed the *wound* once more with cotton flannel soaked in Echinacea preparation and covered it as before with *Echinacea* leaves. The *wound* healed completely without inflammation and little pain. Unfortunately, one of the workmen accidentally trod on my damaged foot with his heavy boot while we were working in the woods shortly afterwards. Naturally it was painful, so painful that, as they used to say in Basle, "I saw fire in Alsace." The wound opened again but with a further application of *Echinacea* it healed in a very short time.

I must admit that this experience with *Echinacea* aroused my enthusiasm for this wonderful plant and I am convinced that it will yet play a great part in the practice of biological medicine. At present it is grown in different parts of Switzerland where the soil seems just right for it. There are gardens in Roggwil, Teufen and in the Engadine. The powerful sun in the Engadine valley creates a good climatic environment for the plants, similar to that of their native Mexico where they are grown in abundance. If medical research would focus its attention on botanic-biological aspects of the plant kingdom, I am sure the discoveries would enrich our own materia medica greatly.

COMFREY (Symphytum off.)

The Comfrey plant grows, for the most part unnoticed, near farmyards. Even in ancient times it was used to heal wounds, broken *bones* and especially leg fractures. Considering its value in these cases alone, it should deserve more attention than it usually receives. It encourages the *healing* process and speeds up the formation of new *bone* cells, which is probably due to the fact that it contains 0.8 to 1% of Allantoin. This is known to promote granulation and the formation of epithelial cells. Cholin is another constituent of the Comfrey plant while other important elements may also be present. They are, as yet, unknown.

Comfrey tincture is an excellent remedy for an injured periosteum, the dense fibrous membrane covering the surface of the *bones,* and it has been used successfully for suppurating *ulcers* (wounds which refuse to heal) and leg ulcers. There is hardly a better remedy to be found for the external treatment of *gout;* the raw root should be finely grated and applied to the affected part like a poultice. If fresh roots are not available, use the tincture instead. The tincture is very effective in relieving neuralgic pains, especially *facial neuralgia.*

Tincture of Comfrey should be rubbed very lightly into the affected parts because gouty conditions or injuries to the periosteum react unfavorably to forcible massage. Following the tincture application, follow up with clay, cabbage, giant sorrel, or goldenrod packs.

Comfrey tincture can be taken internally. This is recommended in cases of fractures, all sorts of injuries and before and after operations. Once the bandages or clips have been removed, the fresh scars can be treated with it. Additionally, healing can be accelerated by drinking vegetable water, chiefly that from potatoes and leeks and the raw juices from the cabbage family.

HORSETAIL (Equisetum arvense)

This little plant is to be found chiefly on the moors, in damp clay pits and forest clearings. In the remote past it was considerably taller, attaining the size of a tree, as the fossilized roots, dug from the earth, prove.

Today we must content ourselves with the small, delicate plant. It has a finely wrought construction and like a tender young fir it stands, pliant yet tough. A flood can knock it to the ground and drag it from its roots, but the little Horsetail takes root anew and stands erect. What gives it this toughness and resilience? If we examine it closely and analyze it, we will find its main constituents are approximately 60% *Silica*, 15% Calcium and the balance other minerals. From this analysis it is evident that *Silica*, as the predominant element, is probably responsible for the majority of its curative properties. Horsetail tea is diuretic and stimulates the kidneys; it also helps overcome spitting of blood, whether it comes from the lungs or the stomach. There is only one other plant that can compete with Horsetail in alleviating this condition and that is Bloodwort.

Silica is of great importance in the regeneration of the *tissue* and so is calcium. Diseases of the *respiratory tract* and the *glandular system* likewise depend on Silica for help. Either an infusion of the herb or an extract from the fresh plant will serve the purpose equally. There is only one other plant so far known, that contains more Silica than Horsetail and that is the

Hemp nettle (Galeopsis ochroleuca) which contains 72%. These Silica plants have a greater variety of uses other than those already mentioned. They are beneficial to the skin and are frequently recommended in baths for various skin diseases.

ARE ALPINE PLANTS OF GREATER VALUE THAN LOWLAND PLANTS?

This question cannot be answered by a simple "yes" or "no", for there are many points that have to be taken into consideration. For instance, I noticed that strawberries grown in my garden in Teufen (3,000 ft.) had less sugar content then the same variety grown in the Engadine (5,000 ft.). I wondered if this was due to the humus in the soil of the Engadine highmoors or to the intensive sunlight. On the other hand, I noticed that the sugar content of the lowland strawberries increased if the summer was a warm and dry one.

We can conclude from this, that warmth and sun are mainly responsible for sweetness. Feeding too must be taken into consideration; our strawberries are given a sufficient quantity of organic lime which would account for their being sweeter than if they received the less nourishment or if the earth was not fed at all. Carrots also seemed to do better in the Engadine than in Teufen and they are sweeter and better flavored. For this we must not only thank the strong, warm sunshine but also the higher elevation of the Engadine, its excellent climatic condition, and the richness of its soil.

Not every high elevation has the same advantages. The Southern Alps have many more hours of sunshine than the Northern. For this reason plants do much better in the southern than in the northern regions. For example, Solidago, grown in the higher Engadine has a better and stronger effect on the kidneys than that grown in the lowlands of Teufen and that grown in Teufen is certainly better than any grown farther north in the districts below an altitude of 1,000 feet.

Scientific experiments:

Some time ago, Professor Fleuck delivered a lecture to the Swiss Association of Apothecaries. This lecture was based upon experiments in which various medicinal herbs were grown at various altitudes but in identical soils. He contended that the therapeutic value of the plants does not always depend upon the altitude in which they grow. Better results were obtained from plants that grew in sheltered valleys, exposed to sunshine but protected from the winds, than from those grown at higher altitudes with plenty of sun but unprotected from the winds.

There are certain plants that do better in the shade or at least semi-shade but this is usually an exception to the rule. As far as the medicinal value of plants is concerned, it will be found that this depends upon a variety of factors. Thus, if a highland herb proves to be more effective than others, it cannot always be attributed to altitude alone. In view of my experience I found this hard to believe, but further investigation brought me around to the opinion that it was the variety of the plant rather than the height to which it grew that mattered. It is evident that different plants demand different environments. Thus if a herb demands an acid soil, semi-shade and plenty of moisture for its maximum development, it is bound to grow poorly in a parched, calcareous soil that receives full sunshine, however high its location.

Alpine plant forms:

The alpine plant is usually richer in its constituents and medicinal value than its lowland relative. Analysis shows that, the lowland yarrow for example contains less etheric oils and is less aromatic than the highland yarrow from the Engadine. There is no question that the soil and the sunshine with its more intense ultra-violet radiation have a great influence on the quality of a plant. Since these factors are usually found in most highland localities, it is my contention that alpine herbs are better than lowland ones and until now that contention has not been disproved.

Professor Fleuck's experimental results were arrived at with little if any consideration of the influence of ultra-violet radiation and this would lead one to believe that these rays are not so important in plant life, at least as far as their principal active elements are concerned. However, there are other constituents to be reckoned with, especially the trace elements which seem to depend upon ultra-violet light to a far greater extent than the more common substances, although little is known about this relationship as Professor Fleuck admitted. To obtain scientifically acceptable knowledge on this subject would involve costly experiments. In any case, the empirically confirmed knowledge that alpine herbs are better suffices for us, until it can be scientifically disproved. What is true about highland yarrow also applies to highland St. John's wort. The tincture obtained from it is a much darker shade than that prepared from the lowland plant. It looks different than the ordinary Hypericum perforatum; its growth is shorter and more compact; and its name distinguishes it – "Hypericum alpinum" – from the other variety. Goldenrod is another plant about which the same can be said. The alpine variety is small and bushy and instead of one flower stem it has 12 to 15. It contains more etheric oils, is more aromatic and therapeutically more effective than its lowland cousin. I am sure you will agree with me that although the highland environment offers better growth conditions, it is nevertheless not so much the altitude that decides the medicinal qualities of plants as much as it is their variety and requirements.

Other noteworthy influences:

It is quite obvious that experiments made with some lowland plants, Belladonna for instance, are less conclusive than those made with plants that grow in both regions. The pureness of the soil has to be considered too, for lowland soil usually has its bacterial flora damaged by artificial fertilizers and therefore cannot offer the same favorable conditions for growth as the naturally fertilized ground of the mountain valley, the homous of which is brought down by the snow every spring.

Scientific research is an interesting profession for the laboratory technician, but when it comes to assessing the therapeutic value of a herbal preparation, practical experience with actual patients wins out every time over laboratory methods. A pure, whole-plant remedy is an intricate complex of active elements, the overall effect of which can hardly be determined by chemical analysis. Some of the elements are even unknown. For this reason, the medical scientist needs the co-operation of the herbal therapist for the final confirmation of his findings, and this can only come from practice and experience.

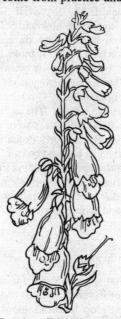

Fox glove (Digitalis purpurea)

WILD FRUITS

ROSE HIPS (Rosa canina)

It is not only the modest but beautiful blossoms of the wild rose, so unjustly called rosa canina or dog rose, that is a pleasure to behold; but the fruit too is beautiful and colorful as it splashes its color across the autumn scene. Even in the winter they remain like little mandrakes in their white fur capes. Many a hungry bird has enjoyed its berries when everything was covered with ice and snow. As a food, rose hips are very good for many reasons. It contains natural fruit sugar which is as sweet as any jam and in recent years it has been made into a preserve or spread and is very tasty. It is nourishing also for it contains mineral nutrients such as calcium, silica, magnesium and phosphorus and incidentally, phosphorus is good for the brain! Rose hips contains a large amount of ascorbic acid better known as *Vitamin C*, and among other things it has a calming effect on the nerves. Since we are considering the rose hip, we will not go into the details of the benefits of Vitamin C at this time, although the fruit does play a large role in treatments where this vitamin is used.

Rose hip conserve is tasty, slightly tart and is not only a food but a medicine, a nerve restorer, conforming Hippocrate's demand: "Let food be your medicine and medicine your food".

It is important to remember that rose hip should not be boiled as heat destroys its remedial properties to a large extent. A slice of bread thickly spread with raw pulp will more than supply the daily requirement of Vitamin C. If the conserve is made from pulp, dextrose or other fruit sugars may be added if it does not seem sweet enough. In any event the final product will be exceedingly healthful, easy to assimilate and provide food of a high caloric value.

343

The preparation of *rose hip conserve* is as follows:

Gather the well-ripened berries of the wild rose, the hips, and spread them out to dry in a dry shady place. Make sure they are not piled up or they will get moldy. When they are nice and soft, put them through a mincer to obtain a thick red puree. Rub the puree through a sieve, which will keep back the pips (seeds), with a wooden spoon. The resulting paste, rich in Vitamin C, should now be mixed with honey or dextrose to taste. That's all there is to it! Although uncooked, the mixture will keep well, preferably in the refrigerator. For therapeutic purposes take a teaspoonful a day. This will be of much greater value than any of the manufactured Vitamin C pills you could possibly take.

Rose hip kernels make a wonderfully relaxing *tea*. Where do you get it? Having made the conserve you will have kernels, skin and some pulp left over. These can be dried slowly and used for making tea. This tea has the most delicate flavor and can be served with lemon or milk. It is rich in Silica and is an excellent kidney remedy. Seriously ill people who cannot take any other herb tea can take this one with safety.

BARBERRY (Berberis vulgaris)

Wandering through the valleys, bright with the autumn sun and colors, you will find not only hedgerows of wild rose berries, but also many sprays of Barberry berries. So many people pass by this wild fruit never realizing it has wonderful healing powers. It is bushy and grows to a height of three to six feet. Certainly this colorful plant with its bunches of oval-shaped red berries nesting among yellow flowers and pale green leaves, is a delight to the eye and a tonic to the nerves. No other berry contains as much *Vitamin C* and many suffering from "nerves" could benefit enormously by filling their mouths with barberries, chewing them slowly and then swallowing them.

A raw barberry conserve, made from well ripened berries is rich in Vitamin C, malic and citric acids. In preparing the

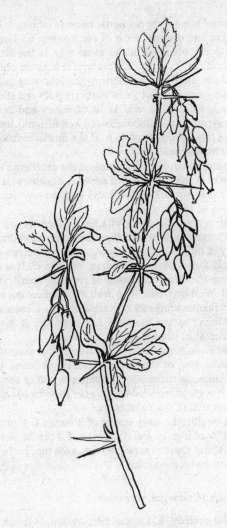

Barberry (Berberis vulgaris)

conserve, avoid using a copper kettle because copper acts as a catalytic agent and destroys most of the Vitamin C. The juice and the pulp are obtained in the same way as the rose hip puree. Experiments have shown that best results are obtained if the rest of the preparation is done in the following manner:

Add ¼ cup raw sugar to 1 lb. of barberry pulp and stir well. When sugar has dissolved, add ½ lb. of honey and ½ lb. of grape sugar syrup. Stir the mixture until well blended and then pour in glass jars as you would jam. If the mixture is too thin, add a little more sugar.

Experimental research has established the excellence of this nature remedy in the treatment of nervous disorders. It has a wonderful effect also on the *kidneys* and on any scorbutic tendency such as *bleeding gums*.

If our bodies are deficient in Vitamin C, then we are much more liable to succumb to infectious diseases. In addition to the barberry, a thorny bush with orange colored berries called the *Sea buckthorn* is also very high in *Vitamin C*. It is found growing along the coast and banks of rivers in many parts of Europe and Western Asia. The fruit of the Sea buckthorn (Hippophae rhamnoides) can be prepared into a conserve in the same manner as the barberry and rose hip. It makes a delicious syrup also, slightly on the tart side.

There is absolutely no doubt that Vitamin C is necessary to the vital functioning of the body because it is found in the endocrine glands, in the suprarenal capsule, and in the pituitary gland. It is recommended that cancer patients eat a lot of foods that are rich in this substance.

To insure health, the daily intake of *Vitamin C* should not be less than ¾ of a grain and it is better if it can be obtained from such natural sources as raspberries, rose hip, barberries, sea buckthorn and lemon juice.

HAWTHORN (Crataegus oxyacantha)

That splendid remedy, Crataegus preparation, is made from the hawthorn berries which hang in bunches from the thorny bushes by the wayside or in the meadows. When I was a child, my friends and I called them flour berries. We did not know anything about them, beyond the fact that they were good to eat and of course we ate them because there was nothing else to eat at the moment. Certainly we didn't need those berries in our childhood, for Crataegus is a *heart remedy* which is very valuable in cases of weak heart muscles. When *hardening of the arteries, high blood pressure* and especially a hardened and constricted coronary artery is diagnosed, there is no doubt that Crataegus is the best, the most harmless and the most reliable remedy that can be taken. Arnica, mixed in proper proportion with Crataegus, has benefited many *elderly people,* even to the extent of lengthening their lives.

The Crataegus mother tincture is a successful remedy in *Angina pectoris,* when heart cramps occur. These cramps are usually accompanied by stabbing pains in the region of the heart resulting in difficult breathing and a weak, irregular pulse. In this case, where immediate relief is necessary, take 5 to 10 drops every half hour. When the pains subside and the cramps have eased up, then take 5 drops, three times daily in a little water or juice.

ROWANBERRIES (Frutus sorbi)

In the autumn, the Rowan tree produces beautiful red berries. If you spread these berries out in a shady place and dry them, you will have a reliable remedy for *hoarseness.* Just chew the berries and the hoarseness will quickly disappear. Also, following the procedure for rose hip, barberry and Sea buckthorn, a very tasty conserve can be made that is rich in vitamins and minerals.

JUNIPER BERRIES (Fructus juniperus)

These are well enough known in pickled red cabbage and usually are removed and left on the side of the plate. In olden days everyone knew that these berries were used for flavoring and that grandfather often chewed them first thing in the morning. Old herbalists say that the eagle lives to such an old age because it feeds on juniper berries. They contain a delicate etheric oil, and although they contain sugar, they do not taste sweet because the bitter constituents over-ride the sweet.

Sufferers from *rheumatism* find that juniper berries are an excellent remedy because they help to increase the excretion of uric acid by way of the urine. Be careful how you use it. Too much may irritate the kidneys. In *nephritis* and similar kidney conditions, Juniper berries should be taken in Homeopathic doses, Juniperus communis 1x or 2x.

In cases of *asthma,* i.e. excessive mucus secretion, juniper extract should be alternated with barberries and rowan berries. Oedematous conditions and acute inflammations of the *bladder* will respond to juniper in the form of infusion, essence or extract. Juniper berries added to breakfast cereals stimulate the appetite, strengthen the stomach and benefit the glands.

A SELECTION
OF HOMEOPATHIC REMEDIES

In an age in which the predominance of synthetic drugs has almost completely overshadowed any other remedies in the treatment of the ailing and afflicted, natural remedies have been all too often neglected as instruments for healing and until recently, had been relegated to the kitchen as flavoring aids. But times are changing rapidly. Europeans, Orientals and Latin Americans have never abandoned natural medicines and have been instrumental in reviving interest in many of the old healing methods accomplished through the use and applications of herbs.

The subject of homeopathic remedies is so vast that we present only a small selection of what would otherwise fill many volumes.

ACONITUM NAPELLUS (Aconite)

It stands proudly in the field, this tall friend, which can be as dangerous as it is helpful. The beautiful Aconite is given many names, i.e. wolfsbane and monkshood, and is native to the Swiss Alps. There you will find it on the alpine meadows, where the ground is rich, in damp hollows between low bushes and in thinning woods right up to the highest growing conifers, the creeping firs.

Every part of the plant, including the subsidiary tuber, which is developed from the root for the following year's growth, is very poisonous. The whole plant is used to make tincture. If one took large quantities of this tincture, it would result in certain death due to cardiac paralysis and damage to the spinal cord. But, diluted a thousand or one hundred thousand times, this dangerous plant becomes one of the best and most reliable homeopathic medicines.

Aconitum is the best first aid in cases of *inflammatory diseases* which usually are accompanied by fever. In *infectious diseases*, especially when the skin is hot and dry, Aconitum in the third and fourth decimal potency has a rapid and very good effect.

It diverts the toxins from the blood and the tissues to the skin and encourages *perspiration.* A rush of blood to the head, such as occurs during the *change of life,* is best dealt with by lower potencies of the remedy, as for example 10x. Aconitum is, in the language of Homeopathy, an acute, sudden, violent remedy. Its sphere of action is therefore chiefly in the beginning of an *acute disease* when fever, mental anguish, palpitations, etc. are present. It can cure only *functional* disturbances and has no effect after pathological changes have occurred. When perspiration has established itself, the patient usually calms down and, when this happens, treatment with Aconitum can be stopped and Belladonna 4x taken instead. These two homeopathic remedies should be in everyone's medicine chest, for they are more frequently used than any other medicine. The tinctures must never be used as they are dangerous. Although some doctors use them for neuralgia caused by chill, for gout and rheumatism, there are more harmless remedies available which are just as effective.

Aconitum is a mydriatic, i. e. it dilates the pupil if it is instilled into the eye. Belladonna has the same property and it is the Atropin in this plant which is used in orthodox medicine for that purpose. To achieve the best results, Aconitum should be given in the third or fourth decimal potency (3x or 4x); five drops in a glass of water taken at one hour intervals will suffice.

ATROPA BELLADONNA (Deadly Nightshade)

This beautiful plant with its thick stems and leaves is somewhat like the tobacco plant; but its greenish red-brown blossoms indicate that it is neither the tobacco plant nor the *winter cherry* or *Chinese lantern,* which has a juicy red berry that is slightly acid, but the famous as well as infamous belladonna.

The ripe, shiny berries entice children to pick and eat them – with fatal results. Belladonna has been associated with witchcraft by the peasants since before the Middle Ages and Satan was thought to be its cultivator. But in considering this plant we cannot overlook its many benefits even though aware of its evil qualities. As with humans, plants can have good and bad characteristics and this is especially true of belladonna, which, as well as being a killer, is also famed as a life saver.

Belladonna is partly responsible for the rediscovery of the law of similarity. Dr. Hahnemann once found himself unable to prescribe treatment for a very sick woman, until an unconscious child was carried in to him. The child's face was suffused by a bluish-red color and Hahnemann realized immediately what had happened when the father showed him the pretty berries he had snatched from the child's hands – Belladonna poisoning! Then the doctor noticed that there was an extraordinary resemblance in the appearance of the woman and the child; both had a bluish-red flush in the face. The causes were different but the results were the same! In a flash the doctor recognized the importance of his observation: "Simila similibus curentur" – the ancient hippocratic teaching and the law of similarity. As soon as he had given the child something to make it vomit, he went out with the father, took a branch of

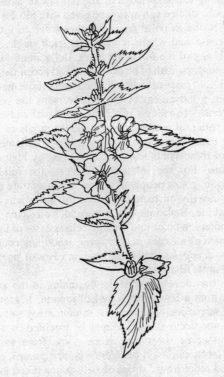

Marsh mallow (Althaea officinalis)

the belladonna with blossoms and fruit, and squeezed the plant into some water. By diluting it to about 4x he prepared this yellowish-green liquid into a medicine which he gave to the sick woman. Noting her reaction, the doctor followed up with a second dose and a few more until the woman was out of danger. Thus, the child's belladonna poisoning saved the woman's life and at the same time brought about a deeper understanding and knowledge of another law of nature.

Belladonna diluted can always be given with success where a condition is due to poisoning – whether from an internal or external cause and where it manifests itself in the nervous system. In any of the following cases, Belladonna 4x is indicated: *Headaches*, rush of blood to the head accompanied by a racing pulse; in cases of *delirium* when every movement of the body, even a movement of the eyes worsens the condition; when the crisis of an illness establishes itself with sudden force; when the patient is sensitive to light and the pupils are dilated; when the mucous membrane is dry, hot and inflamed – and any one of these symptoms is accompanied by high fever or temperature. For the intellectually alert, the full-blooded active person, young people who have to concentrate mentally and draw heavily on their brains, or for those who lead an intellectual life, Belladonna 4x is a wonder medicine.

Belladonna is a quick and reliable help in cases of infectious diseases such as *measles, scarlet fever, whooping cough, conjunctivitis, erysipelas, boils,* and even in cases of *pneumonia,* especially in its first stages.

Cramps that develop suddenly, beginning in the anus, are relieved within a few minutes by Belladonna. If grandfather exhibits a suspiciously red face, the same remedy will avert an imminent *apoplectic fit*. Auntie may be troubled by neuralgic pains, brother or sister may come home from work with *stomach, intestinal, liver, bladder* or *biliary cramps*, and they will all find relief from 5 drops of Belladonna taken in a small glass of water.

Dosage: The generally used potency is 4x. Seldom is it necessary to strengthen the potency to 3x. Typical Belladonna cases should not receive potencies below 6x.

COCCUS CACTI

This is an excellent remedy for *whooping cough* and is often combined with Drosera in the form of whooping cough drops. If this is used prior to the onset of the characteristic symptoms, such as a prophylactic, the whoop may be aborted.

It is extraordinary that Drosera, which is a carnivorous plant and Coccus Cacti, are both remedies which have little to do with plant life. To obtain the raw material for this whooping cough remedy one must travel far; to Algeria, the Canary islands, or even to Central America where many cactus plants are to be found especially in desert areas and stony wastes. The search goes on to locate a genus of cacti called "Opuntia coccinellifera" and on it, one will find a small insect about 3 mm long, which feeds on the juicy flesh of its host. The insect has a broad shell and leaves behind it a trail of red stain. Do not be shocked to learn that this is the female cochineal louse, which is the raw material for the wonderful homeopathic whooping cough remedy called Coccus Cacti.

Students and followers of Dr. Rademacher's teachings have found that Coccus Cacti has a very good effect on the *kidneys* too. Observations made in a Vienna clinic confirm that all kinds of spasmodic blocking, respiration blocking and pneumo-tubercular *coughs* also benefit from it. In the great Homeopathic repertory by the well-known American authority Kent, Coccus Cacti is recommended for diseases of the central nervous system. Physicians in earlier times used this remedy in material doses, i.e. the mother tincture, for severe kidney disorders, but Homeopathy generally employs the 3x to 6x potencies.

GUAIACUM (Resin of Lignum Vitae)

In Paracelsus' time, merchants brought home a sort of wood that was supposed to contain a healing resin. Medical men of those days seized upon this medicine as women might fall for a new fashion. This wood was extraordinary, for it sank in water and this made it different from any other wood hitherto known. It was found in the West Indies and South America and, when heated, pure resin flowed from it. It became a remedy for those who suffered from lung problems.

Today, Guaiacum is one of the best medicines for *pharyngitis* if used in the 1x potency. Five drops on a little sugar cube, taken every one or two hours, will almost certainly have eased the symptoms after two or three doses. It acts almost as a specific in such cases and unpleasant smelling sputum or perspiration is usually a sure indication for its use. Stabbing, tearing pains in the joints, with *gouty* deposits in them, have been relieved not only with the attenuated tinctures, but also with ointments and embrocations which contained this medicine. Used with *Lachesis,* Guaiacum will bring quick relief for those who suffer from *tonsillitis.*

KALIUM IODATUM (Iodate of Potash)

This is one of the remedies that is greatly misused by orthodox medicine insofar as it is given in large material doses which always produce bad physiological reactions. Prof. Bier has promoted the success of this remedy and has proved that it is one of the best *expectorants* for *catarrhal conditions* and that it will even cut the development of such catarrhs short. Those who are disposed to *rheumatism* and *"colds"* will find it a most excellent help, even if their cases have already become chronic. *Bronchitis* and *pneumonia* will be favorably helped by it as well, providing expectoration is still present. It should be generally given in the 4x potency. Best results are obtained when it is combined with *raw pine bud syrup* or *Imperatoria (Masterwort).*

LACHESIS

Do not be shocked, dear readers, when I tell you that this remedy is made from snake poison, taken from a rattle snake

(Lachesis muta) whose bite if unattended means certain death. Homeopathically potentized, however, Lachesis is a most valuable remedy.

Thanks goes to Dr. Constantin Hering for the discovery of this remarkable remedy which has saved more lives than have ever been lost through the bite of the rattle snake. *Malignant diseases, blood poisoning, septicaemia, fungus hamatodes, chronic ulcers, boils, carbuncles, smallpox, scarlet fever,* severe *measles* and other disorders just as serious, can be safely and reliably cured with Lachesis. Whenever a disease is accompanied by a bluish, purplish appearance of the skin, by blue-black swellings, you can be sure that Lachesis 12x will help, if not cure the disease. It is predominantly a left-sided remedy, i.e. it will cure problems located on or in the left side of the body. Therefore, when some female disease affects the left side chiefly, Lachesis should be considered as a remedy.

After a serious illness, when all sorts of toxins are circulating in the bloodstream, Lachesis can be of great service.

Where *typhus* is concerned one will find in Lachesis a most useful and reliable help. After an apoplectic seizure, especially in cases where the left side is paralyzed, one can give Lachesis as well as Arnica with great success.

In cases of *pulmonary abscesses, gangrene of the lung,* or very bad *tonsillitis,* Lachesis can help where all other remedies have failed. I have often seen tonsillitis completely disappear after an injection of Lachesis 10x, without any ill effects. It is good to remember it in cases of afflictions of the *throat.*

This remedy should be kept in every home, for whenever a serious illness tends to induce *blood poisoning,* it is an irreplaceable remedy as well as a necessity. The safest potencies to use are 10x or 12x.

MEZEREUM DAPHNE (Daphne)

The last grubby streaks of snow are lying between the rockroses in the upland meadows, when we come upon the bright red blossoms of the Daphne. The homeopathic remedy

Mezereum is prepared from the bark of this attractive but poisonous plant.

It is a wonderful remedy for *shingles,* facial *erysipelas* and those itching little blisters with a red base, that become worse when scratched. For deep *ulcers* on the *calves* there is hardly a better remedy to be found. The respiratory symptoms of this remedy include a cough, which is aggravated by eating or taking a warm drink, a feeling of constriction across the chest, which occurs especially during the night, dry and irritated mucous membranes and intense thirst with burning pains in the throat. Raw nasal discharge also comes within range of its action. In acute diseases it should not be given below 3x.

SEPIA

If I were to describe all the merits of this wonderful homeopathic medicine, merits quite unknown to the orthodox section of the medical profession, you too would become enthusiastic about it. Just because it is obtained from the cuttle fish is no reason to turn one's nose up at it.

Anyone who knows the Mediterranean or has visited other southern seas must have come across these unusual creatures with their little sacs that spew forth an inky liquid. Formerly painters used this for ink just as it came from the cuttle fish. Today the chemical industry produces a dye known as sepia.

Sepia is one of the best medicines for *females.* Frail women who tire easily after only a short walk or who perspire freely have their best friend in Sepia. It helps the over-worked, the tired, the sad, and those who complain of *backaches.*

Chronic *skin eruptions* that itch and burn, little *blisters* around the joints, desire to sleep during the daytime and *insomnia* during the night, *vertigo,* a weak memory and many other conditions are alleviated or cured, if the medicine is taken for a certain period of time. The potency depends upon the sensitivity of the person; robust ones can use a lower potency, while those with a more delicate constitution may require higher potencies.

TARANTULA CUBENSIS

It is hardly conceivable that the poison of the hairy Cuban spider should possess such remarkable curative powers when homeopathically potentized, but the fact is, it does.

Furuncles, whitlows or any other gathering on the fingers or under the nails, *panaritium* (a whitlow that remains chronic and destroys part of the finger) and small *abscesses* on the hands and feet, are miraculously cured by this remedy. In most cases the affected parts are characterized by a bluish color and cause severe, burning pains. To produce immediate effect, the injection method is recommended. Safest potencies are from 8x to 12x. Tarantula cubensis should not be confused with Tarantula hispanic (Spanish spider).

URTICA (Nettle)

The fresh plant extract from the stinging nettle is homeopathically known as Urtica mother tincture. As well as glycoside, tannin-like substances and formic acid, it also contains a quantity of silica, calcium, phosphorus, iron, sodium and sulphur.

In *arthritic* ailments, inflamed joints of a gouty nature, and diminished urine with increased sedimentation, and *bladder* irritation, Urtica provides a very reliable remedy.

In such cases, the elimination through the skin assumes an acrid character accompanied by an unpleasant odor. This takes place as a result of decreased kidney function and may in time lead to a skin irritation that itches and burns, especially at night. Dosage: Ten drops of the Urtica mother tincture in a glass of water should be sipped during the daytime when relief is desired. In addition to Urtica, the kidneys can be further assisted with Solidago tea. Both remedies can be taken at the same time, alternating one with the other.

357

SOME EXAMPLES
TAKEN FROM BIOCHEMISTRY

CALCIUM FLUORATICUM (Fluorine)

If your *teeth* hurt when you eat hot or cold foods, if they feel a bit loose, or if the enamel becomes brittle and chips off easily so that bacteria can enter through the crevices and carry further destruction into the internal structure of the teeth, then it is time for you to remember Calcium fluoraticum. Silica however, should be taken at the same time because it is equally important in the construction of the teeth.

It is not surprising that our Wallisian mountain peasants possess such beautiful teeth because the whole rye bread they consume is a rich source of Calcium fluoraticum. This mineral is of importance in the connective tissues and for this reason should be taken after operations so that granulation such as scar formation can take place without interruption. The thought suggests itself that a deficiency in Calcium fluoraticum in the system must play some part in the predisposition to hernia.

Interesting observations have been made with this mineral in connection with hard swellings of the tendons and ligaments, dilations of the tendon sheaths, glandular tumors and hard cyst formations. It is gratifying to know that, besides other remedies, such simple medicines as Calcium fluoraticum will have an equally advantageous effect on these conditions. It would of course be unreasonable to expect more from a given biochemic remedy than it usually accomplishes, because it must not be forgotten that disease is hardly ever due to the deficiency of a single cell-salt. Besides a major deficiency, there may be minor deficiencies that have to be corrected before the most urgently required remedy can unfold its curative action to the fullest extent.

It has been found that *cataract* of the lens of the eye is usually associated with a deficiency of Calcium fluoraticum and that it will, in conjunction with Kalium chloride and other therapeutic measures, often cure this disease.

Sclerotic deposits on the tympanic membrane which may give rise to *deafness* and *"head noises"*, painful *whitlows* and *itching, eczematous* diseases of the skin are also relieved by taking the remedy for a period of time. Used with Yarrow or the "Hypericum-complex", the treatment will improve the elasticity of the walls of the veins and will for this reason, be invaluable in cases of *hemorrhoids (piles), varicose veins* and *phlebitis* (inflammation of the veins).

Teething problems in babies require Calcium fluoraticum in alternation with Calcium phosphate. Mothers can preserve their figures after the birth of their babies and prevent a pendulous *abdomen,* which is due to a relaxation of the abdominal muscles and ligaments, if they take Calcium fluoraticum or an Urtica preparation, which contains the former, regularly during their pregnancy.

Dosage: Calcium fluoraticum is generally given in 12x and sometimes in the 6x potency. Normal dose is two 2 grain tablets 3 times daily.

NATRIUM MURIATICUM (Cooking Salt)

Pharmaceutically known as Natrium chloratum
or Natrium hydrochloricum

The type of person most likely to benefit from Natrium Muriaticum can be described as follows: puffy with watery looking skin, thin, in spite of having a good appetite, feels the cold very acutely especially along the spine, easily exhausted by mental and physical work, cannot stand the heat of the sun, inclined to headaches or migraines, easily agitated. If one tries to comfort such persons, they become bad tempered and easily angered. Their bowels function badly and the stool is dry and crumbly. In the case of women these symptoms are accentuated during and after their periods, which incidentally are irregular. A typical aversion to bread can be noted. There either seems to be a great yearning for salt or a definite aversion to it. Those who have any of these characteristics will find Natrium Muriatricum a most excellent and quite harmless remedy.

It has an instantaneous effect on infants and small children, especially when there are disturbances of the *bowels* or *liver*, and it is an excellent remedy for *worm* problems if taken regularly for a long time.

Those suffering from *Basedow's disease*, a swelling of the *thyroid* gland, will find immediate relief by taking Natrium Muriaticum. In vasomotor disorders, palpitations with a feeling of faintness, irregular pulse, such as every third stroke out of rhythm, the medication has a very good effect.

Exanthematic *skin diseases* with watery secretions, *acne* and skin conditions associated with dry mucous membranes, respond to treatment with Natrium Muriaticum.

Dosage: In cases of *constipation,* a low potency such as 3x is indicated. All other ailments will benefit from a higher potency from 6x to 30x. Nervous and high-strung persons always do better on the higher potencies.

NATRIUM SULPHURICUM (Glauber's salt)

Glauber discovered this salt in 1658 und it still bears his name today. Although it is water soluble, it is absorbed with difficulty by the intestines and, if its curative powers are to be utilized, it has to be attenuated to the sixth decimal potency.

One of its most important effects is to increase the secretion of bile into the duodenum and thus aid in the digestion of fats. Natrium phosphate splits up lactic acid into carbonic acid and water, leaving a residue of water to be removed from the system; and Natrium sulphuricum performs this work. Each molecule of this cell-salt has the power to take up and carry out of the organism two molecules of water, while Natrium phosphate, previously mentioned, regulates the quantity of water in the system.

Natrium sulphuricum's action also extends to the *blood*. In the case of *haemophilia*, which is characterized by lack of coagulation of the blood, Natrium sulphuricum will improve this condition if it is taken over a long period of time. *Yarrow* is another remedy that will benefit a hemophiliac or "bleeder".

Diabetes can be favorably influenced with Natrium sulphuricum if taken in conjunction with the fresh plant extract of Tormentil root. Other indications include *liver* problems, *jaundice,* an inflamed *bile duct* or an *inflammation of the small intestines.* For "early morning *diarrhea"* with flatulence, it is a specific but should be alternated with doses of clay water. Metabolic disturbances, having their origin in some *liver disfunction,* are greatly improved with Natrium sulphuricum 6x, two tablets taken three times daily.

In cases of *obesity* and *dropsy* and special kinds of *asthma,* so-called chronic malaria, and the well-known spring rashes from which mostly adolescents suffer, Natrium sulphuricum brings quick relief. This medication should be taken from time to time by people who have a sallow complexion or a slight tinge of yellow in the whites of their eyes, and who often suffer from slight depressions too.

Nursing mothers should not take Natrium sulphuricum because it lessens the flow of milk. On the other hand, at the time of weaning it has been found to be of great help.

SILICA (Pure Flint)

Silica is found in plants, usually in the stalks of grain or grass and gives them the ability to stand up against the wind. This excellent remedy is valued as much in biochemistry as in homeopathy, and I will try to outline its most important uses as briefly as possible.

Silica is used for *suppuration* of every kind but only when it has established itself properly or is already dispersing. In the beginning Hepar. sulph. 4x should be given so as to encourage the elimination of pus. The healing process should be left for the Silica to accomplish.

In Northern lands, Silica is used by the peasants for every sort of suppuration, especially for *boils.* For suppuration of the bone, tonsil abscesses, dental fistula, indeed for any sort of fistula, Silica is a slow but certain remedy for these problems and it has been known to correct hair and nail problems.

Give Silica to lymphatic-scrofulous children with swollen *glands;* there is no better remedy than this for changing the whole constitution of the child. As a rule these children are thin, or else puffy with a swollen stomach, a very poor appetite, and little stamina as well as a very uncertain disposition.

Those who suffer from *lung problems* and *scrofula* should take Silica with a homeopathic calcium preparation. It is very good for the skin and the connective tissues, and is successful in the treatment of hand and foot perspiration which has an unpleasant odor and causes the skin between the toes to become sore and macerated. Problems arising from suppressed foot sweat can be dealt with satisfactorily by Silica, but it is probable that the sweat will be re-established. This is something to be welcomed of course and should be correctly treated; increase elimination through the skin and the kidneys and in time, foot sweat will disappear without harmful consequences.

People who are always cold and shivery, even when they are active, might try Silica for a couple of months. It will improve oxidation, and their vitality and joy of living will gradually return.

Nodular lumps in the *breast*, even though malignant, will benefit from the continued use of Silica. *Wounds* that refuse to heal will improve if Silica is sprinkled over their surfaces. This external method of treatment has proven its value in *leg ulcers*, but it should be given internally as well. Apart from its medicinal value, women will find that it improves the hair, making it glossy and another plus for Silica is its encouragement and promotion of a clean complexion.

Dosage: Two tablets of the 6x or 12x potency three times daily. Some physicians use 30x with good results.

SEASONINGS

THE ONION (Allium Cepa)

As a food, the onion is known to be rich in Vitamin C, and taken regularly and in small quantities, it is an excellent remedy for the nerves.

Chopped up or grated raw, it is the simplest "drawing" agent readily available. In cases of *headache, toothache, earache, inflammation of the eyes* and especially after a chill, an onion compress on the back of the neck can relieve and very often does disperse the pain entirely.

When a person is feverish with a congested, burning head, an onion compress on the soles of the feet is very helpful; and if the heart is affected, a compress on the calves of the legs will give quick relief, or at least act as an auxilliary to another remedial treatment. For *gout* and *diabetes* as well as for *hardening of the arteries,* the onion as a food is a vital standby.

Homeopathically, Allium Cepa is the best remedy for a running, watery *head cold.* Very often it is effective just to leave a halved onion on the bedside table, so that the odor can be breathed in. Cut a thin slice off every morning and evening and if this does not affect a cure, it will, nevertheless, bring relief.

For flatulent *colic* in the umbilical region and for infants and children who have *bladder cramps* along with a reddish, smarting urine, Cepa is a harmless and reliable remedy. If you do not have extract of Allium Cepa in your medicine chest, cut a thin slice of onion, put it into a glass of warm water for a few seconds, remove, and take a few sips of the water every hour. You will be astonished at the relief this will bring.

GARLIC AND ONIONS (Allium Sativum and Allium Cepa)

Today, if we visit the great pyramids of Egypt, we undoubtedly would be unaware that the overseers of the Pharoahs were not only responsible for the construction of these great architectural masterpieces but additionally they faced the problem of feeding a great army of workmen engaged in the work. Herodotus, the Greek historian, relates that during the time of the building of the Cheops pyramid 1,600 silver talents or about two million dollars worth of garlic, onions and radishes were purchased to support the workers' strength. Garlic and onions were sacred plants to the Egyptians and they attributed all manner of magic skill against machinations of evil spirits to these simple plants. The Greeks and Romans also used the roots for healing. From the Bible we learn of how the Jews gave great prominence to garlic as a cure for many ailments, as they do even today. Perhaps the garlic plant is partly responsible for the endurance and tenacity of this people. These descendents of Shem, as a Semitic race, seem to suffer much less than other races from hardening of the arteries and poor functioning of the lymphatic gland.

Like all foods that have a penetrating smell and a strong taste, garlic should be taken in very small quantities, otherwise it could be harmful, especially to the kidneys. Garlic as well as onions provide an essential oil extract which, when refined, is known to contain glycosides which in turn decompose into sulphur compounds. This etheric, sulphurous oil is without a doubt responsible for the therapeutic effect upon the *skin*, the *scalp* and in particular upon *dandruff* and *falling hair*.

Garlic can be also recommended for the treatment of worms. The basis of this treatment is grated cloves and minced garlic stirred into a half pint of milk. Drink the mixture. This mixture can also be used as an enema. For added strength, you may put the garlic grated into a wormwood infusion and this may be used as a drink or as an enema.

Half a garlic clove placed between the gums and cheek will often take away a *toothache*.

GARLIC MILK

This is an excellent remedy for *sciatic* pains. Also, if taken over a prolonged period of time it will also cure foot perspiration.

A garage mechanic who had suffered from *sciatica* for a considerable time, and for whom the doctor could not offer any help, was advised to drink garlic milk daily. He took the advice and within a few days, the sciatica was greatly relieved. At the end of a fortnight the pain had disappeared completely.

Garlic milk may be prepared cooked or uncooked. In the raw state, uncooked, it has a more potent effect. Cooking lessens the smell somewhat and the effect is still quite good.

To prepare: crush the garlic – there is a garlic crusher available in most department and speciality stores for this purpose – add it to the uncooked milk, or if you wish the garlic may be added to heated milk. To receive the maximum effect, one should drink a half pint of this mixture daily.

Of course, not everyone reacts in the same way and not every remedy produces the same results in every person, but, in the case of a bad *sciatica*, it is well worth giving this simple remedy a trial. According to the individual, one of three different treatments should produce results: formic acid treatment, adjustments by an osteopath or chiropractor, or garlic milk. Since garlic milk is the more readily convenient, why not try it first and if it works you will benefit and save time and money.

HORSERADISH (Nasturtium armoracia) also, (Cochlearia armoracia)

It is a pity that horseradish is so little known and, as a result, its very individual and pleasant flavor is all too often neglected in the kitchen. Did you know that raw carrot salad, which because of its sweetness does not appeal to all palates, can be pleasantly seasoned with a little grated horseradish? Even grated horseradish by itself is a wonderful additional dish on the dinner table.

The healing properties of horseradish are very little known. Curative properties consist of an essential oil, asparagine. In addition to its use in treating *bronchial pulmonary infections,* it is an excellent aid to digestion. Also, in the treatment of *septic wounds* that tend to heal with an ugly scar, which other medicaments have failed to overcome, horseradish tincture is proven to be most excellent. Not only does it give quick relief but also cures completely.

For home use, tincture of horseradish may be prepared in the following manner: grate fresh horseradish, mix with pure alcohol and let stand for a week or so. Then filter it through gauze or muslin. The resulting tincture then can be used on *wounds* as an antiseptic. It will prove to be somewhat "stingy" but nevertheless, effective.

Grated horseradish also can be used in place of onions when those, applied as a poultice, have not had the desired effect as in the case of *headaches,* etc.

Horseradish syrup:

If a *catarrh* does not yield to other treatments, try horseradish syrup. Prepare by adding sugar or honey to the grated horseradish. Mix well and press thorough muslin. The residue should be cooked with a little water and sugar and then added to the previously obtained syrup. This provides a strong remedial mixture. The syrup is also indicated for treatment of *weak lungs, bronchial* and *respiratory* problems.

Always mix a little grated horseradish with your salads. In addition to making the salad taste better, horseradish will reduce your liability to *colds* and *chills.*

For *older people,* horseradish as well as garlic is a most excellent medicine. It regenerates the blood vessels and reduces *blood pressure.* If you are over forty, you should give this serious consideration.

BLACK OR SPANISH RADISH

The radish is the best possible *liver* medicine that you are likely to have about the house. Taken in small quantities, it can relieve certain liver disorders, *gallstones* and many kinds of *digestive problems*.

Radish syrup:

Finely grated radish, sprinkled with cane sugar so that it makes a syrup, provides a good medicine for *bronchial catarrh*. First press the grated radish through muslin and then add sufficient sugar to form a thick syrup. Made this way it should keep for weeks. Take a few teaspoonsful every day. This is inexpensive and a reliable help in the treatment of persistent *whooping cough*, also. For those who do not want to take the time to make the syrup, or those who are unable to obtain radishes, radish syrup can be bought, prepared in much the same way.

In cases of *gall disorders*, 10 drops of raw radish essence in a tablespoon of water, three times a day, are sufficient to give relief. You may use this radish essence for *whooping cough* and *bronchial catarrh* in conjunction with the syrup. Sip throughout the day ten drops in a glass of water sweetened with honey.

VARIOUS REMEDIES AND TREATMENTS

Herbal packs:

Herbs which favorably influence the function of organs when taken as teas, tinctures, extracts, will still benefit us, even if we apply them simply as external packs. Kidney herbs such as Birch leaves, Goldenrod, Horsetail, can be minced and applied to the region over the *kidneys*. These external remedies will favorably add to the effect of the same remedies taken internally.

The lymphatic and blood vessel system especially will benefit from such treatments as sorrel, giant dock and rhubarb leaf packs. They will dissipate swellings and congestions much better than commercial plasters and ointments.

Care must be taken not to employ the leaves of such poisonous plants as Rhus tox. and Belladonna, as they can cause inflammatory conditions of the skin. Poisonous plants, it must be remembered, are safe only in the hands of a professional expert. In the case of the well-known cabbage leaf packs, which are helpful in treating numerous ailments, a strong reaction can easily be controlled by reducing the time the packs are allowed to remain on the affected area.

Cabbage leaf and other herbal packs:

The curative properties of the lowly cabbage are becoming more widely known now, although the use of them is by no means a new idea. Dr. Blanc has written a brochure on the subject and many poor people have benefited by this inexpensive remedy since then.

Alternated with clay packs they have been used with success for *cancerous growths.* It sometimes happens that the condition becomes aggravated at first, but after a while, amelioration usually takes place.

Many a chronic illness can be made to yield with *cabbage* and *clay packs* alternated, and cases are known where the surgeon's knife could be avoided by their use.

Some *skin diseases* clear up when soaked wheat is applied. The wheat is put through a mincer and then mixed with marigold or horsetail tea to make a pulp.

TESTIMONIALS CONCERNING THE EFFECT OF CABBAGE LEAF PACKS

Very often the orthodox doctor goes to no end of trouble to help a patient, but unfortunately, without success. When a simple, natural remedy like cabbage produces a cure, we are astonished at how natural active forces, without depending upon laboriously collected human knowledge, can bring about near miraculous effects.

A 62 year old patient who suffered considerably serves as a good illustration of just one of many interesting cases. An infection was aggravated by eating sprayed cherries and resulted in the development of a small lump on the person's tongue. The doctor removed it with cautery (silver nitrate) and found it necessary to prescribe, in addition, eight days of radium treatments. After three weeks the patient left the hospital with a paralyzed tongue.

After another five weeks had passed, a large swelling appeared on the neck. It seemed like another operation would be necessary to remove it. Discouraged over the prospect of having another operation, the patient kept postponing it. Another eight weeks passed and the pain became so great that the circumstances made another operation out of the question. To treat the ailment 43 X-ray treatments were given. After this treatment, the patient felt weak and thought death was inevitable. At this point the doctors had given up hope of curing her. The wound would not heal and constantly exuded pus. After nine weeks the patient asked to return home from the hospital and her family and relatives continued the treatment. Every ten minutes the dressing on the wound had to be changed and a special ointment applied. But with all this kind attention, the pain could not be relieved.

An acquaintance who had read of *cabbage leaf packs* in my monthly paper "Health News" recommended this treatment and within four days after trying it, the pus was discharging freely and the terrible pain had disappeared. In spite of suffering from chronic constipation and headaches, the patient felt much better and soon was delighted to be well again, after a year and a half of illness. It is hard to believe that cabbage can achieve such success, but it is indeed so, and if this patient had not taken advantage of the treatment, her condition would not have improved at the rate she was going.

Here's another example: A worried mother wrote asking for advice on how to treat her child's swollen neck glands. Having followed the treatment prescribed, this is what she wrote:

"The trouble was soon put right by the remedies and *cabbage compresses.* Cabbage, in general, seems to be a marvelous thing. Our 13 year old son who is 5'10' tall and whose voice has already broken, seemed as though he would not be able to get rid of his cold before he had to go back to school on Monday. He then complained of a really bad *headache* and yesterday afternoon of a pain in and above his right eye. I was afraid of *sinus trouble,* so I put a cabbage compress on his head just above the eyes, and left it on for two hours. Off he went to school and came back cheerfully in the evening, for the pain had completely gone."

It is quite peculiar that the humble cabbage should have such remarkable healing powers and can give such unexpected relief without any side effects or harmful aftereffects. This can be explained insofar as cabbage not only supplies curative elements to the tissues, but also eliminates toxins and other harmful substances from these same affected tissues.

CLAY AS A HEALING FACTOR

From earliest times, clay has been used to cure many ailments and today it is once more finding favor. Among other things, it is particularly recommended as a treatment for *tumors.*

Also, doesn't the account in the Bible book of John tell how Christ used clay to cure a blind man? At John 9:11 the account reads as follows: "He (the blind man) answered and said, A man that is called Jesus made clay and annointed my eyes and said unto me: Go to the pool of Siloam and wash: and I went and washed, and received sight." Even though this may have been a symbolic act, we should not lose sight of the fact that earth or clay was used and that the Teacher of Nazareth surely knew of the healing elements of nature. Primitive people treat many illnesses with clay, veterinary surgeons make use of clay too, beauty specialists recommend it to make women beautiful and wrinkle-free by means of clay facials and sportsmen use it for *strains and sprains.*

A combination of clay and herbs can accomplish many wonderful things. Usually the clay is mixed into a paste, to which the hot herb infusion is added to form a poultice. The poultice is then applied to the affected part of the body. Thus a double-action of clay and herb results in a more potent effect.

If you want to get the best out of a clay treatment, you must be certain that you understand how clay works. There are those who use clay where linseed should be used and this is quite wrong. For instance, *clay* should not be used on a boil to collect the pus and draw the boil to a head. *Hot linseed compresses* will do this job far better, for the action of clay disperses and it never draws or gathers.

Directions for the use of clay

According to the time of the year, clay poultices may be used or applied either hot or cold. Those who are sensitive to cold should use a hot poultice – a hot herb bag may be placed on top of the clay to help retain the heat. The effect of a cold clay pack, if desired, may be modified in the same way.

For a small *clay poultice,* a tablespoon of clay, mixed with a herb infusion to a thin paste, will suffice. Spread the paste about ¼ inch thick evenly onto a piece of gauze or linen and place on the affected part. In cases of inflammation, especially *inflammation of the nerves,* St. John's wort oil mixed with the clay can work wonders and has the added advantage of keeping the poultice soft and easy to remove. Clay, as it dries, becomes brittle and hard and its removal can be unpleasant for those with sensitive skin. In such cases it is advisable to keep the clay moist. It is recommended that the *clay poultice* be applied at night, for then it will not be in the way and will leave one free to go about one's business during the day.

There are certain instances, usually in the case of chronic ailments, where it is advantageous to apply *clay and cabbage poultices* alternately. Since we know that *clay disperses* and *cabbage draws together,* the alternating actions will produce effects similar to those of a counter-irritation. This is often desirable in chronic *rheumatic* and *arthritic conditions.*

Taken internally, clay has a remarkable effect on *diarrhea* and inflammation of the intestinal mucous membranes and whatever medication is taken for these problems, it should be added to the clay water.

Everyone could profit physically with an intestinal cleaning twice a year and the best clay to use for this purpose is the white, sand-free kind, although yellow clay is quite suitable also. Such a course of treatment should last a week at a time.

Choice of herbs

For application to *tumors* an infusion made from Horsetail or Oak bark produces good results when mixed with clay. *Inflammation of the nerves* react favorably to a mixture of Balm and clay; and for *rheumatic problems,* an infusion of eucalyptus, juniper needles or wild thyme with clay is recommended. Never boil these aromatic teas, as their technical description "infusion" means to "steep" in hot liquid.

When ready they should be strained and then mixed with clay. If you infuse the herbs in a little cloth bag, this will be most useful to lay on top of the clay poultice when it is in position. As previously explained this will help retain the heat longer.

THE CURATIVE PROPERTIES OF CHICKEN FAT AND CHICKEN FLESH

The following story confirms the efficacy of an old nature remedy: A woman tried to lift a heavy pot with boiling water from the fire and in doing so, slipped. She sustained scalds and 2nd and 3rd degree burns over a considerable area of her body.

Fortunately, her husband remembered his mother's treatment for all *burns* and *scalds*. She always used raw chicken fat. He proceeded to spread the fat over the parts of the body that had been scalded. The burning pain was relieved and his wife quieted down and was able to sleep that night. Within a few days the pain had completely gone and new skin was forming over the burned area. Not only was the woman's life spared but she was spared much pain. Fresh chicken fat is an old nature remedy and is one of the best treatments for severe burns and scalds.

Another experience with chicken fat is just as interesting: In a lonely farmstead, a young man hurt himself badly while felling a tree. The axe went right into his knee and cracked the knee cap. He dragged himself to the house with difficulty. There was no doctor for miles around and, of course, there was no such thing as a telephone. His father could not think of what to do. Meanwhile the boy's leg had become very swollen and discolored. The lymph glands in the groin swelled and became painful. *Blood poisoning* had set in already.

The mother then remembered that her grandmother had always used chicken fat in such cases. So she killed several chickens and spread the raw fat on the whole leg as quickly as possible. The doctor, whom the family finally succeeded in contacting, could only come the following morning. As a traveling country doctor he did not consider the chicken fat treatment strange and appeared well satisfied with the condition of the boy's leg. He took the patient with him to the hospital for surgical treatment and in a short time the leg was completely healed. The mother was convinced that she had saved the boy's life by rubbing on chicken fat as soon as the blood poisoning became evident.

Some doctors may smile ironically if they were to read of such simple nature remedies. However, they should not forget that these remedies have been known and used for hundreds or possibly a few thousand years as reliable remedies and they have outlasted many a modern day wonder drug which is hailed at first appearance and then discarded later on in favor of another wonder drug. These natural treatments are always near at hand and invariably provide help when other remedies fail, and will continue to do so long after many of the present day products of the pharmaceutical industry have been discarded and forgotten.

Chicken Flesh as a Styptic

No less interesting is the story that a Berlin doctor, who was attached to the famous hospital "Charité", told me. A person suffering from *haemophilia* had to have a small operation and the doctors were worried about stopping the bleeding. A peasant who was a patient in the hospital happened to hear of their anxiety and when one of the doctors passed by his bed, he said in his blunt peasant way: "I know of something that will stop the bleeding and it is better than all the strong smelling ointments in the hospital." The doctor, who had formerly been a country practitioner for many years and had often obtained valuable information from his patients and knew their ways, treated the peasant seriously. "Well, what would you say was good for stopping bleeding?", he asked. "Chicken flesh would help, doctor, but it must be put on absolutely fresh and warm", replied the peasant, and the conversation ended there.

More out of curiosity, but perhaps with a little faith, the doctor got hold of a chicken before the operation. After colloidein injections and everything else had failed to stop the bleeding, as a last resort, he cut a piece of flesh from the chicken, laid it while still warm on the small incision. As if by magic, before the unbelieving eyes of the other doctors, the bleeding stopped!

WHEY CONCENTRATE

Milk has always been regarded as a remedial food and also has been applied externally in the form of packs in cases such as

374

inflammation of the gall bladder. While curd-packs are well known, *whey,* which constitutes the serum of the milk, is the remedy mostly used. It contains most of the mineral nutrients, while cheese, from which whey is derived, is valued chiefly on account of its high protein and fat content. The rennet used in the manufacture of cheese doubtlessly plays an important part in the therapeutic effects of the whey. Milk itself is a whole food which implies that it contains all the necessary elements to sustain life. Among these elements are protein, carbohydrates, fat, minerals, vitamins and trace elements. Since cheese chiefly contains the proteins and fats only, *whey,* the by-product of its manufacture, still has considerable nutritional value.

It is, therefore, of no little wonder that in former times royalty and the famous from France and other countries made special journeys to Switzerland to take the world-renowned "Swiss Whey-cure". Usually the visitors were afflicted with metabolic problems such as obesity, circulatory congestions, intestinal ills, pancreatic deficiencies, etc., although whey-cures were prescribed for a multitude of other conditions as well.

The benefits of whey-concentrate are many. *Digestion* can be greatly assisted if a teaspoon or a tablespoon of whey-concentrate is added to a glass of mineral water. It makes an excellent drink as well. Of course, if you dislike mineral water, ordinary water will do just as well for diluting.

Whey-concentrate appears to regulate the secretion of *gastric acid,* for it reduces an excess of acid and increases its quantity when there is a lack of acid. It also benefits *diabetics* because the lactic ferment stimulates the pancreas. Thus, it is without a doubt one of the best drinks these patients could wish for. Regular use of *whey-concentrate* will lower the *blood sugar* level and, at the same time, reduce the quantity of sugar in the urine. The results are not overnight; it will take several weeks for these effects to manifest themselves, but with patience and persistence a positive change for the better will be realized.

The activity of the pancreas is important in cases of *obesity*, as it influences the fat metabolism and, as in the case of gastric secretions, whey concentrate regulates rather than one-sidely stimulates its function. This implies, of course, that underweight persons will benefit from whey-concentrate just as much as overweight ones, because their powers of assimilation will increase while they drink it.

Whey-concentrate also can be used externally and has proved to be more valuable in the treatment of *pimples, eczema* and *crusta lactaea* than many more expensive preparations. For the most part, eczema can be treated by dabbing on undiluted whey-concentrate solution and the blemish eventually will disappear. At the same time, as a supportive treatment, take whey-concentrate preparation internally, as it will help the success of the treatment.

Externally, *whey-concentrate* preparation can be used as a first aid antiseptic on *scratches, cuts* and small abrasive wounds, for it is a remarkable disinfectant. It is often prescribed by doctors as a throat gargle in the first stages of *tonsillitis*. Also, painting the throat with it can be very beneficial. In fact, if you do this in the early stages, you may well avoid the disease altogether. It has been found to be the best remedy for *mycotic diseases* such as the itching of the skin between the toes and the nails. *Athlete's foot* is one of the most prominent of these diseases. Dr. Devrient of Berlin says that whey-concentrate preparation is the quickest and most reliable remedy that he knows of for these conditions.

Many years ago, I drew attention to my experiences in the treatment of internal and external cancer with whey-concentrate. Frequently, the mere swabbing of external *malignant growths* has proven very effective. I remember very vividly one special case of a cancerous growth on the calf of the leg. When the surgeon had removed it, he told the nurse in attendance that he felt doubtful about the wound healing. We swabbed the wound with a whey-concentrate formula and, to the surgeon's astonishment, it did heal. Other successful treatments have been achieved by giving whey-concentrate preparation orally and locally and I am happy to say that Dr. Kuhl, having made his own experiments, now acknowledges the importance of lactic acid in the treatment of cancer.

Of course, I do not wish to say that these lactic acid preparations are a panacea or universal remedy for cancer, but they certainly have brought the treatment of the disease a step further along the road. Because the whey-concentrate formula has a fairly high percentage of natural lactic acid, it is of immense value in the cancer diet. As a drink, diluted with mineral water, it acts both prophylactically and curatively.

It, therefore, is indeed a great pleasure to see how the experiments and observations carried out over a long period of years and published in our journal are now being confirmed.

The discovery of *whey-concentrate* formula as a successful treatment for all the aforementioned internal and external problems establishes it, beyond a doub¹, as the one thing you should have in the medicine chest if you do not have anything else. It will come in handy more often than you think.

THE POTATO AS A REMEDY

Raw, grated potatoes, mixed with a little milk, are an ideal remedy for the following conditions: retarded healing of *wounds,* wounds that form *"proud flesh"* instead of normal *scar tissue* or secrete obnoxious, putrefying matter, *swelling, bruises, rheumatism of the joints, inflamed muscles* and *inflammation of the periosteum of the bones.*

Potatoes boiled in their skins, mixed with a little raw milk while they are still hot and applied as a *poultice,* are beneficial to those who have a poor reaction to cold applications. Those who benefit from cold packs, on the other hand, should use the raw grated or pulped potatoes.

A remarkable effect can be obtained by alternating three applications on three consecutive days. On the first day, a *potato poultice,* on the second day, a cabbage poultice and on the third day, a clay poultice prepared with Horsetail infusion and St. John's wort oil. If you continue to apply these for some time, even the worse swelling will yield.

Raw potato juice is well known as a treatment for *gastritis*. For *stomach ulcers* drink the potato juice diluted in warm water first thing in the morning. The juice of a small potato will do. If you find it difficult to drink potato juice, add to a warm cereal, taking care not to cook it with the cereal – add it after. Eaten with cereal, its unpleasant taste completely vanishes.

Potato juice and a mild, *fiber free diet* will cure the most stubborn *gastric ulcers,* if attention is given to proper mastication and thorough insalivation of the food one eats.

Old potatoes should have their sprouts carefully removed because they contain a poisonous substance called Solanin. These sprouts should neither be fed to animals, nor used as food or as a remedy.

Potato juice is highly alkaline and is a very effective antidote for *uric acid* conditions such as *rheumatism* and *arthritis*.

COMFREY (Symphytum off.)

A mucilaginous tincture prepared from the fresh root of the Comfrey plant, taken orally, will benefit *arthritic conditions* and *circulatory problems*. It regulates the *blood pressure* inasmuch as it will lower *high* blood pressure and increase *low* blood pressure. More important than its internal, is its external use. Applied in the form of an ointment, a raw pulp, or as a tincture, it will alleviate *gout* and *pains in the joints* which manifest themselves when degenerative changes in them begin to occur, as flexing the joints, when a grating noise can be noticed. Naturally, it is important to adopt a strict diet as well for the cure must, in the first place, come from within, that is from the bloodstream. There is no reason for arthritis sufferers to lose hope if they use Comfrey and plan a well regulated diet. Even if the condition is no longer amenable to a cure, its progress will have been arrested.

Inflammation of the nerves may also be treated with a Comfrey preparation. In fact, wherever there are painful parts in the body, or wherever there is any sensitivity to pressure which manifests itself in the peripheral nerves, Comfrey can be recommended as a simple, natural and successful remedy.

It is extraordinary what a regenerating influence Comfrey preparation has on the skin. *Wrinkles, "crow's feet"* or *aging skin* which has been damaged by chemicals in cosmetics will be regenerated by its continuous use. Within the limitations of age, it is possible to have a firm, youthfully fresh skin. As a beauty treatment, therefore, a Comfrey preparation should have its proper place on the dressing table. It really can be considered as a healing remedy, because true beauty is not just painted on but identifies itself with good health.

Comfrey preparations will have a soothing and healing effect upon *pains in the face,* whatever their origin. *Abrasions and cuts* which take a long time to heal, *blood blisters* and *blood effusions* will respond favorably and benefit greatly from the application of this remedy.

Hypericum Complex taken internally and Comfrey preparation applied externally will produce excellent results in cases of *phlebitis. Open leg wounds* respond to a local application of Comfrey preparation. First, dab the affected part and, if it stings too much, just dab the surrounding area until the pain subsides. Gradually dab the affected area again until the whole area has been covered.

The Components of Comfrey Preparation

To obtain a therapeutically balanced preparation, the fresh plant extract of St. John's wort is added to the Comfrey root. The former extract is well known as a remedy for the blood and for wounds and as such, helps to intensify the effect of Symphytum. Hamamelis and Sanicula have similar therapeutic indications but, unfortunately, the latter herb does not grow in many areas. Goldenrod is another wound herb that contains etheric oils, tannin and saponin, which probably account for its healing action in inflammatory conditions. Arnica, which may be found anywhere in Switzerland at a height of over 8,000 feet, has long been recognized as an aid to heal wounds and bruises and it is mentioned with praise in the oldest of herbal records. *Contusions* with extravasation of blood into the adjoining tissues, is corrected by an extract from the root which will encourage proper capillary circulation. The mucilage obtained from the seeds of the quince is another ingredient of Comfrey preparation. This mucilage is a valued component of good skin preparations and should be properly called an "herbal glycerine", because it regenerates the skin to a remarkable degree. Houseleek, a final composition to Comfrey preparation, is still to be found growing on the roofs of old houses in Switzerland, especially the thatched ones. It may not be a welcome guest today, but in olden times, householders knew how to take advantage of it to cure *inflamed eyes, burns, ulcers* and *wounds,* for which it is known to be a cooling and healing medicine. All these natural remedies combine to make Comfrey preparation a truly remarkable remedy that should be in every medicine chest.

STEAM BATHS AT HOME

Steam baths are useful to disperse *congestions,* to make the *urine flow* again when retention occurs, to relieve *cystitis* (inflammation of the bladder) and similar conditions which are bound to benefit from an improved circulation. Most are easily prepared at home. First prepare a steaming hot infusion of hayflowers, camomile or wild thyme, ready to pour into a large vessel, across which a narrow plank or board has been placed on which you can sit. As steam takes some time to do its work, guard against cold by covering yourself with towels or sheets from head to foot. If the plank is found to be uncomfortable, you might use some sort of wicker chair instead. If you do not have one, it may be possible to cut a hole out of the seat of an ordinary chair so that the steam can rise from underneath. In any event, you must keep your body warm. Keep adding more hot water and herb infusion so that the steam continues to rise. Such a steam bath is very effective, inexpensive to construct, and serves a very good purpose.

HIP-BATHS (Sitzbaths)

Hip-baths are very useful in relieving many ailments, but few people know anything about them such as how they should be taken, what are their effects, and for what conditions they are indicated.

The purpose of a sitzbath is to relieve congestions to which women are especially prone. They usually manifest themselves as *cramp-like conditions* and *venous problems* and a sitzbath is a most excellent treatment for these.

In the course of normal events sitzbaths are usually taken in the evening but urgent cases may call for more frequent applications during the daytime as well. The temperature of the sitzbath should always be about blood heat. If the bath is too hot or too cold it may cause head congestions. In this particular case, cold hip-baths serve purposes other than those we are concerned with here.

The addition of herbs in the form of infusions can be recommended, for it would be a pity to take so much time and trouble to prepare a hip-bath if full use of the other beneficial factors were not taken into consideration. The best herbs to use are hayflowers, wild thyme, juniper needles or eucalyptus leaves. Which ones to use depends on the effects desired. Some of the aromatic herbs are stimulating while others have sedative properties. Lemon balm, for example, will help a patient to enjoy a peaceful night's sleep, while other herbs might make him feel active and lively.

The best vessel to use for a hip-bath is, of course, one specially designed for that purpose. Lacking that, an ordinary bath tub will do but the water should never be allowed to reach above the navel when you are seated. Such a "half bath" does not make one feel so weak as a full bath and it will not harm persons with weak hearts.

A warm room is essential for such a bath. The time spent in it can vary from 15 to 30 minutes and, generally speaking, it is the half hour bath that produces the best results. The water must be kept at the same temperature, accomplished by adding more hot water as necessary. The feet should be kept in the water or, if a smaller vessel does not permit this, the patient should be warmly wrapped with wool blankets.

THE IRON AS A HELP IN NEED

With the help of an ordinary household iron the efficiency of St. John's wort oil can be increased to provide greater absorption by the skin. Neuralgic and rheumatic pains and aches resulting from a chill can be alleviated by rubbing the affected parts with St. John's wort oil or covering them with a piece of cloth that has been soaked in it. A dry cloth should then be placed over the oiled skin or the oiled cloth, and gently ironed over with an iron. If electric, set for "synthetic fabrics", or if it does not have such a marking, set for the lower end of the heat scale so as to avoid a steam burn. The heat of the iron will thin the oil and force its absorption into the pores of the skin thus intensifying its therapeutic effect. But, beware! Care must be taken that relief is not obtained at the price of a burn. Test from the lower settings first and exert extreme caution!

POWDERED LIME-WOOD CHARCOAL

Those who suffer from *gastric acidity* or an infection of the gastric mucous membrane, as a consequence of jaundice or liver trouble, should certainly take this powder in a little milk, as it is very effective and perfectly harmless.

RED SNAIL SYRUP

When in a serious condition, everything else having been tried without success, red snail syrup, however unattractive it may sound, should be considered as a last chance. Diseases in which germs play a part, *ulcers,* (even those of the stomach) and *lung infections,* greatly benefit from it.

Its preparation is simple. Place a layer of red-forest snails in a dish, cover with a layer of sugar, then further layers of snails and sugar until the dish is filled. The sugar should be about the same weight as the snails although you can use a little more sugar. After a short time the sugar begins to dissolve the snails. Then you should add about a third of the dish with alcohol. If this is not enough to dissolve the snails completely, add more alcohol and strain the mixture through a sieve. A tablespoon, or in serious cases a liqueur glass full of the syrup, which by now is indeed very much like a liqueur, should be taken every morning before breakfast. The success of this treatment is so extraordinary that even doctors who have taken the remedy are quite amazed.

Though the preparation and perhaps even the idea of this syrup is rather repugnant, such feelings can be disregarded when grave necessity arises. Peasants, who are less fussy about such things, are very pleased to avail themselves of this remedy. A young farmer who had stomach ulcers and was spitting blood would not consent to medical attention nor take any nature remedies. He did consent, however, to take snail syrup with the result that, today, he is once more able to farm his family property.

Chronic bronchial catarrh also has been cured by this remedy and another example of the wonderful healing properties of this syrup is the story of a man who was suffering from some form of a lung disease. The doctors had despaired of curing him. He tried the snail syrup and in a short time was quite well again. Many other successful examples prove that it is better to take a remedy, the thought of which is revolting, than to accept defeat in matters of health and perhaps even suffer death as a result of neglect. Of course, if you don't know what the syrup is made of, you will not worry at all, for it really doesn't have such an unpleasant taste.

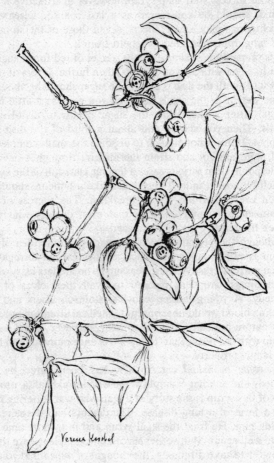

Verena Kimbel

Mistletoe (Viscum album)

NUTRITIONAL QUESTIONS

NATURAL FOOD

It is certainly difficult for a housewife to feed her family along scientific lines, for even an expert in the field of scientific nutrition would find it impossible to prepare a diet which takes into consideration calories, minerals, proteins, fats, vitamins, trace elements, etc. in their individually required amounts and qualities. Theoretically, he may be able to compile a satisfactory diet sheet from his own point of view, but who can assess what each particular individual really needs in the way of nutritional factors?

In fifty or a hundred years from now we could look back at the things we now think of as necessities for our bodies and we would probably be surprised at our ignorance of the elements which go into the making of a healthy diet.

How much simpler it would be if man, instead of letting himself be deceived by all sorts of dietetic adventures that prove disastrous in the end, would accept the idea that a wise Creator has already provided us with all the nourishment we require. If we look upon our food as something prepared for us by Him, for our well-being, then we know we have at our disposal all the known and unknown food elements we need. They will contribute all that is necessary for our bodies.

Primitive people are more sensible than we are in this respect. They take their food just as it grows and prepare it very simply, thus preserving its nutritive value. Doesn't that give our ailing society cause to think on these things? New drugs are being discovered every day, but do we see a decline in the incidence of disease generally? Far from it. Certain diseases are becoming more prevalent than ever, especially those that are connected with metabolism of the cells and the central nervous system. Among the most notable, cancer and multiple sclerosis. These two diseases are practically unknown among the natives of various "uncivilized" societies.

Degenerative changes in the cells of the body occur chiefly among those who live on a denaturalized diet. There are other diseases as well that cannot get a foothold in other countries simply because the inhabitants live more naturally and therefore have sufficient resistance to them.

It is only whole food that offers real sustenance and protection and this is shown by the example that whole rice provides. Everything offered by nature consists of an integral whole and if, through human folly, only a fraction of it is removed, whatever it may be, we are deprived of something that would otherwise provide us with complete health.

WHOLE RICE

Let us look at a rice grain. The inner kernel consists, as in all other grains, of starch. This is turned into the commercial flour we all know. Starch is a carbohydrate and as such, a calorific or heat producing food, without which we cannot live. It would be unwise to throw the starch away and use only the parts of the grain which, as we know, contain elements relatively more valuable than starch. It would be unwise, because the proportion in which starch is associated with other substances is intimately related to the needs of our bodies. To change these would be equivalent to altering the proportions of the ingredients of a perfect recipe. What the result of such an act would be can easily be imagined.

Besides starch, bran is found in the grain; also layers of gluten, various minerals and trace elements. Research has shown that only the most minute amounts of these trace elements are required, yet, if they are missing altogether, serious interference with the various functions of the system takes place.

Another vital part of the grain is the germ. Fats, proteins, phosphates and vitamins are found in it. It is especially the vitamin E in the germ that is of great importance, because it regulates the functions of the sex glands and therefore affects reproduction.

Some may argue that the indigestible residue of the grain, the cellulose, serves no valid purpose and that we could do without it very well. Is this really so? True, it has little food value, but its action, a purely mechanical one, is nevertheless a necessary one for the intestinal tract. It cleanses its lining which is studded with tiny microscopic processes that assist assimilation. These hair like processes are apt to become clogged up if the food ingested consists of too much material lacking in roughage. It is here that the cellulose containing bran comes in. Its particles scrape along the intestinal walls, cleaning away the filmy adhesions and stimulate at the same time peristalsis, the wavelike contractions of the intestines that press their contents onward and so prevent constipation.

The importance of the bran and the germ of the rice has been drastically demonstrated when Orientals began copying the West in refining their staple food, their rice. A disease known as Beri-Beri became rife among them and after all the known medicines had been thrown into the combat against the disease proved useless, a colonial doctor, Dr. Eijkman, discovered that rice bran alone was the only thing that cured the disease. This definitely established the fact that Beri-Beri was a deficiency disease, an avitaminosis.

Fortunately, our diet is much more varied than that of the Eastern nations and such pronounced deficiencies rarely occur, although most of us suffer minor ones which is a good argument in favor of changing over to whole cereals. It is incomprehensible how students who have been shown films and experiments showing what happens to pigeons when they are fed on refined rice, can continue to eat the very food that is responsible for such devastating results. Why spend time in tireless research if the findings continue to be ignored by the consumer?

Natural rice, also known as unpolished, whole, brown rice, contains nine and a half times more minerals than the polished, refined rice. It should be prepared in the same way as the latter, only it needs to be cooked much longer. Ordinary white rice usually requires 15 minutes cooking time, whereas brown, unpolished rice requires 45 minutes to an hour to cook. It should only be cooked in as much water as it requires to soften and absorb, so that the nutritional elements are not wasted or lost. Rice can be served in a number of ways: as a dessert or pudding, as a savory with tomatoes, as a typical Chinese or Arab dish. In fact, there are a number of recipe books on the market that have excellent rice recipes and even one, published by a nationally known brand of rice, has nothing but recipes for different kinds of rice dishes.

WHEAT

What was said about the rice grain also applies to the wheat kernel. Its most valuable constituents are to be found, not in the inner part, but in the outer, the bran. Like rice, the wheat grain should be used in its entirety as flour or flakes, the latter being especially suitable for soups and now used in the internationally known Swiss muesli, a tasty breakfast cereal combination. Although muesli is usually prepared with oats, wheat is just as suitable. It is soaked overnight and then put through a mincer, together with some raisins or sultanas, and this serves as the basis for muesli. Honey, a little lemon juice, ground almonds and a variety of fruit, depending upon the seasonal availability, should be added. Out of season, a variety of dried fruits may be added. Berries are an ideal addition. If one is constipated, mix soaked linseeds into the muesli so as to encourage bowel function.

The best way of using wheat is to keep it moist and warm so it can germinate. When the *sprouts* are about a quarter inch long, the wheat is ready to be used in the same way as you would use the ungerminated one. It is important to remember that germinated wheat should never be boiled or in any other way prepared by heat, because it would lose its health-giving qualities. Eaten raw, in salads, it will build blood and generally strengthen the whole body. For *anemic* persons, germinate the wheat on cloth (muslin or some similar material) exposed to the light, so that the sprouts form chlorophyll and become greenish instead of remaining white.

Bread and cakes should be made from the fresh wheat or any other fresh cereal, for they are far more nourishing than anything made from bleached flour. The oxygen in the air is harmless as long as the grain remains whole, but as soon as it is milled into flour it begins to destroy the highly active ferments. If eaten fresh, raw and if possible germinated, the whole goodness is derived from the grain in its entirety. A sick person derives infinitely greater benefit from the "live" food than from the most expensive medicines and this is proven by the reaction to each.

VEGETABLES

The health value of vegetables depends upon the soil in which they are grown. Sick soil will produce sick plants and if we want healthy vegetables the soil must be restored to its proper health. Much is being taught nowadays about organic farming, biological soil cultivation, compost gardening, biodynamic soil health, etc. so that those acquainted with the principles of organic soil cultivation will know where to buy their vegetables if they cannot grow them themselves. If you live in the country, take advantage of the various edible plants growing wild in the woods and the fields. *Wild leek,* for example, is a prize, because it is one of the best blood purifying vegetables and also regenerates the *blood vessels* and lowers *hypertension. Old age* with its blood pressure problems, brought on by the loss of elasticity of the arteries, can be effectively helped with brown rice, wild leek and mistletoe tea, if taken on a regular basis.

Dandelion salad, so rich in vitamins, cleanses, stimulates and aids the liver to do its job. Every spring this delightful salad should be on the table. To prolong the season, dig up some roots growing wild and plant them in a trench in your own garden. Fill the trench with compost, forest soil and peat and then dress the top with a layer of pine needles. The roots will begin to sprout as soon as the weather turns warm and if you are blessed with a "green thumb" you will doubtless be able to obtain a continuous supply of green or blanched leaves throughout the growing seasons.

Watercress is often found growing wild also. As it is rich in iodine, it will be welcomed by your thyroid and all the other endocrine glands that will benefit from it. Thyroid problems such as palpitations, enlargement of the gland itself, lack of vitality, etc. can be improved with watercress, especially if a little Yarrow and St. John's wort is added to it. The delicate bitter taste of yarrow is by no means unpleasant if it is not used excessively and, with St. John's wort, it is very effective in the treatment of the venous system. The healing plants are so easily collected from the meadows and the woods. Even if one is not troubled by any ailments, these plants should be used as a prevention rather than a cure. If you have a garden area, the cultivating of culinary herbs such as savory, tarragon, thyme, marjoram, sage, chives, dill, lovage and many others will be found most rewarding. Either fresh or dried, they provide welcome changes for the palate throughout the year and they act as immunizing agents to protect us from disease.

MANURING

Manure is an essential part of any healthy garden. Compost, bone meal, forest soil, peat, loam, and stone meal, all can be used, according to your particular soil's need. Artificial fertilizers should be avoided. The keeping qualities and the flavor of produce grown and produced in organic soil is vastly superior to those grown in inorganic fertilized soil. Liquid manure and animal dung should not be applied directly to the soil, but should be incorporated into the compost heap which will improve the quality. The compost heap also will mature quicker, if layers of yarrow or pine needles are used in its construction. After the first year, no new material should be added to the heap; it should merely be turned over to let the air to get at it. Vegetables, which require nitrogen, will do better if the compost has bone meal added to it, while legumes like peas and string beans that are rich in potassium grow better with wood ash compost. If we are to benefit from the minerals in the plants we should avoid boiling them, as the minerals pass into the water which is discarded. It is better to steam the vegetables or, if cooked in water, use barely enough so that hardly any is left when cooking has been completed.

RAW VEGETABLES AND THEIR JUICES

Raw vegetables and particularly their juices possess greater curative value than heat prepared vegetables. Deficient digestion and assimilation require raw juices rather than processed ones. *Cabbage juice,* for example, will improve and often cure such conditions as arthritis, stomach ulcers and metabolic problems. *Raw potato juice* is another excellent remedy for *stomach ulcers* and is excellent when taken in combination with cabbage juice. Raw juices can be diluted with warm water or, if one prefers, they can be added to soups and stews after cooking. Boiled cabbage frequently produces indigestion and flatulence, while raw cabbage will be found to produce no such consequences. White cabbage can be made into Sauerkraut and this should be eaten raw as it tastes better that way and is more healthful. Cabbage is rich in calcium and will overcome this body deficiency.

Although juices are excellent curative agencies, they should not be taken exclusively, as our digestive tract also requires cellulose if it is to remain in proper working order. Juices are potent and as such should not be taken in excessive quantities over long periods of time. Raw vegetables demand good teeth and should be thoroughly masticated and properly insalivated which promotes half the digestive process. The fibers and cells must be broken down if they are to release their nutrients. The reason why many people cannot tolerate raw vegetables is, not that they are indigestible, but that they have not been properly masticated and insalivated. Acid fruit juices need to be neutralized by the alkaline saliva first, before they reach the stomach. Vegetable juices, at least most of them, are alkaline in themselves, and can be more easily tolerated. Liver and kidney patients usually have little difficulty in digesting vegetable juices.

A GOOD NATURAL DIET

A good natural diet consists partly of cooked and partly of raw foods. Cancer and similar constitutional diseases require an almost exclusive raw food regime, because this is the only measure that will get to the root of these pathological problems.

Those who have lost the ability to digest and assimilate raw foods should begin with small quantities of raw juices first and gradually increase them. Then start taking small amounts of finely grated raw vegetables and fruit. Increase the intake of these until you are once more able to eat the foods in their natural state. If there is no need to change over to an exclusive raw food diet, nevertheless, it would be beneficial to incorporate small quantities in your daily meals.

Vegetables and fruits should not be served at the same meal, but be taken separately. If you break this rule you are likely to be bothered with flatulence, although nutritional experts like Dr. Bircher-Benner of the famous Zurich Clinic do not consider it a major mistake. Experience has proved that most people will do better if they keep these two foods apart. Our taste buds would hardly find a mixture of radishes and strawberries acceptable! Cereals, organically grown and stone ground if possible, are good companions to both fruit and vegetable dishes.

MILK

When milk is free from impurities, it is a valuable food. Since, however, there are many sick cows and since the main cause of the sickness is tuberculosis, milk cannot be recommended without reservation. In cases of cancer, arthritis and many other serious illnesses, it is better to avoid milk altogether.

Good milk provides valuable proteins and fats. The question as to whether one should drink it sour or sweet has never been solved; some say one thing, some another. There is obviously more nourishment in fresh, raw milk direct from the cow. Sour milk has lost the milk sugar which, through fermentation, has been transformed into lactic acid. Although of reduced calorific value, sour milk is nevertheless easier to digest and more beneficial to the intestinal flora which it regenerates. From this it will be seen that both kinds of milk have their advantages.

EGGS

Eggs should come from healthy, naturally fed, free running poultry. Eaten raw, they are more healthful than any other way. Since it is quite possible that eggs contain infectious agents, great care should be taken in choosing one's supplier. Duck eggs are known as carriers of the infamous paratyphoid bacillus, although the hens themselves may appear to be quite healthy.

Eggs, however, are rich in lecithin, which is a nerve food. They can be beaten raw into soups after cooking or mixed with honey or some other natural sugar and eaten in this way. The yolks are rich in protein and it is here that most people make the mistake of assuming that it is found chiefly in the egg white. This applies particularly to German speaking people, whose language promotes the perpetuation of this mistake, as "egg white" is known as "Eiweiss" in German which also means "protein".

Eggs, unfortunately, have the disadvantage of being the cause of the formation of uric acid. This gives rise to the release of sulphuric acid, which can be noticed in the breath after one has eaten boiled eggs. Persons with arthritis, cancer or rheumatism should abstain from eggs in all forms.

CHEESE

Cheese is rich in protein and fat but does not really belong to the category of natural foods, because it does not contain all the elements of the milk from which it is made. Cheese cannot be recommended without discrimination to everyone because it is such a highly concentrated food. In Switzerland and Holland where great amounts of cheese are manufactured and consumed, the incidence of arterioslerosis and cancer is high. If, for reasons of health, you have to adopt a special diet, you will do well not to include cheese in it. Laborers doing heavy manual work can eat cheese with greater impunity than those with sedentary occupations.

MEAT

Meat has universal appeal and, providing it is fresh, can be called or classed as a natural food. Veal and beef are probably best, while pork, sausages, tinned and otherwise, should be shunned. Saltpetre (sodium nitrate) is used as a preservative in most canned meats and also to give a red color to the meat and the result is anything but healthful. The same applies to smoked meats which contain certain amounts of harmful phenols and other poisons. For cancer patients, meat is prohibited in any form, and should be avoided.

SUGAR

Beware of white refined sugar which is bereft of all mineral salts and invites kidney diseases. It upsets the mineral balance in the system and particularly calcium. It has been declared, quite mistakenly, that brown cane sugar contains sulphur and after all the trouble that has been taken to introduce it into a healthy diet, this mistake should be rectified. A superior sugar is found in the sweet fruits, such as raisins, currants, dates, apricots, pears, etc. and these are the fruit sugars that should be used to sweeten all foods. Care must be exercised, though, as many commercially distributed dried fruits have been sulphured and otherwise treated which is a danger that must not be overlooked. Read the labels carefully and they will tell you whether the fruit is naturally dried or if it has been sulphured. Dried fruits that have a dark color usually are not sulphured while those with a bleached appearance or a lighter color are suspect. The best sugar is found in and obtained from grapes. However, not everything sold under the name of grape sugar or dextrose is the genuine sugar obtained from grapes. More often than not it is a synthetic product possessing the chemical formula of grape sugar, but not its therapeutic and nutritional qualities and properties. It is manufactured by hydrolysis, not from grapes, but from maize or corn starch and even from wood and other similar sources. That such an imitation, however perfect from the chemical point of view, can have little in common with the original article, is obvious.

HONEY

The energy contained in honey is illustrated in the Bible record in the case of King Saul's son, Jonathan. Thoroughly exhausted from battling the enemy he saw some honey and tasted it and immediately his eyes "began to beam".

It is extraordinarily interesting to study how that little wonder, the bee, makes its honey. We marvel too at the diligent industry of the bee as we watch its flight over the flowering countryside, but it is not this which I wish to speak about right now. Our interest, at the moment, lies in the remedial and nutritional value of honey, which earns for itself a high mark in natural medicine. In days long past honey was well known for its healing properties and as time passed on they were forgotten. The rediscovery and scientific explanation of the value of honey, however, enables it once more to assume its place among natural remedies that it formerly occupied. A doctor writes in a medical journal about having successfully used honey in the treatment of diphtheria. A 25% addition of honey to another remedy proved antiseptic and prevented the diphtheria bacilli from propagating.

Honey plays an important part in the dietary approach to *hay fever*. Years ago, country folk recommended eating honey and also chewing the honeycomb. The scientific explanation accepted today is that the benefit received was probably from the pollen in the honey and the wax. Now on the market and available in the health food stores is an ample supply of *bee pollen* for which many other things are claimed. There is no doubt that honey does have curative powers or properties and the Bible mentions it as a source of "healing to the bones".

Dr. Muller asserts that potential carriers of the diphtheria bacillus can render themselves much less dangerous to their environment by the systematic consumption of honey. "Carriers" are those who harbor the micro-organism of a disease, but are not necessarily affected by it themselves, although they constitute a source of infection for others.

CANNED FOODS

Foods, canned or tinned, cannot be recommended under any circumstance, if the fresh equivalent is available. They have received so many chemical additions, have been deprived of most of their health-giving elements, that there is no place for them in a natural diet.

Home canned foods are probably less harmful and can be tolerated when there is no availability of fresh foods and thus they would be a supplement to the usual fare.

SPRAYED FRUIT

There is very little that can be said in favor of sprayed fruit. It may be poisoned with lead, arsenic and other chemicals so as to make it inedible. It can cause serious upsets to the body, although it need not necessarily bring on an acute case of poisoning. Chemical insecticides may be cumulative and small but continuous doses, sooner or later, can lead to pathological conditions.

If in doubt, in any case, fruit purchased in the market should always be properly washed and cleaned and it is a good idea to peel the fruit if spray spots can be seen. Many fruit orchards are sprayed with chemicals to which have been added a substance with a special adhesive property so that the rain cannot wash the spray off the fruit.

Very valuable elements are found in and under the peel and, therefore, it is much better to exercise discrimination as to where you buy your fruit and look for those organically grown, if at all possible.

CONDIMENTS (Seasonings)

Among these, nutmeg and pepper should be avoided and their place taken by natural health-promoting herbs, vegetable extracts, and most importantly, yeast extract. As a pure culture, yeast extract is about the best you could use, for it tastes pleasant and is rich in vitamin B-complex. It can be used in various ways, as a sandwich spread, as an addition to soups and stews, but it should never be boiled.

A PRACTICAL HEALTHFUL DIET

By this time it should be self-evident to every reader that a practical, healthful diet should consist of natural foods in their natural state. Various ailments will disappear without medication of any sort, if we feed our bodies in the proper manner. One does not have to be a learned dietician to realize that the "divine recipe" embodied in every fruit of the earth cannot possibly be improved upon by man if it is to remain a health-promoting food. If we contemplate on the unhealthy state of mankind in the civilized world, we must conclude that he apparently thought himself wiser than the Creator by changing, refining and otherwise adulterating the food that was offered him in the most perfect condition possible.

A Protein-restricted diet

This is of paramount importance in all metabolic and digestive disturbances, in *arthritic* and *gout* conditions. This diet should be adopted for some time, at least, until it has accomplished its purpose. Protein is found chiefly in meat, eggs, cheese, milk and milk products, peas, beans and lentils. Vegetarians also should reduce the intake of milk products and legumes. Those having previously enjoyed a mixed diet ought to refrain from eating pork and sausages and restrict the diet to beef and veal. Eggs may be eaten raw, but arthritics who suffer from an excess of uric acid would be better off leaving them alone. Women whose ovaries function inadequately may take raw eggs in moderate amounts.

Much better than cheese is curd, known as cottage, soft or white cheese, because it has none of the disadvantages of other high protein foods and additionally assists the function of the liver.

One should avoid high protein foods for the evening meal because they usually are the cause of a restless sleep during the night. The same applies to dinner which should not be served in the evening but at midday, as it consists generally of foods that require longer periods for digestion than breakfast or tea.

FRIED FOODS

These are responsible for sclerotic and liver disorders and should have no place in a sensible, healthy diet. Although vegetable oil may be better tolerated in frying, it is the animal fat that is so detrimental to health. If you must fry, use soy, safflower, nut or olive oils, never animal fat oils.

DIET SUGGESTIONS

To impose no burden upon your system and support any treatment you may be taking for the good of your health, you would do well to conform as far as possible to the following suggestions:

Breakfast: Bircher-muesli consisting of soaked, raw or germinated wheat, fruits that may be seasonally available, dried fruit, honey, lemon juice, grated nuts or ground almonds. A level teaspoon of ground linseed can be added, if constipation is a problem. Whole grain or crisp bread with butter, nut-butter, honey or rose hip conserve sprinkled with wheat germ (which can also be added to the muesli) can be eaten after the muesli. For a drink make a cup of rose hip kernel tea or cereal coffee. For a sweetener use honey or grape sugar and top your drink with cream rather than milk because it contains more fat than protein. For a liver patient, milk or almond milk will be found to be more tolerable.

An occasional fruit juice breakfast is beneficial and grape, orange, or grapefruit juice can be recommended. Grapefruit juice is especially good because it stimulates the kidneys, the liver and the glandular system.

Impeded liver function can be assisted with raw carrot juice and wheat germ sprinkled between a butter-crisp bread sandwich. This would of course take the place of the muesli. If this does not satisfy, sandwiches listed under "supper" can supplement this kind of breakfast.

Dinner: Depending upon the season, a great variety of salads may be served. The dressing may be prepared with *whey* concentrate or lemon. Whey concentrate is a great aid to digestion and should be given first consideration, but never use *vinegar.* Another tasty dressing can be made with sour cream or *yogurt* and herbs such as savory, marjoram, thyme, parsley may be added to give a zesty flavor to any one of the dressings. Cabbage, in any form, is best eaten raw in a salad because cooked cabbage causes flatulence. Cabbage salad is not only well tolerated, but it is also very healthful and should be on the menu often.

Some starch containing food should follow the salad. From a dietetic point of view, rice is the best. It has a good effect on the blood pressure and helps to regenerate the veins. For variation, substitute potatoes, cooked in their skins, either boiled or baked. Potatoes can be harmful to the liver when fried and should be avoided. Whole wheat also provides an excellent dish and should be prepared like rice. Other carbohydrate foods that are good are millet and buckwheat.

Those who like soup should have vegetable soup mildly flavored. Meat soups are not particularly healthful for they promote uric acid in the system and really should not be considered in the normal diet. Vegetable soups, on the other hand, are very healthy for sufferers of arthritis. A really delightful soup can be made from fresh herbs, raw vegetable juices and raw vegetables finely grated. Finely chopped nettles, wild leek and other health herbs will improve the taste of the soup.

For those who like meat, beef or veal may be added to whatever dish they have chosen but this should be considered as just a small addition to the main meal, for it is best to restrict oneself to a minimum of the protein containing foods.

A sweet course or dessert has no place in a health diet because it encourages fermentation. If you cannot overcome your desire for fruit or some other naturally sweet food after the dinner, postpone eating it until at least four o'clock in the afternoon. It is better, however, not to make a habit of such in-between-snacks because it is better to eat little rather than much food. A small amount of good food goes a long way towards good health.

Slow eating and thorough insalivation enables you to obtain the maximum value from your food; it prevents the pancreas from being overburdened and the formation of intestinal gases.

In place of soup, substitute vegetables juices or natural unsweetened yogurt. Sugar or fruit juices do not go well with the lactic acid of yogurt. If you wish to increase your weight, by all means take the soup.

Supper: I would call the evening meal supper rather than dinner, and this meal should be light instead of heavy. A light meal will be well digested before it is time to go to bed. This evening meal may be the same as breakfast, but it does not have to consist of sweet dishes and fruit, although a fruit salad makes a pleasant change, especially if served with any of the whole cereal breads. A good mixture is one made from ordinary oat flakes with currants and chopped nuts and fruit, although these last should not be too heavily indulged in, especially at the end of the day. True, they are nourishing, but the sooner one learns to be moderate in his diet, the better his body will feel. If you tire of ordinary nuts, for a change, have you ever considered pine kernels; they have a very pleasant taste and are a welcome change. Crisp bread and whole grain bread with a little butter or nut butter is a good companion for fruit salad, but if you have a problem with your liver, consider using honey or rose hip puree instead of fats.

As a change from fruit, a meal of sandwiches followed by a salad can be very good. If you wish to drink something with it, have some cereal or fruit coffee with cream or milk. Liver patients should have a glass of carrot juice instead.

Sandwiches: These can vary considerably. Use whole grain bread or crisp bread lightly spread with butter and then with yeast extract, some good vegetable extract or perhaps a mild curd cheese. According to the foundation of the sandwich one can make a variety of additions such as chives mixed with curd or, if you like garlic, mince it and spread it on the buttered bread. Garlic, chives and watercress go very well together in making a tomato sandwich and so will finely chopped onion in place of the garlic. Grated carrot and horseradish also make a tasty sandwich. Radishes, too, are a welcome addition to the spring sandwich menu, but they should be used sparingly because they are quite strong and can overstimulate the liver. Small cucumbers are delicious in a sandwich as well as tomatoes, which enrich the meal with many vitamins.

General Advice

A health diet should always be so arranged that it does not cause unnecessary disturbances to the system. This can easily occur when an over-enthusiastic person attempts to hurry things up and to overdo a good thing. Special attention to the requirements of the individual organs should also be taken into account. The liver and the pancreas cannot tolerate an excess of fats or sweets, the kidneys revolt against too much salt and other sharp condiments and similar factors have to be considered in respect to other organs.

In the case of salt, it has been shown, that sea salt is vastly superior to mined stone salt because unrefined, it contains many of those substances and trace elements which are naturally found in a healthy bloodstream. And if the sea salt is further enriched with herbs, then a condiment results which is without parallel for seasoning. For those who have catarrh or similar infections, there is a sea salt made that is enriched with eight different antibiotic fresh plants, which produces similar effects to those of penicillin without the danger of the body becoming resistant to it or causing damage to the intestinal flora. As in all cases of herb seasonings, they should never be boiled in the preparation of the food but should be added when the cooked food is taken off the fire. Boiling will destroy the majority of the active ingredients of this seasoning.

By using sea salt with fresh plant mixtures one has, not only a good flavoring, but a reliable prevention against internal problems. Of course, sea salt should be used in small quantities and those who suffer from nephritis or cardiac problems should not ever use the sea salt.

402

Strong seasonings should be reduced to a minimum. This does not mean to say that food should be dull or tasteless. Far from it. If vegetables are steamed instead of boiled, they retain all their rich flavor and by making use of the many kitchen herbs that are at our disposal, the palate will have no reason to fault the taste of the food.

That salads should not be salted goes without saying. As suggested elsewhere, lemon juice or whey concentrate are excellent for making the dressing. By adhering to a correct diet we can do much to help whatever natural remedy we may be taking to achieve success. There is little point in swallowing medicines or taking water treatments if, at the same time, we pay no attention to the food we are eating. Actually, our diet should be the first thing to come under consideration since it is useless to take remedies to cure, for example, uric acid, if at the same time we encourage its formation by eating eggs and other concentrated protein foods. It is senseless to take kidney and blood purifying teas and steam baths to eliminate metabolic waste from the system, if we continue to live on the diet that is responsible for our problem at the same time.

Manure is for the plant what food is for man. If the manure is of the wrong kind, lush growth may occur in the corn fields, but no grain will be forthcoming. If we eat the wrong kind of food we may become heavy and perhaps appear strong, but in reality we would become weak and without energy. Food has only one purpose – to sustain life and health. Therefore we should eat to live and not live to eat. What, in the past, we have eaten for no better reason than that it was pleasant to the palate, must, in the future, be considered from the point of view of food's purpose. It is in this way only that we can expect to benefit to the fullest from the food we eat. It is only with persistence that health can be achieved, for it required equal persistence in the wrong kind of eating to make disease possible. We should all remember that health does not depend upon our physician but to an equal degree upon ourselves. To a larger degree we are our own doctors and in the final analysis we are what we eat.

FASTING

One of the best remedies to maintain general well-being that is at our disposal is fasting. If we do not feel well because we ate too much, if our stomach is disturbed because we have eaten unsuitable food resulting in sickness or diarrhea, then fasting is a most natural remedy. Under a similar situation our domestic animals have more sense than we do; in such situations they refuse all food. Dogs and cats usually eat grass, so as to bring up the mucus and follow this with at least a day's fasting. Animals know they must not eat again until they feel well. Instinct tells them. These natural health regulations are followed even more closely by wild animals. They, too, know of no special remedy beyond fasting if they are ill. They just lie down in the shade and rest and fast until they feel well again.

When a person fasts the body has an opportunity to rid itself of harmful metabolic accumulations. From time to time it is a good idea to plan ahead to have a fruit juice day and follow this by two days of taking only water. But, before beginning the fast, make sure the bowels are empty. Linseed or a herbal laxative will help make this possible. Or perhaps you prefer to use a camomile enema. If you have no liver problem you can now begin the fruit juice fast either with orange, grape or grapefruit juice. During the berry season you can add berry juice to the list. Any waste left in the body will thus be disposed of and your organs will begin to function better. Should you begin to feel sick during the fast, you will be well advised to speed up the elimination by encouraging skin function – cold friction baths will open the pores of the skin and stimulate circulation, while deep breathing exercises will likewise help. Short walks in the woods and along country lanes will soon restore a feeling of health and well-being.

If you get very hungry, chew a few raisins slowly and thoroughly. The Bedouins wandering in the desert can live for days on a few dates, because they get the fullest value out of this humble meal by chewing thoroughly and thus predigesting it properly. In the same way we can help ourselves during our period of fasting. Spit out the skins of the raisins and just make good use of the grape sugar.

Never enter upon a fast while disturbed or worried about the outcome of some problem of a personal nature because, fasting and worrying do not go together. You should be in a reasonably happy frame of mind, undisturbed and calm. Happiness is a natural medicine that stimulates the endocrine glands and keeps them at the peak of their efficiency. This is one reason why the increasing tempo of modern life with all its problems and worries can damage our health to a great extent. For how long should one fast? That should be determined by the needs of the individual. Two or three days should be sufficient; but, having gone beyond the third day, it is perhaps a pity to stop, when the most difficult time is behind us. The first three days are like climbing a mountain with all its initial difficulties. Having scaled the most difficult part, the worst is over and the going becomes easy. An eight day fast, taking only fruit juice, will provide a complete spring clean-up for your body, but if you suffer from arthritis you will find it necessary to continue the fast for another week or even longer.

Remarkable men like John the Baptist, and a still more remarkable person, Christ himself, fasted; not perhaps to cleanse their bodies, but certainly to achieve the utmost mental concentration. According to the Scriptures, Christ fasted for 40 days. Of course it would be quite unlikely that anyone could better that record, nor should he try to. However, it is a well known fact that, when great demands are made on the mind, fasting will help to make one's thoughts crystal clear, one's understanding precise and accurate. A modern day example is that of Mahatma Ghandi who made some of his most profound observations while fasting.

People who suffer from Basedow's disease (exophthalmic goiter) or tuberculosis should not undertake to combat these two diseases by fasting. Such a course would definitely be harmful. Be very careful, therefore, about recommending a fast to others, just because yours was successful and led to better health. A long and complete fast might prove dangerous to people with certain types of heart trouble, although drinking fruit juice would make it less strenuous, because the body is being nourished to a certain extent while the work of cleansing is going on. If a liver disorder is suspect, take vegetable juices rather than fruit juices. Carrot juice is particularly good in such cases. But, each case, as we see, should be considered individually and in some emotional cases it may not be advisable at all.

When on a fast, if using medication, take a third or even a quarter of the normal dose of any remedy. Your system, in the process of being cleansed, already works more efficiently and will respond to medicines much more promptly than usual.

During the fast it is necessary to attend to the normal rhythm of movement and take adequate rest. Avoid extremes in one direction or the other. For instance, do not spend your days on the couch or bed, in the mistaken belief that you must conserve your energy while not eating. On the other hand, do not enter into strenuous sports or extra hard work either, just because you feel new life and vitality streaming into you, as is quite likely to happen after a week or more has passed. This may sound ridiculous to the uninitiated, but it does happen in many instances. The point that is being stressed is that, while fasting, lead a life of moderation in all things, except eating.

"FATTENING-UP" METHODS

Although it should be sufficiently well known today that fattening-up procedures are anything but sensible, and contrary to the findings of modern nutritional research, they are still occasionally recommended. Lymphatically affected children with swollen tonsils and shadows on their lungs are overfed during their stay in our mountain health resorts to such an extent that upon returning home they complain of excessive tiredness and occasionally succumb to jaundice or some liver trouble. The increase of weight by means of milk, butter and rich foods is no longer the accepted procedure of the progressive physician, by which he assesses the health of his patient. The stuffing regimen gives rise to something like an optical illusion. Fat, solid bodied children somehow create the impression of being in the best of health. That this isn't always so is borne out by past experience and common knowledge. Excessive feeding usually affects the liver because the diet contains too much fat. This in turn leads to other metabolic disturbances which in the end have to be reassessed and corrected by a more sensible diet. Stuffing may be all right for the geese of Strasbourg to provide pate de foie gras for the epicure's table, but it has no place in the fattening-up of children or adults for that matter. The resistance to infection is nearly always lowered after such a feeding process and, all in all, nothing is ever gained by it.

HOW MUCH FOOD DO WE NEED?

I have often been asked how much a grown-up person should eat. Should one accept the system of calories as a measure of one's need or should one use another measuring stick?

Like most systems, reckoning in terms of calories is not the ideal system, and, therefore, should be considered as a purely theoretical guide. An exact system of calculation is not possible since one's need for food depends on so many different conditions that the adoption of a strict and definite system can do more harm than good. Weight plays an important part in determining how much food one should eat. Theoretically speaking, a stout person should require more food than a slim one. It is possible, however, that the thin person has a more vital nature and burns up more energy than the fat, placid, calm man, and in this case our system already ceases to work.

A happy, jolly type needs less food than a discontented, unhappy person, because cheerfulness leads to better glandular functioning and consequently to better digestion and improved assimilation. In other words, the happy person gets more out of his food than the other type. There is much truth in the saying, that one does not live on what one eats but on what one digests.

Someone who works in the garden with a spade and a fork needs different food than someone who sits in an office all day. Climate must be considered too, according to whether one lives in Sweden, Switzerland, South Africa or California or the West Indies. One's need will change from the point of view of climate, quality and quantity. On no account should one depend on a system that will probably change like the whim of a fashion. The only reliable guide is furnished by the body itself. Its demands in terms of likes and dislikes will automatically change with circumstances. I fared well by listening to its voice when I lived in the temperate zone of tropical lands. The underlying principle is that if you take care to eat only natural foods – wherever you are – you cannot go far wrong. You will know when to eat, when to drink and when to stop, if you follow your inner urges and interpret them correctly. In this manner you will develop those finer instincts which nowadays only the primitive races possess. A mineral or vitamin deficiency will automatically give rise to a desire for foods which contain these missing elements. That such a "system" is superior than any invented by man need hardly be emphasized.

OUR BREAD

Bread has always played an important part in the nutrition of man and his age old request, "Give us this day our daily bread" illustrates to what extent he depends upon it. We may have an abundance of other foods, but bread still remains the foundation of our diet. How much we disliked having it rationed out to us during the World War years. Things have changed since then and a large part of the population is once again eating the snowy loaf of commerce that goes under the name of bread, much to the disadvantage of our health.

Real Bread

It has always pleased me when, here and there, on my travels, I have been served with bread as it was once made in my own country, from the whole grain. I found that the Red-Indian women prepared their bread from grain that they had ground themselves with a stone mill. Arabs, Berbers and other African people, also the hill peasants of Greece, still retain the custom of making their bread from whole grain. Some use wheat, some, rye, others, barley and each of these breads tastes good and provides the body with all the goodness of whole grain. It is because cereals contain the majority of the elements needed for the construction and preservation of the health of the organism. They abound in minerals, ferments (enzymes), vitamins and other life-giving nourishment.

Wherever you find good whole grain bread, you will find that the health and resistance of the people consuming it, is higher than those living on white bread.

One cannot imagine Ruth (of Bible fame) having gleaned the valuable ears of corn from Boaz's field, only to turn it into refined flour. The Bible states that she ground the whole corn in a stone mill, added honey to it and made cakes from it.

Correct Baking

We know from the history of ancient Rome that the legions were issued a certain quantity of wheat every day. Wheat can be kept almost indefinitely without losing any of its value, but this is not the case with flour. As soon as the external sheath has been broken and the grain has been milled, the oxygen in the air begins to take effect, and the longer the flour is kept, the more it will lose of its value. The enzymes are probably the first to suffer from such exposure. These are active ferments like, for example, diastase that comes to life during the process of germination and changes the starch of the grain into sugar. An interesting observation will illustrate this. Make freshly ground cereal into dough and knead this well with your hands. You will notice that the hands become quite red as hyperaemia is produced. It is the active ferments that are responsible for this and they are found only in the bran and the germ. If you make dough from the same flour that has been stored for some time, this reaction will no longer occur to the same extent, if at all, because the enzymes have died off during the long storage. That is why it is better to use a stone mill for grinding, mix and bake immediately. Thus the value of the enzmes will be preserved and the bread will be more nourishing.

The Milling Process

The manner in which wheat is ground is quite important. Some time ago I visited an old miller, who showed me an ancient stone mill beside the beautiful new machines he had just bought to replace it. Without my saying anything and before we had a chance to discuss the matter, the miller began to tell me that his old mill had produced really good flour, while the other two modern machines seemed to take all the goodness out of the grain. At first I thought this was rather exaggerated, but in the light of subsequent observations I was forced to agree with him.

The ancient Romans who knew something about metallurgy were certainly in a position to make metal rollers or discs, if they had not been convinced that the use of stone was more advantageous. Every metal mill, if it develops too much friction heat, does something detrimental to the flour which ultimately is reflected in its taste. It is not unusual for metal to do this. It is known that copper destroys most of the vitamin C in the food that is brought into contact with this metal. Similar effects take place with other materials such as aluminium. Thus it is understandable how metal mills could affect the taste or composition, or both, of whole grains after processing.

SOLUTION OF THE BREAD QUESTION

All these considerations urged me to find a solution to the bread question which would comply with all the things I have mentioned. With the help of a master baker, I have carried out experiments on bread baking for six months. I decided to use not only wheat, but also rye, on account of its rich flourine content. As a rule, the bread we eat is mainly made from wheat, but rye is particularly important for the teeth and bones. In the Swiss canton of Valais, where much rye bread is eaten, good teeth and excellent bone formation stand out as a characteristic among the people. Rye is the main grain of the people of Northern Europe, especially Scandinavian countries, and it is the principal cereal of the Russians. Good bone formation and good teeth are notable physical attributes among these people.

On the other hand, wherever white bread is now consumed, deficiencies have developed to such an extent that dental caries and other ailments affecting the teeth and bone structure are very much in evidence. On account of the definite link between white bread consumption and poor dental health, I decided to bring out a natural bread that can be compared favorably with the one eaten by primitive people or races. This bread is called "Flake bread" and contains 80% rye, 20% whole wheat to which has been added rice bran because of its richness in vital mineral elements. Unfortunately, for the most part, we are used to refined rice instead of the whole brown rice and it is advantageous to increase the efficiency of the bread with the latter.

It is too early to assess the effects of "flake bread" but it is being consumed extensively in Switzerland, Holland, Germany, Austria and Australia. It is reasonable to assume that those who consistently eat this bread and at the same time follow a natural diet of healthful foods will eventually benefit from it. It is important to remember that nature does not work according to the dictates of our palates, our moods and our appetites, but rather according to its eternal laws.

RAW JUICES

While living in New York for a short time during 1950, I used to drink freshly squeezed orange juice regularly at the same "health bar". Whenever I went there I was amazed to find Americans drinking cabbage juice from enormous glasses. I had known, of course, of the benefits of raw *cabbage juice* in certain disorders for a long time, but I also knew that it was a rather unpalatable drink. Later I came across an article in the Toronto Magazine Digest which extolled the virtues of cabbage juice in the treatment of *gastric ulcers*. Dr. Garnet, the author, based his article upon experiments with Vitamin U (U standing for Ulcer) which, according to him is probably responsible for the curative effects of this juice. He may not know that raw potato juice is even better and quite likely he would find Vitamin U in it as well. Another researcher advances Ragnar Berg's explanation. He asserts it is the alkaline properties of raw juices that neutralize the free acids in the system and so establish the condition for a successful treatment of many ailments including gastric ulcers.

Empirical Knowledge

It is not so very important to know exactly how a cure takes place. The mere knowledge that juices can cure is infinitely more valuable than any scientific explanation advanced in this connection. Science, after all, only confirms the discoveries made decades ago. These cures existed but had to wait until man discovered them, bearing out wise Solomon's observation that "there is no new thing under the sun". About 55 years ago, as a young man, I lectured upon this subject and drew attention to the value of raw juices without, however, succeeding in convincing the audience. Today it is easier to convince because science has, in the meantime, confirmed our assertions of the past. It is and will remain a fact that raw potato juice and cabbage juice will heal *gastric* and *duodenal ulcers*.

Even more interesting is the observation I made in connection with raw potato, cabbage and carrot juice in the curing of gout, rheumatism and allied conditions. If these juices are taken in conjunction with a strictly natural diet, most of the diseases will eventually yield to this treatment.

412

A Special Diet

Before breakfast take half a glass of raw potato juice diluted with warm water. The breakfast itself should consist of whole wheat that has been soaked in water for two or three days. It can be made more palatable with the addition of a good vegetable stock or butter. Crisp bread with butter and wheat germ will complete your breakfast. If the *bowels* need special attention, add psyllium or freshly ground linseeds to the wheat. If the liver isn't functioning properly, drink a glass of raw carrot juice. Chew all food and insalivate it thoroughly. Lunch: A good, strong vegetable soup with a cup of raw cabbage juice added, after the soup has been taken off the fire. Then a dish of unpolished rice, whole wheat, buckwheat or millet, steamed vegetables and a salad. Never use vinegar to make your salad dressing. Use lemon juice, sour milk or whey concentrate instead. If you feel nervous and tired out, take a beaten raw egg and add it to your food every second day. On no account should the eggs be cooked because this would destroy most of their vitamins and, in addition, lead to uric acid. Only raw eggs have a place in a curative diet, never eggs cooked. *Supper:* This can be along similar lines to the breakfast. The whole wheat dish can be varied by taking oat flake porridge or preferably raw, soaked oats, put through the mincer. Instead of fruit, use fruit juices only on this special diet.

If strictly adhered to, this diet will cure a *stomach ulcer* within a month. *Gout* or any rheumatic complaint will disappear within two or three months. Avoid anything in the way of sausages, pork, canned foods, white sugar, white flour and anything made from white flour. As a matter of fact, these items should be crossed off your list for the rest of your life. If you must, you may start eating meat again after six months, but only beef or veal. Carry out this diet suggestion faithfully and you will find the most difficult case of gout will disappear.

Natural remedies will, in the majority of cases, hasten the healing process. Never lose sight of the fact that the healing depends fundamentally on the raw juices. Since these juices, with the exception of carrot juice, are not too palatable, try mixing them in a soup and add just before serving. The juices may be warmed in a double boiler so as not to cool the soup too much, but do not boil the juices.

Persons with severe cases of stomach ulcers should drink at least two cups of the juices daily.

Proponents of nature cures and nutritional therapy have been advocating the use of raw juices long before scientific research had ever thought of investigating them. Now that "raw juice therapy" has become "respectable" in the eyes of orthodox medicine, patients will thereby be assured of its practicality and be willing to persevere in taking the treatment until the hoped for results are obtained.

It is not surprising that it was in America where the drastic methods of treatment were evolved and practiced, for, it was there, that the greatest crimes against food have been committed by commercial interests, with disastrous results to the health of the nation. Perhaps it was the prospect of becoming slowly crippled by arthritis that galvanized many sufferers into action, accepting a raw juice diet rather than face the life of an invalid.

The Compatability of Juices

It is often assumed that it is permissible to combine fruit and vegetable juices, such as orange with carrot juice. This, of course, is no better than to eat fruit and vegetables at the same time which, as mentioned previously, is apt to cause fermentation and flatulence.

Generally speaking, one juice can be mixed with another of the same kind so that the best way is to take potato and carrot juice at one time and orange and grapefruit juice at another. Sipping is much better than drinking and little sips, properly insalivated will avoid flatulence or any other digestive disturbance. If you have difficulty with the acid juices and find them difficult to tolerate, you can neutralize them somewhat by taking a bite of crisp bread with each sip of juice. Fruit juices can be mixed with muesli while vegetable juices are best incorporated in soups and stews after they have been cooked.

DISADVANTAGES OF "RAW FOOD" CURES

High blood pressure, venous ailments, etc. demand a change in the viscosity of the blood and this can be accomplished only by means of a protein reduced diet. Meat, cheese, eggs and other protein foods have to be cut down to a minimum in such cases. It is, however, not always easy to change over to a fruit diet. Elderly people are likely to be troubled by the fact that the gastric acids do not always mix well with the acids found in fruits. It is then advisable to eat some crisp bread, toast or cereal with the fruit as the starch contained in them will neutralize the acids to a certain extent and render them more acceptable to the stomach.

Those who change to a raw food diet must take into consideration that the digestive organs will not immediately adapt themselves to the change from a mixed or one-sided protein diet. A little time and patience is needed before a really successful changeover is achieved and one must give the body all the help it needs during this time. Using a motor car as an illustration, a driver knows that he cannot change from a high octane gas to a low octane one without first making adjustments to his carburetor. Similarly, the stomach must be adjusted to the new diet and many of these diet changes are not successful simply because this point has been neglected or insufficiently considered.

FRUIT AND VEGETABLES AT THE SAME MEAL

I am constantly reminded of the fact that problems arise when fruit and vegetables are eaten at the same meal. The following account proves this sufficiently:

"There has been much talk recently about modern diets and lecture upon lecture has been given on the subject. My daughter and I went to an interesting one given by Dr. Bircher. The speaker was very insistent that, before each meal, fruit and raw vegetables, or a salad, should be eaten. So my whole family started a regimen of eating an apple each, before dinner every day. The result seemed to be that my goiter scar, now eleven years old, was dreadfully painful for three or four days and a small swelling developed. The pain diminished considerably although it did not disappear entirely. I should also tell you that on the evening of the lecture, I hurried a little and for the first time in my life, I was conscious of my heart beating rather rapidly and ever since I have felt sick almost every day. We have now stopped eating an apple before our meal for it seemed to give us flatulence as well."

This account emphasizes the following points: It is certainly good to serve a dish of raw food before the principal meal, but stick to one variety of food – before a vegetable meal eat raw vegetables and before a meal composed of sweet dishes, you may eat fruit. However, Dr. Bircher's theory may apply to healthy people whose organs function properly but if there is the slightest tendency towards dysfunction of one or more organs, the simultaneous consumption of fruit and vegetables at the same meal may encourage disturbances.

A urinalysis of the above letter writer showed that her liver and pancreas were subnormal and undoubtedly it was for this reason that she suffered from flatulence when she ate fruit and vegetable at the same meal. If no complication exists and the digestive juices can accommodate fruit under these circumstances, then Dr. Birchers's theory would be correct.

In a personal interview with Dr. Bircher, he told me that he could find no scientific reason for separating two classes of foods. But, the question arises: "Why eat mixtures of foods that have proven to disagree with you?"

VITAMIN A AND VITAMIN E

At one time there was absolutely no cure for *conjunctivitis* and for dehydration of the cornea. Conjunctivitis, as we now are aware, is the result of Vitamin A deficiency. While it was more common in infants and small children, adults also have been known to be afflicted.

Vitamin A deficiency also predisposes one to lung ailments, pneumonia, inflammation of the middle ear (Mastoid), to suppurations and the development of abscesses, etc. Where do we find this important vitamin? In butter, in cod liver oil, in dandelion leaves, nettles, parsley, savoy cabbage and in carrots. Fruits which contain Vitamin A are apricots, dates and rose hips.

A Vitamin A deficiency can quickly be overcome by taking cod liver oil, rose hip conserve and date sugar. Anyone whose assimilation is poor should take the condensed juice of biologically grown raw spring carrots. This has the added advantage of being a liver medicine as well.

It is unnecessary to buy expensive vitamin preparations when natural foods serve the purpose much better. For example: one gram of human milk contains 2 to 5 international units of Vitamin A. The same amount of black currant juice, 3 to 5 units, and rose hip conserve, 60 to 100 units.

Vitamin E: Although the effects brought about by a deficiency of this vitamin in the past has not received sufficient attention, by now the majority of health-oriented people are well acquainted with the merits of Vitamin E. Since the opening of the Shute Foundation Clinic in Canada for the treatment of heart disease and a host of other ailments through the use of Vitamin E and the subsequent publication of his book, "Vitamin E for Ailing and Healthy Hearts" a whole new field of Vitamin E therapy has been introduced. Since many books have already dealt with this subject in great length, suffice it to say that among other things, beside the heart, Vitamin E has received high recommendation for improving the circulation of the blood, to prevent aging, and as an excellent remedy for burns and blood clotting. It is also called the fertility vitamin and a deficiency of it can lead to serious interference with the function of the reproductive glands and may result in sterility.

Since the secretion of the reproductive glands, the so-called hormones, are to a large extent responsible for one's general well-being, vitality and pleasure in work and achievement, it is obvious that Vitamin E, which influences the formation of these hormones, assumes a major role in the maintenance of health.

Raw wheat germ is the richest source of Vitamin E and this wonderful food has been neglected for too long a time. In the autumn, a dish of berries sweetened with honey and covered with wheat germ should be a dish on everyone's table. Since this book considers natural foods, less emphasis is placed on the manufactured variety of vitamins for obvious reasons.

THE VALUE OF
CANNED AND BOTTLED FRUITS

A short letter came over my desk a few years ago with the following query:

"Lately I read in a book on diet reform, that sterilized fruits are only nutritional ballast. I have been wondering about this, because during the past year I have bottled a quantity of fruit, thinking the home bottled fruit had greater food value than the tinned fruit."

Answer: "I would like to answer your inquiry publicly because it is of interest to everyone. It is quite true that in sterilizing fruits and vegetables by the heat process, many of the vitamins are destroyed. However, the statement you read in a book about sterilized fruits being nutritional ballast for the body is absolutely untrue. The actual nutrients such as carbohydrates, sugar, starch and the minerals remain unchanged and for this reason, sterilized fruits and vegetables do have considerable food value, assuming that a natural process is used in sterilizing. It is quite a different story with commercially preserved fruits and vegetables. The bleaching, shaping and chemical preservatives added, definitely has a direct effect on the food value after processing and this it is sad to note, is mostly negative."

If, from time to time, I have spoken against preserved foods, it is because it so often happens that just for the sake of convenience, factory preserved foods have been used when the meal could, with a little extra effort, have consisted of fresh fruits or vegetables. Canned foods are used all too often by hospitals and sanitoriums and it has become a normal thing. If sick people are to get well, they must have health giving nourishment, which can be obtained at its maximum value only in fresh foods. For this reason one should eat fresh foods as much as possible during harvest time. Eat your vegetables raw in salads as much as possible and eat fruits and berries by themselves or in muesli or fruit salad. Anything that cannot be used should be sterilized and bottled when fresh so that provision is made for the winter.

It is not necessary that everything you eat have a high vitamin value. The important thing is to make sure that you do not leave out anything essential when planning your menu. Let's suppose that, for lunch in the winter, you have yogurt which contains vitamins and some fresh carrots, turnips and cabbage salad. To this you may add preserved vegetables, followed by potatoes or unpolished rice. The body will then get its vitamins from the fresh vegetables and other nourishing foods from the canned or bottled materials. Thus, you will be not only well, but correctly fed.

Sterilize and bottle all leftovers from your garden produce, but do not make the mistake of depriving the children of fresh fruits and berries just because you want to preserve them. I remember as a child having to watch the black currants and raspberries I longed to eat, being prepared into jam. Parents, in their eagerness to preserve forget about the value of fresh fruit.

419

COPPER UTENSILS – Their disadvantages and dangers

Years ago, copper utensils were used to a considerable extent in hotels, restaurants and were considered a prerequisite to any well-to-do home. With the knowledge we have today, it is easy to do without copper especially when it is known that it destroys Vitamin C. Rose hip puree and barberries for instance, are both rich in this vitamin but if prepared in copper kettles, will lose much of their vitamin value. On the other hand iron and enamel covered pans have no effect on the vitamin content. Also, copper oxydizes easily and forms verdigris which may cause poisoning. It has been observed that the use of copper utensils leads to gastroenteritis – gastric inflammation with involvement of the intestinal mucous membranes. That the liver may be affected as well, is obvious, because everything assimilated from the digestive tract finds its way through the portal circulation to this organ. Jaundice, anemia, damage to the kidneys and minor disturbances in the central nervous system, can often be traced to the regular absorption of metallic oxides and salts from copper and aluminium utensils.

Health Considerations

Facts regarding metals should be reason enough for us to examine the materials we use in the kitchen from the point of view of health, and eliminate all metals which may have an adverse effect upon it. Homeopathy employs copper (Cuprum met.) in potencies as high as 20x and if such fantastic attenuations still affect the body, how much greater must be the effect produced by the physical uses of such utensils?

It is interesting to note the effect of copper upon Infusoria (a class of protozoa found in infusions of decaying matter). If copper filings are immersed in the liquid containing them, they will be destroyed without the copper undergoing any material change. The reason is that copper acts, in this case, as a catalyst.

This should lead us to mistrust copper. And aluminium is in the same category. If we wish to cook health giving foods we will have to make sure that the pots and pans we cook in meet the proper standards. It is difficult enough to steer one's way through the maize of dangers which beset our foods such as preservatives, chemical adulterations, sprays, etc., all of which destroy the nutritive value of our foods. One should, therefore, take care not to add to the general lowering of food standards by cooking with utensils that are harmful.

BE CAREFUL WITH STONE-FRUITS

Persons who have liver and pancreas problems must take care not to eat stone-fruits such as peaches, apricots, etc. in any great quantity for, if they do, they will probably pay for it in a very short time with discomfort and pain. Stone-fruits should never be eaten on an empty stomach. Slow eating and thorough insalivation of the fruit is necessary. Crisp bread, rusks, or whole grain bread will diminish gastric reaction to the hydrocyanic acid. Healthy constitutions used to raw foods can probably digest stone-fruit very well and can eat it at any time; but sick or delicate persons should not risk eating them. If the latter should happen to eat some by mistake and upset the gastric and intestinal mucous membranes, they can get relief by taking a tablespoon of clay in water, morning and evening for a few days. Should excessive gastric acidity develop, take a teaspoon of wood ash before each meal and the disturbance will quickly go away.

SPRAYED FRUIT

As more instances of poison from sprayed fruit come to our attention, it would be well to consider the different aspects of this evil.

Some people do not react immediately to poisons such as lead, arsenic, copper sulphate, DTD, etc. used in sprays;

others are more sensitive and immediately show signs of poisoning upon eating such fruit. When buying fruit one should make sure it hasn't been sprayed. It is common to find blemishes or an occasional brown spot on unsprayed fruit but they do not affect the properties of the fruit as far as edibility is concerned. If uncertain as to whether a fruit has been sprayed, the greater part of caution is to peel it, foregoing the phosphates and other valuable materials which lie immediately under the skin. It is better to do without the minerals, however valuable, than to risk poisoning.

It is hoped that poisonous spraying will eventually stop as there is always the possibility of discovering a harmless insecticide that will help increase crops without the risk of harming the consumer. Experiments carried out with herbal sprays, containing extracts of horsetail, yarrow and monkshood, have given very satisfactory results and investigations are continuing. Spraying with tobacco extract is now a recommended way as it is much less harmful than chemical sprays.

BERRIES

If it were known how rich in vitamins berries are, they would figure far more in our everyday diet. Most of them contain a considerable amount of Vitamin C, the importance of which is fully realized in bleeding gums, the first signs of scurvy; also in loose teeth, a tendency to chills and a predisposition to hemorrhaging.

Black currants are richest in Vitamin C although they have a curious taste which not everybody likes. But, if you ate two ounces of these daily, you would provide your body with sufficient Vitamin C for 24 hours. Raspberries, red currants, cranberries and nearly all other berries are excellent sources of the same vitamin.

Vitamin A is supplied by various other berries. 100 grams of bilberries (similar to blueberries) contain as much as 1.6 mg. per 100 grams. The principal source of Vitamin A among the vegetables are carrot juice and watercress.

A deficiency of Vitamin A shows up in skin diseases, pathological changes in the hair, teeth and nails, softening of the cornea, obesity from glandular malfunction, Nyctalopia (night blindness) and other conditions.

Although much has been done, said and written about vitamins, the last word on the subject is far from having been spoken. We are catching a glimpse of the intricate interplay between vitamins, ferments and hormones. Vitamin B_1 is an indispensable component of the yellow respiration ferment; Vitamin A, the opponent of the thyroid hormones and so on. Hyperthyroidism can thus be checked by eating plenty of food containing Vitamin A, such as the berries mentioned above.

Experience has shown that berries are good for the liver. In pancreatic disturbances, bilberries will do much to restore order. Whereas stone-fruit, pears, etc. can have a harmful effect, berry fruits can be eaten by most people without any harmful effect. The one berry that has to be watched is the strawberry. Many people are allergic to strawberries and they can also affect the kidneys, although much depends upon the fertilizers used in their cultivation. If the right manure or compost is used, that is a nature compost, bone meal and natural lime, then they may not cause reactions such as nettle rash, etc. If you are allergic to cultivated strawberries, try the wild ones, because there is a difference.

Lymphatic constitutions will frequently have reason to complain of swollen glands, and anyone thus afflicted should make the fullest use possible of all available berries. They may help them to reduce their liability to infectious respiratory diseases. Mothers-to-be will similarly benefit from berries. When there are sufficient vitamins and minerals in the blood, most of the ailments associated with pregnancy, including *morning sickness,* can be avoided. Vitamin C is especially important during this time.

Allergic ailments and the weariness often felt in the spring will be greatly reduced by eating plenty of berries. Of course, we are referring to berries in their fresh, uncooked or raw state. Use as many of them as possible before preserving the surplus. When making jam take care to use unrefined brown sugar, for white refined sugar is a calcium robber. The sugar contained in fruits is, of course, the most valuable of all and the berries are very rich in it. Since extra sugar must be used in making jams, let it be brown sugar with at least 10% to 20% grape concentrate added, to give it still greater food value.

RHUBARB

I am often asked if rhubarb is harmful as a food. There are some good things to be said about it, namely that it is rich in vitamins, acids that can be of value in certain cases, and, of course, it contains various essential minerals.

The great disadvantage, however, is that it can be very harmful to the kidneys, especially when there is a tendency to kidney stones. One should be very careful with rhubarb as well as asparagus and brussel sprouts as all three of these are excessively acid-forming. Although they are good if taken in small quantities, they can have a very injurious affect on the kidneys if eaten in large amounts. Care should be exercised by anyone suffering from kidney stones, or gravel, rheumatism or arthritis, and they should touch these foods lightly.

Further, the manure used for rhubarb is important. If artificial or unfermented liquid manure is used, the rhubarb can become actually poisonous. It is indeed lamentable that what is advantageous to the farmer, becomes a disadvantage to the consumer. Therefore as someone once said " caveat emptor" (let the buyer beware).

SUGAR DEFINED

It is necessary to clarify certain problems connected with the various kinds of sugars because, for example, it has been said that brown sugar (unrefined cane sugar) is sulphur treated and therefore no less detrimental to health than the bleached, dyed and refined white sugar.

424

White sugar is dyed solely to enhance its whiteness. This is done on the same principle as in a laundry when blue is added to the rinsing water to make the linen appear whiter than it actually is. Refined sugar keeps indefinitely and therefore needs no preservatives. It is "blued" for the eye and for no other reason.

Refined sugar like refined flour is a product of advanced civilization, an unnatural "food" and is a contributory factor to ill health. Brown sugar, on the other hand, contains various minerals which are alkaline-forming and, at least, make some contribution to health, and the allegation that it has been treated with sulphur is untrue.

The best sugar is and always will be that found in fruits, either fresh or dried. Raisins, sultanas, dates, figs, apricots, etc. are excellent sources of this kind of sugar. Since it does not need to be digested, but is assimilated in the same form in which it is ingested, it is the best and quickest source of energy.

If you wish to sweeten your morning dish of muesli you do not need either sugar or honey, as currants, raisins or any of the fruits mentioned will amply sweeten your breakfast dish. A point to keep in mind when buying dried fruits is to make sure that the fruit has not been bleached or treated with sulphur. Grape sugar and honey are excellent nutritious sweeteners. Lacking these, condensed sugar cane juice (called guarapo by Latin-Americans), pear, peach syrup and similar sugar forms, which have not been refined, can be used with confidence.

The so-called grape sugar or glucose, made from maize starch, does not belong in the category of natural sugars. A chemical formula which sounds as though it were derived from grapes, gives it a misleading name and does not entitle it to be called a natural food. The "grape sugar" that is sold over-the-counter in powder or tablet form is a misnomer.

What exactly is *grape sugar*? The sugar which has been extracted from grapes, of course, the reader must think. The chemist, however, considers grape sugar as a carbohydrate which come from sources other than grapes. If you ask him for grape sugar, you will get a fairly sweet white powder, labelled "grape sugar" or glucose. This product is made from maize and has little to do with grapes. Of course it supplies calories, it gives energy, but it lacks the nutritive and curative value of the genuine element extracted from grapes in a concentrated syrup. This syrup can also be extracted from raisins, sultanas and currants and is almost identical to that extracted from fresh, vine ripened grapes. It is the very best sweetening available and not even honey can take its place because some people cannot tolerate it whereas practically everyone can tolerate real grape sugar. Infants and children and seriously ill adults suffering from metabolic disorders should use only grape sugar to sweeten their drinks. It oxydizes in the system without any waste and therefore does not impose any additional burden on the organism. Unlike white sugar, grape sugar is not a calcium robber. It should be part of the diet of every convalescent and those with weak hearts or frayed nerves because of its soothing assimilation. Herb teas sweetened with grape sugar encourage proper sleep and will quiet the nerves after a hectic day. Although grape sugar is rather expensive, it really pays for itself in that it is readily absorbed in the system and does provide definite health benefits.

GELEE ROYALE (Royal Jelly)

Not everyone knows that a bee's life is restricted to 28 working days and that the egg cells which normally produce working bees, can, when fed with a special substance, develop into queens. These queens are considerably bigger than the other bees and the interesting thing about them is that they live 60 times longer than the worker bees. A very special fluid is collected by the workers for those cells which ultimately produce queens. This phenomenon has been the subject of extensive scientific investigation by medical researchers, but the understanding of its exact nature still eludes them.

It is quite possible that ancient races knew something about this, as we frequently find references to "ambrosia", "nectar" and wonder foods in their writings and it is not unreasonable to assume that they were referring to what is now called "Royal Gelee". Unfortunately no references as to how this "ambrosia" was obtained is to be found, so that our assumption must necessarily remain speculative.

There is no doubt that Royal Gelee possesses biological qualities of the highest order, for it enables the queen to lay as many as 2,000 eggs daily, and this with a single fertilization. This is a marvellous biological achievement which cannot be found in any other living creature.

Scientific periodicals have devoted much space to this subject through promotional cleverly disguised advertising and for a time the response was tremendous, demonstrating a need for a biological safe natural tonic.

A few years ago the daily press reported that the Pope had recovered from a severe illness after his personal physician, Dr. Galeazzi, prescribed Royal Jelly as a tonic for him. It also was reported that Dr. Paul Niehans, eminent Swiss endocrinologist and originator of the Cellular-therapy, was of the opinion that Royal Jelly vitalizes the glandular system in a similar manner that an injection of fresh endocrine cells does.

At the Second International Biogenetic Congress, under the chairmanship of Dr. Galeazzi, most of the papers read, dealt with the research findings on Royal Jelly.

Further reports explained that it not only vitalizes and rejuvenates through the endocrine glands, but also successfully combats *whooping cough* and *asthma* in children. Other diseases will also benefit from a regular intake of Royal Jelly and it is thought to be one of the best prophylactic measures against a predisposition to cancer.

PAPAYA Origin and Action of Papain

In the lush forest growth of Florida are found not only thousands of Cabis-palms and many other tropical plants, but also, a great number of wild Papaya. This delicious fruit constitutes not only a food for the Indians living there, but also a medicine. In addition, the leaves, stems and fruit, which contain a substance that breaks down protein, is widely used to tenderize meat. Meat wrapped up in papaya leaves and left standing overnight will become real tender and tasty. The substance which tenderizes is called Papain and commercially it is sold under various trade names today, as a meat tenderizer.

This handsome plant, which looks like a little palm and has big leaves similar to those of a fig tree, grows mostly in the western hemisphere and is found in Central America, the islands of the Caribbean and parts of South America, as well as in Florida. Not only does the papaya have a deliciously distinct taste but its delicately shaded salmon-colored fruit is an excellent aid to digestion. It has also been observed that the natives who eat it seldom suffer from intestinal worms and this is not surprising because the papain digests proteins in the food and also any unwelcome inhabitants.

Because the ripe papaya fruit is perishable it cannot be transported over long distances. However, it was discovered that the unripe fruit, the stems and the leaves contain more papain than the ripe fruit and this solved the problem of shipping. A papaya preparation is now available for combating digestive weaknesses and for the *elimination of worms* and it is one of the safest remedies known. In the past there have been many problems in finding a safe worm medicine. According to the third edition of Prof. Eicholz's "Pharmakologie" it is noted that even experts consider the usual worm medicine risky and far from harmless, for he writes: "The toxicity of all worm medicines should induce the prescriber to consider, whether it is not preferable to tolerate the presence of parasites, than to take the risk of poisoning the patient." If this is of concern to pharmacists, how much greater the concern should be to the patient. However, with the papaya preparation no one need fear, for it is beneficial to digestion and aids in the assimilation of proteins.

Worms are by no means to be taken lightly, whether they are *oxyuris,* the little thread worms that cause an itching irritation in the anus, and can be found by the thousands in the colon; the *ascaris,* inhabiting the small intestines, the *trichures,* found in the colon or any other kind of *intestinal parasites.* They are all very harmful, and lead to severe disturbances in the composition of the blood causing conditions such as Eosinophilia, Anemia and Chlorosis. Not infrequently, the liver can be damaged. The chief factors responsible are probably the metabolic toxins of the worms. The papaya preparation is a protein digestion, botanical enzyme that dissolves the cuticle of the ascaris, oxyuris and trichures and with the aid of intestinal fermentation, will completely dissolve them.

COFFEE

The product of the coffee plant has general acceptance all over the world with the result that millions of tons are consumed annually. Because of its composition, it is not surprising that many people concerned with their health are talking about it in forums, in the press and by means of other media. *Coffee* can damage our health, for it has been shown to have a definitely injurious effect on the nerves. Although I disapprove of the regular use of coffee, I have drunk coffee on occasions where I was going to drive for some distance at night in order to stay awake. However, if one is not a regular coffee drinker, and only takes it occasionally as a stimulant, its immediate effect is surprising. If, however, you have been drinking coffee regularly, the effect it not apparent.

Arabian Coffee:

I established an interesting fact with regard to Arabian coffee. It surprised me that it can be prepared in a way that is much less harmful than the coffee made in the European or American home, and that its stimulating effect was hardly noticeable. The Arabs serve their coffee, as the Turks do, in little cups and it is also served with the grounds. As a rule, they prepare it when the guests arrive and they never store it once it has been roasted and ground. It is usually served very strong with the grounds and sugar. In comparison with regular coffee and cream, this coffee seemed less stimulating. In some way the unfavorable effects of the coffee appear to be eliminated by the Arabian method of preparation. I later learned that the grounds contain certain substances that neutralize the etheric components such as caffein to a certain extent and also weaken the stimulating properties of the coffee.

Caffein extracted Coffee:

I would rather drink coffee prepared the Arabian way than to destroy its natural flavor by extracting the caffein, which may not be the most harmful substance found in it. As other components of the coffee affect the health adversely as well, many different opinions are encountered on the subject.

To rid the coffee of its caffein, inorganic substances such as Benzol or similar coal tar derivatives are used. This gives rise to the question as to whether the decafeinated is really better for one than regular coffee.

Coffee percolators

The coffee percolator is not the best way to prepare coffee because it loses much of its taste and aroma. One obtains a dark brew which frequently tastes a little bitter, and even with sugar and cream, one feels a little bit cheated from the point of view of quality. Those who insist on drinking coffee should prepare it another way, perhaps by the drip method. Additions or adulterants to coffee do little to improve its flavor or its ill effects. The real answer seems to be that most coffee drinkers should give it up completely for the sake of their health. There is a way for them to do this easily.

430

CEREAL AND FRUIT COFFEE

Efforts to find a satisfactory substitute for coffee have been going on for over fifty years with the result that there are good cereal and fruit mixtures on the market today, which have many advantages to health and none of the disadvantages of the bean coffee. Aside from the contents, the cereal and fruit coffee, when drunk with milk, is ingested much better, turning into a fine flaky rather than a lumpy curd in the stomach. For nervous, sensitive and high-strung people, who should abstain from coffee altogether, the cereal coffee is an excellent substitute.

A Rev. Kneipp, who was a nature healer, introduced a malt coffee which is still being sold, although many other *coffee substitutes* have since appeared, which are in many ways superior.

Cereal and fruit coffee enjoys increasing popularity as it offers more health value than malt coffee. The next time you go to the health store look for it and try it. At first it may be necessary to get used to it but after a very short time you will acquire a taste for it and learn to enjoy it to the benefit of your health.

It is not unreasonable to suggest that a healthful diet should be accompanied by a good coffee substitute, which is pleasant to the taste and has none of the disadvantages of regular coffee. A confirmed coffee drinker might think that it would be impossible to get used to a substitute, no matter how badly the former affected his health. Those who feel like that should try drinking their coffee with a slight addition of the cereal and fruit mixture at first and gradually increase the substitute and decrease the regular coffee until eventually he is drinking only the cereal and fruit coffee. From then on, the palate will come to prefer the new substitute and the heart and nerves will benefit tremendously by it.

WHOLE WHEAT AND OTHER CEREALS

However intensively one may campaign against the use of white flour and other refined foods, there is still far too little attention given to the fact that cereal, deprived of its germ and bran, is no longer a health food, but one that can lead to a variety of diseases. Vitamins, minerals, highly valuable oils, etc. are no longer naturally present in refined flours. As a result, it is not the least bit surprising that the standard of health in most "civilized" society is low, despite the abundance of other varieties of food. The food of our grandfathers was by no means ideal but it had the advantage of being a whole food. It was for this reason that they were able to keep in comparatively good health although their fare did lack variety. In the country, bread was baked in the home and this good, old-fashioned cereal bread formed the basis of their daily diet which, however simple, was extremely nourishing and lacked few of the essential elements necessary to good health.

Whole wheat, without a doubt, is one of the best foods for man, and it should be used in its entirety. It can be soaked and then steamed with a little butter or oil, onions and a variety of herbs. Soups, stews, casseroles, porridge, breads, rissoles, etc. can all be prepared using wheat.

Whole rye and barley can be used in the same way although they are not quite as palatable as wheat. But, the imaginable housewife will never be at a loss as to how to prepare the many cereal dishes that are not only palatable but healthful.

WHEATGERM

Wheatgerm, those little yellow flakes, so necessary to good health, are far too little valued and used. If mothers only knew how wonderfully nourishing and curative they are, they would serve them every day in one way or the other.

Wheatgerm contains a first-class protein and much oil. More important, however, is the Vitamin E it contains. The protein plays a vital part in keeping our nervous system healthy and the Vitamin E is responsible for the efficient function and development of the heart, the organs in general and particularly the procreative organs. Although the ovaries and testicles discharge elements that make new life possible, they also discharge their secretions into the bloodstream and, therefore, belong to that category of organs known as the endocrine glands. Dependance on vitamin E assumes greater importance in the correct functioning of these glands. Very often *Vitamin E* is an aid to *conception* as 100 grams of wheatgerms contains as much as 30 milligrams of pure Vitamin E, providing an especially important additional diet to women. Vitamin E is recommended to help overcome a tendency to premature birth.

Bang's disease has been successfully treated with vitamin E preparations and there is none better than the oil of wheatgerm. For years, farmers have observed that the feeding of good bran, that contains the germ of the wheat, reduced the incidence of disease and contagious abortion in cattle.

Girls and women who become obese because of ovarian subfunction should take, not only herbal sitzbaths, but also wheatgerm, as this will stimulate the ovaries, increase the metabolic rate of the body and so dispose of unwanted fat. In addition to taking wheatgerm in the form of Vitamin E, a diet of watercress, lettuce and soyabeans, should constitute part of one's meals for added sources of natural vitamin E.

Thus there are many reasons why mothers should see that the family eats wheatgerm regularly. Among other things, it will ensure that the children's most important glands will develop properly. It has a delicious taste when sprinkled over muesli and in soups. Wheatgerm as a concentrated food is really a necessity and it is a natural food to strengthen the heart and body in general.

GERMINATED CEREALS – A TONIC

Those who have spent money on expensive tonics will be pleased to learn that there is something much cheaper and very much more effective than the reputedly invigorating tonics, pills and potions from the pharmacist or chemist. I am referring to *germinated cereals,* whether wheat, rye or barley. All that is necessary to make them sprout is moisture and warmth. Place a wet cloth on a plate, sprinkle it with cereal and put it in a cupboard or similar warm place. Be sure to keep the cloth damp, or germination will be retarded or stopped altogether. When the sprouts have grown to a length of about a quarter of an inch, the grain can be minced and used as a foundation for muesli or added to flour for breadmaking.

As soon as germination takes place, the ferment diastase becomes active and transforms the starch into a malt which requires less digestion than starch. If you chew the germinated grain thoroughly you will note its sweet taste which is the malt. This is rich in diastase, and these enzymes are a wonderful and strengthening food. It can be eaten together with linseed as is done in Sweden, where the dish is called "Kruska". It aids in the digestion of other starchy foods and is recommended for those who have poor assimilation and have trouble gaining weight. It will also enrich the blood especially if mixed with carrot or grape juice. Dr. Bircher also recommends germinated cereals to his patients, as he states he has always obtained excellent results with them.

BUCKWHEAT (Fagopyrum)

Those travelling down to Puschlav during the war observed in the districts adjoining the Italian frontier many fields sown in buckwheat, a crop which is almost unknown to this day in our district. Our southern confederates were more artful than we. It seems that flour, semolina and other cereal products had been requisitioned by the government and rationed, while buckwheat, which could take the place of the customary cereals, was free. They therefore started to grow buckwheat which is very nutritious and grows on marginal, sandy soil and grows rapidly to maturity within three months. For this reason it is cultivated in northern climates where seasons are short as in Siberia. The plant attains a height of one and a half feet, has reddish white flowers and provides a good supply of nectar for bees. American buckwheat honey is known far and wide.

The French name "Blé Sarasin" seems to indicate that buckwheat must have been brought to France from the south by the Saracens. The Russian name "grezicha" could indicate that the Greeks introduced this valuable food into their neighboring lands. In many parts of Russia, buckwheat is the national dish and the people prepare a most delicious oven baked buckwheat.

Whole *buckwheat* can be cooked in the same manner as rice and buckwheat gruel is excellent in soup and baked dishes. The flour makes what is called a short pastry and can be mixed with wheat flour. The resulting texture of the pastry is as though it were mixed with a lot of butter.

German biologists have discovered that buckwheat reduces *high blood pressure* and this has been confirmed by American scientists. An extract of buckwheat is claimed to combat high blood pressure and arteriosclerosis. Unpolished rice has the same attributes as buckwheat in this respect. It would be to the advantage of *older people* if they would change their menus a little, so as to include more *brown rice* and *buckwheat* and fewer eggs, legumes and cheeses for these two cereals have a rejuvenating effect on the blood vessels, especially the arteries. Intake of protein and salt should be reduced to a minimum as one advances in age.

BUCKWHEAT DISHES

Whole Buckwheat: Cook the buckwheat in a little water or vegetable stock, then make a sauce from two teaspoons of whole grain flour, finely chopped herbs and unseasoned tomato puree. Add to the buckwheat some steamed onions and a little oil and cook until the grains are soft.

Cold Buckwheat: Prepare buckwheat as above, let cool, pour into a dish and garnish with tomatoes and parsley and serve with a green salad.

Fried Buckwheat: Prepare buckwheat in the same manner as above, then add onions, garlic and marjoram. Cut into small shapes and fry in oil on each side until golden brown.

CONTRIBUTORY CAUSES OF DISEASE

In the search for contributory causes of gout, arthritis, cancer, multiple sclerosis, liver and kidney diseases, investigators must sooner or later arrive at a consensus: that it is not a singular, specific cause that sets in motion the pathological changes which ultimately result in a classified disease, but that it is rather a multitude of great and small daily sins against the laws of nature and health. That hereditary factors can be responsible for the predisposition to certain diseases is indisputable. Mental and physical strain, over-work, constant hurry, irritations, fears and worries, play a part in the causation of diseases too, and may trigger conditions that would otherwise have remained latent.

Poisons finding their way into the system through drugs and unnatural foodstuffs, a vitamin deficient diet and many other factors are recognized as detrimental to health. There is a particular substance that has so far received little attention, and the absence of which may lead to degenerative diseases. I am referring to the highly unsaturated fatty acids which are destroyed by heating, refining, hardening and other factory processes. Lack of these acids gives rise to disturbances in the metabolism of the cells, and that this must have a bearing upon other pathological processes as well, is obvious. A few years ago, little was known about the *unsaturated fatty acids* and few if any references were made to the importance of natural oils and fats in a balanced diet. Not that these fats have a highly complicated chemical formula, on the contrary, they consist of the common elements, carbon, hydrogen and oxygen. But they also contain three types of fatty acids: the saturated, the unsaturated and the highly unsaturated.

If we consume an excess of saturated fatty acids, as found in refined fats and oils, too much energy is required to digest them and for this reason we feel tired and sleepy after a meal. They are chemical compounds, exceedingly poor in oxygen and their consumption would require us to take exercises and breathe deeply – something we feel no inclination to do after eating such foods. The saturated fats are found predominately in animals and have a high melting point, while the unsaturated oils occur chiefly in seeds and have a low melting point. The reason why oils with a low melting point are hardened or hydrogenized is because they are liquid. Firm slabs of fat can be more easily packed and transported than bottles of oil. The hardening process has a detrimental influence on the quality of the fats treated because the low melting unsaturated fatty acids are transformed in the process into high melting stearic acids, which are anything but conducive to health.

Why then, are the unrefined oils, containing highly unsaturated fatty acids, preferable? Because they will combine with the minerals, proteins and oxygen in the body and in this way encourage normal cell metabolism and oxidation. If these functions are interfered with over a period of years, disease will inevitably manifest itself sooner or later. Cell growth becomes abnormal and malignant, the phospholipoids will degenerate and this will lead to thrombosis. The cholesterin will combine with the fats and deposit itself on the walls of the blood vessels and so give rise to arteriosclerosis, high blood pressure and the danger of apoplexy.

Considering all these factors it will be seen how vital it is to change over to unrefined olive, sunflower seed, soya, safflower oils or to the fats from nuts such as walnut, almond, pine kernel and many others. An excellent source of highly unsaturated fatty acids are the sesame seeds which contains

43% of these oils. If you haven't already done so, you should make sure that from now on you will use oil only from the above mentioned sources for your health's sake.

IMPORTANCE OF OIL FRUITS

It surprised me to find that among many primitive people, oil fruits or seeds appeared to play an important part in their diet. Not only do they use the oil, but also the whole fruit which is crushed or chopped up and added to another dish. People living close to nature, uncontaminated by civilization, usually show a very high standard of health which certainly has something to do with their natural diet. We are forced to conclude that natural foods, among which we can certainly count the oil fruits such as oranges, lemons and grapefruit, are of great value and importance to health and well-being.

LINSEED – FLAXSEED

In considering linseed, the seed of the flax, the first thing to note is, that those who are used to eating them regularly, exhibit excellent *liver* function.

Before eating linseed, they should be ground with a small mill or minced. If you buy them already ground, make sure that they are freshly ground because after four or five days ground linseed begins to go rancid. That is why it is better to grind them as you use them to assure their freshness. There are many ways of serving them. They are good mixed with honey, curds or savory herbs. They may be described as a strength giving food and those who have formed the habit of eating them regularly can attest to their beneficial effects.

SUNFLOWER SEEDS

It is to be regretted that these tiny seeds receive so little attention as food for human consumption. They should always be eaten raw by themselves or they make an excellent meal when mixed with dried fruits such as raisins, apples, figs, apricots etc. Also for a super deluxe meal, add to the above, currants and other nuts such as walnuts, cashews, almonds, raw roasted but unsalted peanuts. A mixture of the above supplies all the nourishment one needs and should be considered as adequate food when taking long hikes or on camping trips. Sunflower seeds contain highly unsaturated oils and are rich in vitamins, containing Vitamins A, and B, approximately 25% protein in addition to a generous amount of iron, calcium and carbohydrates. They are easily digested too. Try keeping some on hand in the house and in the car to munch on when a busy schedule makes you late for your lunch or supper. Children love the mixed nuts and fruits and it is much healthier for them to eat this mixture than to satisfy their appetite with candy, cakes or other sweets. Another good idea is to grind the sunflower seed into a coarse meal and then sprinkle them on breakfast muesli or any other cereal you are using. They are one of the best natural foods available and nourish the whole body with the vital elements it needs to keep well. Be sure to make a note of this little seed with giant power – health power – the next time you go shopping for health foods. In baking, try using sunflower seed flour along with whole wheat flour for a real taste treat.

POPPY SEEDS

What has been said about sunflower seeds apply equally as well to poppy seeds. As an article of diet it is worthy of far more consideration than it has hitherto received. One should not be content with making a poppy seed cake once in a while or once a year as they do in Hungary on a certain feast day. Instead of making cake, poppy seeds should be eaten regularly. They do not contain opiates as some people think, as the opium is obtained from the seed capsule of the poppy and not from the seeds themselves. It sometimes happens that fruits or

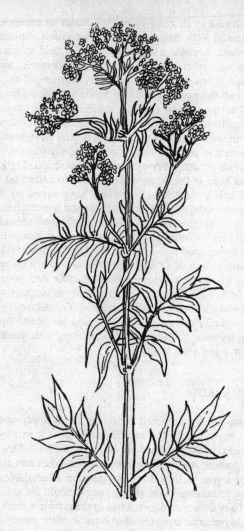

Valerian (Valeriana officinalis)

nuts do have a slight trace of a harmful substance as, for example, the prussic acid in the plum. However, this is no cause for worry. The harmful substance is an integral part of the fruit and, as such, does not act in the same way as the pure, extracted substance would. It is only found in infinitesimal quantities, in what one could say was a homeopathic potency, and far from being harmful, it can actually do some good.

SESAME SEEDS

These little oil-containing seeds of the subtropical sesame plant are comparatively little known worldwide, although in Europe and America they are commonly used. They contain an abundance of minerals such as iron, potassium and are particularly high in Calcium. Vitamins A and B are represented as well as protein and carbohydrates. If your body lacks phosphorus, sesame seeds have an ample supply, containing approximately 300 milligrams per 100 grams of seed.

The highly unsaturated fatty acids are easily assimilated by the cells and thus, oil of sesame finds excellent use in cooking and as salad oil. The same fatty acids also supply the body with oxygen necessary for the combustion of calorific foods and so contribute to proper elimination.

Sesame seeds will be found useful in combating *constipation, suppurations, crusta lactaea, eczema* and even *tumors,* as they form defensive substances in the body. They strengthen the nerves, stimulate heart muscle action and, because of their *Vitamin E* content, can be taken with assurance during pregnancy.

Patients afflicted with *liver* or *gall* problems will welcome not only the seeds, but also the raw oil as well, because both can be easily tolerated. A welcome addition to the diet of children are the different preparations on the market containing, among other things, sesame seeds and honey. These preparations are excellent between meal snacks and have none of the disadvantages of ordinary sweets.

During the 50 years I have been in practice, I have noticed that it is far more advantageous to make use of the whole fruit or seed one eats, insofar as it is practical. Accordingly, one should eat the whole seed and not just the oil extracted from it. If the liver is sensitive and cannot tolerate certain oils, especially those that have been refined, it will accept those unrefined, and better still, those being part of the seed itself.

In the interests of general health the housewife can make that dish of oil seeds and honey that we have previously talked about. In doing so she will prevent oxidation and the deterioration of the food values found in the oil seeds. Creamed into a spread, ground sunflower, sesame or other oil seeds, and honey, is about the healthiest and most strengthening food that exists. It is an excellent food for those who suffer from liver problems, and it promotes healing as well.

THE OIL CURE FOR GALLSTONES

Before even considering an operation, serious thought should be given to the oil cure for the *removal of gallstones,* if the patient is willing and thinks he can take from one-half pint to three-quarters of a pint of oil at one time. Some people assume that the oil cure is effective on account of its entering the gallbladder and cleansing it, but this is not so. The oil merely stimulates the plentiful secretion of bile. One could say it causes a flood which carries the small and medium size stones with it.

The oil used for this purpose should be unrefined (raw). Whether it is the highly unsaturated fatty acids that make it more effective than the refined oil, has not as yet been determined. Olive, walnut, sunflower, safflower and poppy seed oils are all suitable.

Before embarking on the cure, it would be good to take a preparation of artichokes and other remedial herbs to help liquify the gall.

For best results, it will also be necessary to cleanse the bowels first. Soaked prunes or figs, psyllium seed or ground linseed will serve the purpose very well. If they do not move the bowels sufficiently, take an enema of warm water with an infusion of camomile in addition. Hot packs should be applied to the liver area for two hours before and after the drinking of the oil. When the bowels have been emptied you can take the oil. That accomplished, lie down, turn over on your right side and remain in this position for two hours. If you cannot stand drinking the oil by itself try to take it together with coffee or a coffee substitute and if this proves too difficult you will then have to take the required quantity of oil spaced out. This will not be as effective, but at least the liver will be thoroughly cleansed, the smaller stones may be eliminated and the remaining bigger ones may not cause trouble for a while.

However, anyone who is capable of drinking the half-pint of oil all at one time should not be surprised if all the stones are eliminated. This is more likely to occur in cases which have not become chronic where no big stones are present. If a chronic condition has been permitted to occur through lack of treatment and a high fever accompanied by an increase in the number of white blood corpuscles takes place, then surgery must be considered as the only alternative. This is not a satisfactory solution, because after the operation, condensed gall will no longer be available – it cannot accumulate as it previously had done – in the gallbladder that no longer exists. The bile entering the duodenum will always be thin and fresh and if digestive disturbances are to be avoided, a protein and fat restricted diet will have to be adopted forever after. Since the oil cure has produced satisfactory results in literally thousands of cases, according to mail we have received from grateful patients, there is little doubt that it will produce the desired results and certainly this method is to be preferred over the more drastic surgery removal, if it can be avoided, as well as the consequences it brings with it.

WALNUTS

The walnut harvest must be unforgettable for all those who have had the privilege of growing up in the country. It was always a red-letter day for me when, armed with a stick, I was allowed to climb the high walnut trees and beat down the nuts, which though ripe, were not quite ready to fall out of their green outer shell. The bravest climber had fearful moments sometimes when some outer branch would not release its precious burden, and things were neither safe nor easy. Piling them together, then prying the nuts out of their shells, though not the best thing for the hands, was great fun. Such work was not for the ladies with their well manicured and polished nails because for more than two weeks afterward, the yellowish brown stains would still be impregnated in the hands.

Of course we all know the good fresh taste of newly harvested walnuts. Eaten with whole wheat bread and sweet apple cider or freshly extracted grape juice, they are delicious and nutritious. Did you know that walnuts are especially good for those suffering from metabolic disturbances and constipation? When drugstore laxatives do not produce the desired results, walnuts may overcome the problem. Walnuts are recommended for patients with liver problems and, although most people having a liver problem cannot tolerate fats, they will find that moderate quantities of walnuts will agree with them quite well. No need to wait for the holiday season to eat walnuts. They should be eaten all year round. As mentioned before, they are an excellent additive to nuts and dried fruit snacks.

AN INFUSION FROM THE INTERIOR DIVIDING WALLS OF WALNUTS

This infusion is most excellent in cases where the arteries of the cardiac wreath are sclerosed, in cardiac pains and fever. Very often a narrowing of the coronary arteries may be due to chronic nicotine poisoning and in such cases, the physician and friends will have to bring pressure to persuade the person to stop smoking. No doubt a heavy smoker upon seeing the small scar in the muscle tissue of the heart that every severe attack of *angina pectoris* brings, will quit voluntarily. But, if the smoking continues, that person is faced with an infarct – a partial necrosis of the myocardium. Many weeks in bed, resting, may bring about an improvement, which is not to be mistaken for a cure. In the end, instead of a tender pink heart muscle, the patient will be left with one that has an ugly white scar in it. Even so, he must consider himself fortunate, as an infarct can, in some instances lead to a rupture of the heart, which would be fatal. Needless to say, the scars themselves are anything but harmless. One day the last attack will come and the post mortem will then reveal countless tiny scars which bear witness to the suffering that accompanied each seizure and furthermore will reveal the folly of refusing to give up smoking. How many of us would like to pay so high a penalty for our refusal to recognize a true danger when it is presented to us in all seriousness?

Alcohol, nicotine and meat should be avoided by all who are afflicted with *angina pectoris* if they want a chance to keep on living. A preparation from an infusion from the woody, interior dividing walls of the walnuts drunk the first thing in the morning will have an excellent therapeutic effect. Soak the walls of the walnut for four or five days in water and afterwards, boil them for a few minutes. The tea resulting from this will alleviate the pressure and the pain in the chest and will reduce any fever that the patient may have. Amelioration is frequently noticed after the first cup and if the pains continue, the tea should be sipped frequently until they have disappeared.

ALMONDS

A quarter of the total weight of an almond consists of protein and it is in only the rarest cases that it cannot be assimilated by babies. More than 90% of the babies, if placed on an almond diet, would derive greater benefit than from the protein found in cows' milk. Thanks to almond milk many babies have gotten rid of *crusta lactaea, gastric* and *intestinal disturbances.*

Almond puree is eminently suitable for producing almond milk, which should be substituted in the spring when cow's milk does not always agree with every baby, due to the animal's feeding on fresh young grass. Couple almond puree with a good biological preparation of calcium and Viola tricolor in homeopathic form and even the most stubborn cases of *crusta lactaea* will yield. Approximately 60% of the almond consists of oil, which is rich in calcium, and the nerve nourishing phosphates. Almond milk and oil can be tolerated by almost everyone, even those with severe liver problems.

It is necessary to masticate the almonds very thoroughly if the full benefit is to be obtained from them. To make *almond puree* at home, use a liquifying machine to which has been added a little liquid as a starter. Pour in the almonds and run the machine on high speed and it will produce a liquid that can be used in various ways. *Almond milk* is easily digested, rich in Vitamin B and minerals and will benefit the liver and the pancreas. It is the best plant milk in existence.

RICE DIET FOR HIGH BLOOD PRESSURE

It used to be the custom in America to cure *high blood pressure* through a rice diet. A Swiss sanatorium employed the same diet with excellent results. Less encouraging was the fact that patients became anemic at the same time. Mistakes were made in prescribing rice for reducing because the polished rice was used. If natural rice had been used for the purpose of reducing high blood pressure, anemia would not have resulted.

A mono-diet consisting of polished rice is bound to lead to severe deficiencies and this should have been well known, after beri-beri was found to have been caused by a one-sided consumption of polished rice. A mono-diet can be beneficial when the *whole* of the cereal is used. Brown rice contains nine and a half times more minerals than the white, demonstrating the immense value it has nutritionally. Why use white polished rice? During the refining process, not only the external cellulose is removed, but also the germ. Then it is dusted with talcum which may or may not contain asbestos. This results in a beautifully white kernel that pleases the eye, but not the body. It is a guarded secret, but nevertheless fairly well known, that the pharmaceutical companies buy the so-called wastes or byproducts of the refining process to use as ingredients in expensive tonics.

CHRONIC CONSTIPATION

This appears to be a typical ailment of our modern day society that is rarely found among primitive people. It would be reasonable to search for the cause among the unnatural refinements of this late twentieth century life, among which are denaturalized foods, unsuitable clothing, lack of exercise and fresh air, overwork and mental strain. If it were possible to analyze each case for a fundamental cause, no doubt it would be found to be psychological rather than physical. This is well-known in the case of chronic constipation, stomach and duodenal ulcers, heart disease, liver problems and many other ailments. This knowledge has encouraged some scientists to try to prove that the vegetative nervous system which influences the function of internal organs, which today makes excessive demands upon the individual, is not only useless but harmful. They attempted to prove the truth of their assertion by resorting to sympathectomy (severance of pre- or post-ganglionic nerve fibers which control specific involuntary muscles) and vagotomy (severance of the vagus or pneumo-gastric nerve). The disease when due to psychological causes improved. In spite of this, less heroic methods of cure are advised, although the nervous aspect in chronic constipation should receive attention in one way or the other.

We must first deal with any possible physical cause and by means of natural stimuli assure the proper functioning of the kidneys, liver, bile, intestines and pancreas. The physical cause of *constipation* does not always lie in the intestines. A deficient functioning liver or any of the above mentioned organs can also be responsible.

Warm water treatments, either herbal or hip-baths, hot showers, or hot water massage with a brush are excellent for this condition. All constipating foods must be removed from the diet. Foods containing starch must be reduced. Eat little and chew well letting the saliva work well into the food. Linseed and psyllium seeds, since they are mucilage forming, are very good for encouraging intestinal functions. There is little point in overfeeding a weakened constitution, so only increase the quantity when you are sure the body is assimilating it and the constipation is cured.

An intrinsic cause of constipation is a deficiency of cellulose in our food and we blame the food manufacturers for refining cereal products to such an extent that practically no cellulose is available for the intestines to work with. They counter that it is indigestible and useless to the system. This is true and false. It is true that cellulose is indigestible but it does serve an important purpose. The claim that it is useless is false because cellulose is an intestinal "brush" and without it, the 28 feet or so of digestive tubing could not be kept clean.

The intestines need roughage and bran taken night and morning in a glass of fruit juice is good insurance against constipation. Plenty of vegetable salads including lettuce, celery, carrots, cabbage, etc. will produce a healthy condition within the intestines and help them function better. For more direct action, soaked prunes taken morning and evening and carrot juice or fruit juices are helpful. In any event, a natural diet should be followed and anything refined or in any way adulterated should be avoided. Those who have a sedentary occupation should take time out every day for exercise, if nothing more than walking briskly for a mile or so.

A soup which helps combat intestinal sluggishness can be made from freshly ground whole wheat grains with chopped onions and crushed garlic cloves. After cooking these ingredients add some finely chopped parsley and a tablespoon of olive oil. Take this soup in the morning with crisp or whole wheat bread for freedom from intestinal problems. In stubborn cases, add ground linseed to the soup.

HERBAL SOUP

All those who are bothered with *intestinal sluggishness,* who have misused laxatives (herbal or otherwise) and cannot obtain any more effect from them, and those who want to normalize their *bowel action,* will find the following recipe helpful:

Make an herbal infusion such as senna pod or senna leaf tea, strain it and then add sliced potatoes, including the skin, a teaspoon of bran, a teaspoon of linseed and simmer for 15 minutes. Cool and strain and drink the liquid morning and evening. It will cure the most stubborn cases of *constipation.* It works when no other laxative does.

SAUERKRAUT (Fermented Cabbage)

We gratefully accept all the information science can supply us with in regards to the effective substances found in natural foods and medicines. But more important than the long-winded dissertations on the subjects is the practical application of such knowledge – at least to the patient. Anyone who has seen people suffering from *scurvy* will appreciate why foods containing anti-scorbutic elements are so necessary for them. Their diet can be adequate for them in all other respects, but if certain vitamins are missing, nothing can overcome this deficiency.

Apart from lemon, sauerkraut is the best anti-scorbutic remedy and it was sauerkraut that enabled the daring sailor James Cook to sail the farthest seas without any of his men falling victim to scurvy.

In those days, such things as anti-scorbutic vitamins were unknown but through trial and error these men, who observed and understood the ways of nature, eventually discovered the remedy for the disease. On Cook's ship there had to be sufficient barrels of fermented cabbage and it was due to the fact that the men supplemented this natural product with their meals that enabled them to avoid a devastating health disorder.

If your *gums* bleed easily, if the mucous membranes around the teeth are soft and spongy, if you constantly have small ulcers or sores on your gums, if you bleed easily, if your ankles are swollen, if you suffer from a general feeling of weakness and weariness, then you must add sauerkraut to your daily diet and make your salad dressing with lemon juice. The old continental saying that "a spoonful of sauerkraut a day, keeps the doctor away" is true. Raw sauerkraut is a wonderful remedy and should have a place of honor in every home.

Preparation of sauerkraut:

If you want to make your own sauerkraut, which is much to be preferred over the canned variety, follow this recipe: Shred a head of cabbage, not too fine, not too coarse. Place a layer about one inch thick on the bottom of a container, preferably glass or crockery. Scatter the following seeds over the cabbage: juniper berries, mustard and coriander and add a small pinch of salt. On top of this place a layer of sliced onions (onions may be left out if desired). Place another layer of cabbage over this, seasoning, etc. Continue until jar is full. Using a lid smaller than the jar opening, press the cabbage down well. Place a weight on the cover and allow cabbage to ferment. If you want to hurry the fermentation process, add yogurt or whey extract diluted with water. It is important that this preparation is done in a warm room and the cabbage should stand for two or three weeks in a room not under 68 degrees F. After that, place the container somewhere cool so that there is no butyric acid fermentation, which could ruin the sauerkraut. If you prepare sauerkraut without salt you must make sure that you exclude all air from the jar and that everything is scrupulously clean so that it will keep well. Formerly 1% to 2% salt was used, which meant ¼ to ½ lb. for every 20 lbs. of cabbage. Now, however, ½% or less of salt is considered enough as too much salt, it has been found, prevents lactic acid fermentation and inferior sauerkraut would result.

MILK AND DAIRY FARMING

While milk is a valuable food for growing children, it must be free from impurities and pathogenic matter, which it may contain if the animals are housed under poor hygienic conditions. As the quality and the biological value of milk is also dependent upon the feed, one should take care to obtain milk from farmers who do not use excessive quantities of oil cakes and the like, and who do not use artificial fertilizers for their fields and especially a farmer whose veterinary's bill is low.

The best milk sold today is the raw, certifield T. T. milk (tuberculin tested), which, although more expensive than the regular pasteurized milk, is much more to be preferred. Those who cannot obtain the certified or the pasteurized milk, should be sure to boil any raw milk of dubious quality to reduce danger of infection. If you are fortunate enough to live or take your holidays in the mountains where the cows roam freely on the Alps, no such safety measures will be required, for the milk from these animals will be as near to perfect as it is humanly possible. However, human interference can render even the best milk dangerous and the chief source of danger is the systematic inoculation of the herds. It cannot be taken for granted that the assertions of the authorities in regard to the harmlessness of such practices are based on fact.

Consequences of Inoculation

When cows have been inoculated against TB, their milk, on no account, should be drunk raw for at least four or five days. It would be best to discard such milk altogether, at least for human consumption. Unpleasant consequences from drinking this milk may be experienced, such as liver and digestive disturbances, headaches, feverishness. These problems can be counteracted with an Echinacea preparation which will help dispose of the toxins resulting from drinking this milk. Best thing is not to drink it.

Poorly kept stables can result in tubercular cows. However, where cleanliness and hygienic conditions prevail and where the animals get sufficient exercise in the fresh air, the incidence is reduced considerably.

The danger of tuberculosis is often minimized, and although it is true that it is only tuberculosis of the udder that transmits the disease directly to the milk, who would dare to assert that tuberculosis of the lungs, or of any other organ for that matter, would not affect the quality of the milk. Only an absolutely healthy animal can give milk that is safe and wholesome. The milk, derived from the blood, must of necessity exhibit the same deficiencies, and if the blood is diseased, the effects of the milk on the person will be obvious. There still is plenty of room for improvement in dairy farming that can be beneficial to both man and his animals.

AMERICAN DAIRY FARMING

It would be a salutary thing to compare Swiss dairy farming with American dairy farming. The Swiss farmer can learn much from the organization, installations and hygienic conditions and principles found in the average American dairy farm.

452

Of course American dairy farmers have much larger herds and can profit by the use of modern machinery and methods and, because of the scope of his operation, his costs can be written off more rapidly than his Swiss counterpart. But there are many American ideas that the Swiss could apply without much cost or difficulty, thereby improving the health and quality of the milk.

THE ECONOMIC SIDE

There are vegetarians who assert that they can get by quite well without dairy produce. It is perhaps possible in the lowlands where so many fresh vegetables can be grown in the market gardens. A typical example of turning pasture land into arable land is provided by China, where population increases required the conversion of pasture land for the cultivation of more grains and vegetables. Such an arrangement would be impossible to apply to mountainous regions where fruits and vegetables will not grow. With very few exceptions, dairy farming is the only thing that can be carried on successfully as far as food production is concerned. In Switzerland, the best milk comes from the mountain regions and is instrumental in stabilizing the economy of the country through the production of various kinds of cheese and other milk food products.

OVERSTRESSING FINANCIAL CONSIDERATIONS

The subject of dairy farming leads me to consider the mistaken policy of the meat industry, which obviously has much to do with cattle raising. How stupid it seems to prevent a calf from eating hay and feeding it only on milk, so that its flesh will remain white. The idea, of course, is that white meat brings more money than the red meat of veal. This outlook, aided

453

and abetted by the consumer is very short-sighted, because red meat is of better value nutritionally. Since the white meat is more tender, perhaps this is the reason that it is more expensive.

The same principle applies to white bread and other white flour products, showing once more the power of propaganda and how demands are created to spoil the palate so that artificially prepared foods with all their additives seem to taste better, ignoring the fact that they may be greatly inferior to products made from whole cereals. If one continues to eat white bread, soon the lack of cellulose will translate itself into constipation, which in turn, encourages a host of other troubles that will ultimately be dealt with by injections and all sorts of harmful drugs and medicines. One mistake after another is made and, sooner or later, the price for choosing one's food according to the dictates of the palate will have to be paid for by chronic ill health and physical suffering. How much wiser it would be to forego the temporary loss of gastronomic pleasures and adapt oneself to the more healthful foods, which give true taste sensation that really becomes a pleasure to eat, instead of the cultivated taste for the artificial. It is not only the individual who would be the ultimate beneficiary from eating natural health foods, but the economy of the land would gain a boost as well.

YOGURT

The thought of Yogurt recalls to mind the Northern Europeans, in Bulgaria and parts of Siberia, whose longevity and health has been commonly attributed to the fact that they ate this healthgiving food in abundance.

What is Yogurt? One usually gets the answer that it is a kind of sour milk coagulated. In a certain sense this is correct, the difference being that ordinary sour milk contains approximately six grams of lactic acid per liter while yogurt contains about two grams.

The lactic acid fermentation does play a considerable part in the preparation of yogurt, but its particular properties and taste are due to the Maya-bacillus which works in symbiotic association with ordinary oriental lactic acid bacillus.

Is yogurt more healthful than sweet milk? Sweet milk coagulates in the stomach into a curd, simulating the same process as in making cheese. Thus rennet from the stomach of calves is put into warm milk, which thereupon turns into curd. This process imposes upon the stomach quite a bit of work, which it accomplishes only insufficiently, or not at all, if there is a disturbance in the secretion of the gastric fluids or if the stomach lacks tone. People have found it difficult to digest sweet milk if the stomach is not performing well. On the other hand, most people can tolerate yogurt or sour milk quite well. The reason is that they enter the stomach in a predigested form, that is, a fine curd. When children vomit after having drunk milk, the milk returns in big white lumps and this is what causes the digestive problem. When they vomit after having drunk sour milk or yogurt, a flaky fluid will come up instead of lumps. Some children, too, are allergic to pasteurized sweet milk while most youngsters can take yogurt with no ill results.

The greatest benefits from yogurt are intestinal. Yogurt will cleanse the intestinal mucous membranes and encourage the development of a healthy intestinal flora, meanwhile eliminating the pathological kind. This results in better digestion and assimilation of the food. Yogurt should be eaten as the first course of a vegetable meal. To combine it with fruit is less beneficial because it can lead to undesirable fermentation. Anyone inclined to flatulence should avoid taking sugar or sweet fruit with yogurt.

Intestinal putrefaction which manifests itself by bad smelling stools can be overcome eventually by eating yogurt. I emphasize eventually, for there are people who think that an occasional glass of it will rid them of all their digestive disorders. This is not so. If satisfactory results are to be obtained, yogurt will have to be taken regulary over a period of time. It is a good idea to have yogurt in every home, and those who depend upon it for reasons of health will find that it pays to make it themselves. Instructions are readily available at any health food store.

YEAST

Fifty years ago the British experimented with yeast and yeast extract for various expeditions. From the point of view of weight and size, it turned out to be most suitable for its purpose. A man can keep going and last longer on a pound of yeast extract than on a pound of any other concentrated food. At that time the value was known only by the results that were obtained from its practical use. Up until then not much was known of vitamin content. If today yeast is looked upon as one of the most valuable concentrated foods, research and experiments have amply justified this opinion. Most yeast is primarily grown from molasses and has a naturally high amount of phosphorus. Among the various B vitamins can be found B-1 which enables the cell tissue to take up oxygen and burn off carbohydrates. In addition to B-1 yeast contains B-6 and both of these are important to the nervous system. It is high in Niacin and Pantothenic acid and contains many of the Amino acids so necessary to the well-being of the body. Yeast may be considered as something in the nature of a botanic insulin and its beneficial influence on the pancreas, i.e. the islets of Langerhans, certainly warrants this description. Diabetics should use *yeast extract* as a sandwich spread in preference to any other savory paste.

Yeast extract and yeast itself should be taken in small but frequent quantities and those whose intestinal flora is subnormal would be well advised to abstain from "live" yeast and take only the extract so as to avoid flatulence from fermentation. Apart from that, the extract is much more convenient to use as a spread, in stews, soups and the like.

It is well known that yeast taken in small quantities regularly has been demonstrated to have excellent effects upon furunculosis, wounds that refuse to heal, neuralgic pains and similar aches due to inflammation of the nerves. It is also excellent for the treatment of intestinal, metabolic disorders, etc. Due to its high vitamin B content it has been found to be of special benefit during pregnancy. In connection with furunculosis it would be worthwhile mentioning that small quantities may cure this condition, while large quantities can cause the problem, thus confirming the homeopathic principle: any substance leading to pathological conditions when taken in excess, will act as a curative if administered in attenuated or potentized form.

At one time barm or beer yeast was used but due to its bitter taste, which cannot be completely eliminated without altering its health value, it has been replaced by a precultured and special control method, usually using molasses as a base.

COOKING SALT

How much salt do we need? We were taught in school that a person needs or requires 14 lbs. of salt a year in order to survive. Man or beast cannot do without it, although it is acknowledged that certain diseases require a restricted or even a saltfree diet. This apparent contradiction resolves itself when we realize that one's salt requirements need not necessarily be obtained from the crystalline kind of salt, but can very well come from one's food, provided it is consumed in a natural, uncooked state. A case in point is the Asiatic steppe dwellers. They have never heard of salt in crystalline form and, as they could not survive without it, it is obvious that they must obtain sufficient quantities of it from their food. It is impossible to imagine the blood serum, similar in its makeup to sea water, without salt.

In most industrial countries, the intake of salt is usually in excess of the actual requirements. As this is anything but conducive to good health, and the individual has no way of assessing his exact needs, it would be wise to reduce the intake of ordinary cooking salt to a minimum. Instead, eat plenty of fresh vegetables such as leek, onions, carrots, etc. which contain sufficient sodium chloride – the chemical name of salt – to meet the requirements of the body. The fact that fresh, raw vegetables are a source of salt is frequently overlooked and many believe they must use ordinary salt to avoid deficiencies. Many well-known doctors such as Gerson, Riedlin and Hermannsdorfer have stated without reserve, that in cases of tuberculosis of the bones, salt has a markedly bad effect, whereas abstinence from it improves the general condition and stimulates the healing ability of the body.

Those who suffer from kidney ailments know that little or no salt is one of the important treatments if they are to recover rapidly. Even for those in excellent health, it would be sensible to reduce the consumption of salt as much as possible so as to avoid overburdening the kidneys.

Salt as a medicine:

Applied externally, salt is an excellent remedy for a host of ailments or taken orally in the form of biochemic or homeopathic triturations.

Sea water bathing is recommended for glandular disturbances, which so often result in obesity. The thyroid also can benefit considerably from sea bathing and anyone who suffers from goiter or similar thyroid problems will obtain good results from it. If you live in the interior and do not have access to the beach, you can use dry or moist salt packs at home to draw away water from the tissues, and thereby reduce *edema*.

Gargling with salt water is an excellent substitute for the more expensive antiseptics for the throat sold over-the-counter and is probably just as effective. In the case of *catarrh* or inflammation of the mucosa, tepid salt water should be sniffed up the nostrils first and then rinsed with clear water. This simple treatment will reduce one's liability to respiratory ailments. Naturally, if you live near the sea, it would be better to use sea water, provided you can find some uncontaminated.

Sea salt, as opposed to mined and refined ordinary or "Iodine-enriched" salt, can be taken internally advantageously. The trace elements found in sea salt benefit the endocrine glands and normalize both their sub and hyper-function. Obesity is often the cause of glandular sub-function, and in such cases, ordinary salt aggravates the condition by increasing the weight still more. On the other hand, sea salt will reduce obesity. There are dietetic preparations on the market utilizing sea salt with their trace elements and, in addition, antibiotic elements of several different plants. Use of these preparations as seasonings, will have a prophylactic effect against infectious diseases and generally influence the course of any existing ailments favorably.

Salt is an excellent preservative of meat and fresh plant extracts without lessening their therapeutic value. It is also used by homeopaths as Natrium mur. used in different potencies.

CARE OF THE TEETH

It will be agreed, that from a health viewpoint, care of the teeth is more important than any beauty or body care. As a small boy I'm afraid I heartily disagreed with the idea of cleaning my teeth daily. Why couldn't teeth keep themselves clean, I wondered. Of course they could. I had heard of primitive peoples who lived a natural life, close to nature and they had beautiful teeth without brushing them or giving them special care. I was told that, unfortunately, on account of our modern diet and way of living, we had lost many of the advantages that primitive peoples still enjoyed. I was also told that bacteria settles between the teeth, getting into every crevice, and if not regularly removed, would eventually cause decay. However, no satisfactory answer to my question as to how the teeth of primitive races could remain healthy without brushing them, was forthcoming.

Of course, primitive people are exposed to the same tooth destroying germs that we are, but the enamel of their teeth is harder than ours and does not allow bacteria to lodge in their crevices. The excellency of dental health is found in the simplicity of their eating habits. The hard, unrefined food they consume forces them to masticate it thoroughly, which increases the blood supply to the teeth and also cleans them at the same time. The food is more healthful than ours and therefore prevents deficiencies which would sooner or later affect the teeth through the bloodstream and cause them to deteriorate, thereby permitting the germs to lodge which would begin the process of decay.

Natural diet and dental hygiene:

A healthy unrefined diet will supply sufficient calcium, fluorine and other important elements, to keep the teeth in perfect condition. Primitive people have such beautiful teeth because their crude diet supplies all the elements they need to preserve their teeth in a healthy condition, whereas we, with our artificial foods, suffer from all sorts of deficiencies. It does not matter whether you are Chinese, African or Indian or whether you are white, yellow, black or brown because dental health still depends upon a natural diet. The proof of this is found in North American negroes. It is only since they have left their native lands and adopted the diet and customs of their new environment that their teeth have shown signs of deterioration. Thus, dentistry has become part of their every-day lives whereas, a century or more ago, a dentist would have starved for lack of patients.

Should we clean our teeth? Certainly, for we no longer possess natural resistance and therefore have to aid nature mechanically to remove all food particles and germs from the surface and crevices of the teeth.

To insure healthy teeth, we should adopt a natural diet. By so doing we will be taking the first decisive step towards healthier teeth. Because our bodies have now become degenerate through the introduction of modern foods we must completely change our diet to one of eating natural raw fruits and vegetables to give our teeth the care they need. There are still many people who have good teeth, but if an analysis is made of their diet it will be found that they seldom eat sweets and enjoy following a natural way of life. There is a canton in Switzerland where the people, for the most part, seem to have excellent teeth and without a doubt, one of the reasons is that the people of Valais eat bread made from natural cereals.

As a young man, I had bad teeth, due to an artificial diet. I changed it and within three years my dentist assured me that my teeth showed definite signs of hardening. When six years passed, he was congratulating me on my change of diet and said that my teeth were in excellent condition. Now, after 60 years, I still have the same good teeth I had in my youth.

To safeguard the teeth, all refined foods should be avoided. To start with, white sugar and flour should be definitely crossed off your diet. Every school and every dentist's office should have constant reminders of the two enemies of strong, healthy teeth, white sugar and white flour – the main destroyers of children's teeth. Normal, healthy teeth cannot thrive in an atmosphere of candy, cakes, and refined foods in general.

RULES FOR THE CARE OF THE TEETH

A few rules for the care of the teeth might be useful to everyone. First of all, the teeth should be cleaned every day with a good cleansing agent. This can be a tooth paste that does not contain any strong chemicals or it can be baking soda which was a favorite tooth cleanser at the turn of the century. Sometimes a little salt was added to the baking soda for abrasion. Every small sign of decay should be given immediate attention by a competent dentist. This is very important because many persons keep putting off going to the dentist, hoping their tooth problem will go away, but sadly enough, it never does and, in the end, procrastination can cause the loss of an irreplaceable natural tooth. In the modern diet deposits of plaque, which cannot be readily seen, are deposited on the teeth in the form of sticky bacterial matter. If left to accumulate the damage can result in decay and eventual loss of teeth. Daily brushing with a medium to soft brush will remove the plaque and help maintain the teeth in a healthy condition. Small defects when neglected may result in having to kill the nerve if the tooth isn't too far gone. A tooth without a nerve is a dead tooth and becomes a foreign body in the mouth. Blocking out of the nerve is not generally encouraged by dentists as the tooth, being insensitive, has to be watched carefully, for it may precipitate the formation of granuloma, an ideal nesting ground for germs of all sorts. A little thing like that can endanger one's health because the metabolic toxins discharged into the bloodstream can cause a host of ailments. Big problems can come from small beginnings as far as the teeth are concerned. Some of the problems directly attributable to dead teeth are cardiac pains, palpitations when over exerting oneself, kidney and liver dysfunction as well as other organic problems. American doctors are generally credited with the discovery of these problems emanating from germ ridden dead teeth. The sad thing was, that in the case of articular rheumatism, some dentists short-sightedly extracted not only the dead teeth with their granuloma, but also all the other good teeth. This, of course, was later corrected but not until a lot of damage was done.

A railway employee was forced to have all his excellent teeth extracted because a doctor decided they were the cause of his heart trouble. He was unwilling to have this done, but gave in because he was afraid the insurance company would refuse to continue his policy. Unfortunately the removal of his teeth did not cure his heart problem. A nature cure eventually succeeded, but, alas!, nature treatments, however good, could not replace his extracted teeth.

DENTAL TREATMENT

Never deceive yourself in thinking that a small dental defect will eventually correct itself. See your dentist right away. Choose a capable dentist and do not look for the cheapest one as there is no insurance that "cheap is best". Look for one who is highly recommended by friends who have had satisfactory work done, for in the long run it will pay to have the best available dental treatment possible.

A capable dentist, at the first sign of articular rheumatism for example, will X-ray the teeth to see, if by chance, a granuloma is the cause of the trouble. To effectively treat this infection requires professional knowledge and craftsmanship. Some people experience side effects when different amalgams are used to fill a cavity, chiefly among which are mercury and silver. Some material resembling tooth substance should be used to fill root canals and real ivory is obviously the correct material for this. Gold crowns have often proved their worth but they are not suitable for everyone, especially those sensitive to metals. There is no way of knowing beforehand if a sensitivity to metals exists but if problems follow a metal filling, then the patient would be advised to consider many of the non-metal amalgams that are now available.

A good dentist will take great care to see that the crowns and fillings fit well. They must come well up into the neck of the tooth, so that no space is left uncovered, as this would become a breeding ground for germs. The crowns should not be too long either as this might cause irritation and inflammation. The solution to these problems depends upon the dentist's skill. A loose crown can lead to suppurative conditions and an abscess formation which, when prematurely closed in, can cause the most fearful pains imaginable, because of gases that are formed with no outlet to escape. Under such circumstances it will be unavoidable to refrain from using anodyne drugs. A further consequence could be infiltration of bacterial toxins into the system, thus endangering the heart and other organs as well. That is why it's important to go to a really good dentist because his knowledge is indispensible in the proper treatment of your teeth and the avoidance of pitfalls a poor dentist cannot see.

We need healthy teeth to enable us to chew well and this is most essential for proper digestion. Food can be assimilated properly, only if full use of the salivary glands is employed after the food enters the mouth. There are six large and several small salivary glands which secrete various alkaline substances that are of the utmost importance to the whole digestive process. If food particles are sufficiently insalivated, further digestion will be made much easier. The more the teeth are used in chewing, the better chance they have of remaining healthy. For this reason one should not eat an abundance of food soaked or mashed, as this gives the teeth nothing to bite on. Apples are an excellent fruit to eat as they necessitate chewing and their juice is an excellent cleanser. That "an apple a day keeps the doctor away" may sound trite, but it nevertheless is a good tried and true formula as far as keeping the dentist away, although it is no panacea for all dental problems, we realize. A healthy constitution begins with healthy teeth and proper care of them cannot be emphasized too much.

CARE OF THE HAIR

Most people are very careful to give their hair careful attention but many do not seem to grasp the fact that the most important requisite for beautiful hair is internal well-being. There are many preparations available for hair culture, claiming to grow new hair, energize the scalp, replace lost minerals in the hair, etc. A good hair treatment of course, will do some good for the hair as will also certain scalp lotions. However, no matter how much external applications are used, if the internal needs are not satisfied, all is in vain. If the body lacks proper minerals it will be evident in the hair. If our diet is natural and a biological calcium preparation containing silica is taken regularly, it will be a delightful surprise to find that our hair becomes so much better looking.

There are some hair treatments such as scalp lotions that will improve the hair but it is what goes into the mouth in the form of food and food supplements that will have their greatest effect. As a rule, poor hair is the result of a deficiency of calcium and silica. If the hair is very greasy it is usually a sign of a glandular disturbance that can be corrected by taking a tonic designed for this specific purpose. Although a gland tonic will not directly restore the hair immediately, if this dysfunction is corrected it will go a long way toward helping to bring new life back to it.

SCALP LOTIONS AND HAIR GROWING REMEDIES

There are all kinds of scalp lotions advertised and no doubt some may be quite good while others may not be quite so good. However, there is one remedy that never came out of a chemist's laboratory that will certainly have a better effect than most, and which can be easily raised in your garden or is easily procurable from your supermarket. It is the common onion. Onions contain sulphur and this natural sulphur is a very good skin lotion. If you have any *hair or scalp problems,* take half an onion and rub it well into the scalp before washing your hair. The treatment is simple, inexpensive and effective. While onion rubbed into the scalp will stimulate hair growth, in order to achieve still better results, it will be necessary to use another hair nutrient, lanolin, which contains Vitamin F. Obtained from sheep's wool, it is a biologically correct hair oil. In its natural state Adeps Lanae is too tough and too sticky. A specially prepared lanolin cream is available which, when used with onion, brings excellent results.

The plant nettles, in the form of an infusion or a fresh extract, is an excellent hair tonic and especially in the case of skin eruptions in the scalp. Many recommend Birch leaves too, but the best of all, I think, is the onion. If you do not like the idea of using a raw onion, there is an onion scalp lotion on the market in which the onion is deodorized. Naturally, washing the hair regularly is part of the beauty treatment and a protein lotion may be used to soften the hair. If one wishes to have a healthy scalp and beautiful hair, there are plenty of remedies from which to choose.

TREATMENT OF THE SKIN

It is true that Nature itself sees to it that our skin contains the necessary quantity of oil, and for this purpose we have been given our sebacious glands, which work automatically. I have noticed that primitive people have much oilier skin than we have and so it has never been necessary for them to worry about dry skin. For some reason, the sebacious glands do not work as well on people living in industrialized societies and there is a very good reason for this. The fact that we go against, rather than with Nature from the point of view of food, clothing, general living conditions etc. discourages the proper function of the skin and the sebaceous glands. To remedy this we must give our *skin* all the help it needs in the form of a good soothing oil. It is a good idea to always oil the body well before going swimming, whether in a fresh water lake, river or at the seashore. This will help the body to retain its warmth and you will not shiver or feel chilled even if the water is cool. This has been my own personal experience although I must admit I have good circulation and do not chill easily. The oil treatment is especially good when bathing in the ocean as salt water has a tendency to dry the skin, especially when lying in the sun after having bathed.

It is not necessary and does not benefit the skin in any way to smear too much oil on the body so that it looks like a piece of fat bacon. Oil should be used sparingly on the body and massaged well into the skin. Avoid artificially perfumed oils as they may not be as effective due to artificial chemicals used in them to give an odor. Pure olive oil mixed with lemon is a good skin lotion for bathing.

466

If you want to use a prepared oil, look for a skin oil that is made from *St. John's wort oil,* because it is a most excellent skin nutrient on account of the lipoids (substances resembling fats or oils) it contains.

Care of the skin not only requires the use of an oil, but involves common sense in exposing the body to the sun, light and air. Proper skin function is a precondition for proper glandular function and for general well-being.

CARE OF THE FEET

What long and faithful service is rendered by our feet! We take it for granted every day that they will bear the whole weight of our body and take us wherever we want to go. As a rule we neglect the daily foot bath that they so urgently need, as they perform not only a mechanical but also an eliminative function. Everyone knows about perspiration of the feet and although it can become very embarrassing when excessive, it has a function. Excessive foot sweat rids the body of toxins which cannot be eliminated in any other way. Thus, the feet are always on call, and when required, can assume the role of a secondary or emergency channel of elimination. If such a channel is blocked by measures which suppress its function, the toxins will remain in the system where they will cause havoc. I have never found a person with considerable perspiration of the feet suffering from any form of lung trouble. Specialists in lung diseases, whose experience is much wider and deeper than mine, also confirm this. Thus, one forms the logical conclusion, that the beginning of lung problems may be connected in one way or another with the direct suppression of *foot perspiration* or some other eliminative body function.

If your feet perspire, wash them thoroughly at least once a day. This is more important than washing your face, for it does not perspire to the same extent as the feet.

The washing of the feet in the East is almost a ritual because most people wear sandals and they recognize the hygienic and health reasons for it. And so it should be with us. If you wash your feet every day for one month only, you will notice how your general feeling of well-being improves. If you arrive home at the end of a day, tired, depressed, with a headache, try a herb foot bath and see how it will soothe you and give you an entirely different outlook on things. True, it will not solve your problems but it will help you to better face them. For therapeutic purposes take a herb foot bath every second day. Add to the bath wild thyme, juniper needles or any other aromatic herbs and you will be strengthened and refreshed. For further refreshening, after the foot bath, rub well into the feet St. John's wort oil or olive oil as the oil stimulates the skin function, even if used only once a week. This daily care of the feet takes only a few minutes at the end of the day and it pays dividends in good health.

WALKING BAREFOOT

Until a few years ago, when young folks began to go barefoot, the art of walking without shoes had been all but forgotten. In the past it was also associated with poverty and aborigines. However walking barefoot is an exercise that can soothe your entire nervous system. Of course, where you walk is of considerable importance, as it would be inadvisable to do so on city pavements or around the barnyard where nails may cause infections. However, it is suggested that sometimes, in the early morning, take a walk barefoot on the grass still wet with dew and you will immediately realize how good it feels. If you have spent a restless night in bed or if you are overtired and have had great mental strain and your "batteries" so to speak, are running low or your nerves are at the snapping point, you will find, that after a barefoot walk on the grass, your whole nervous system will benefit by it and become regenerated and any tension you may have will be lowered. This renewed strength and energy which Mother Earth imparts to our bodies provides a simple way of unwinding.

Walking barefoot, sensibly employed, is a remedy which should not be despised as the glands are definitely stimulated by this exercise. The ancient Greeks, who were far from being physically degenerate, seem to have known about the energy to be derived from being in contact with the earth. Otherwise the legend of Gäa, who was known as the strength-giving Mother Earth, would not have come into existence. The legend tells of the giant Antaeos, the son of Gäa, as deriving all his strength from her, the earth. His enemies could beat him at wrestling only if they could get him off the ground for then his strength would leave him. The moment his feet touched the ground, his strength would return and he couldn't be defeated. Thus, although only a legend, the strength regenerating powers of the earth are illustrated.

Walking and exercising in the morning dew:

Many will find it easy to walk, run or do their exercises in the still dew-wet grass. Perhaps you live in town and would find it too inconvenient to seek out a green meadow before breakfast but what a lot of good it would do to enjoy this refreshing moment, before the rush of a busy day.

How much to be envied are those who live in the midst of nature, who in early morning carry out their natural exercise of hay-making or general farm work. Even though they may not realize it, these farmers are conditioning their bodies by working outdoors regularly. It would be an excellent restorative to take a holiday on a farm and get up early and join these people in their early morning chores so as to regenerate our bodies which have been worn and wearied during the working year.

Early morning exercises demand from us deep breathing, as this will help to drive out the remaining traces of weariness from our bodies and enable us to start the day's work refreshed.

FRESH AIR

The benefits of fresh air are far too little known and appreciated. One so often enters a bedroom, living room or study and finds the air so heavy that it is almost impossible to breathe. These rooms should be aired frequently. If windows remain closed the morbid air can do much harm. In this day of energy crisis the question might arise as to whether it is wise to air rooms at a time when fuel is so expensive. Most of us have learned in our younger days at school in physics classes, that a fire will not burn if it is deprived of oxygen. That is why a fireplace needs to be ventilated properly in order to make the wood or the coal burn. In the same way our bodies need clean, fresh air in order to work properly. In the case of a sick person, never deprive him of fresh air, even though he may have a fever. If he is properly covered he will not chill. It is lack of air that will do the damage, and retard improvement.

EFFECTS OF SMOKING

When a young person first starts smoking, how very unpleasant he finds it. It is not a question of enjoyment. On the contrary, the young person must fight all the way through nausea, disgust, nervous shock, dizziness, and a general feeling of uneasy aversion in order to overcome the ill-effects of a beginning smoker. Eventually, through dogged persistence, he may acquire a taste for tobacco, but it is far from a natural procedure and the body resists the introduction of nicotine into it.

As with all harmful practices, the person trying to enjoy smoking insists that the enjoyment supersedes the dangers involved. Some may point to their grandfathers, who though constant smokers, lived beyond eighty years or more. The exceptions are quickly put forth but the general average is ignored. It is true that a person with a strong constitution can sometimes stand poisons without apparent damage to health. If there are people who can withstand tobacco poisoning and grow old in spite of it, that does not mean that everyone has such strong powers of resistance. On the contrary, millions are killed prematurely by nicotine, narcotics, alcohol and other intoxicants.

What are the dangers inherent in nicotine? It is the arterial system in general and the coronary arteries in particular that are affected by smoking. If the addict has constitutionally weak blood vessels to start with, the danger of smoking is all the greater for him. The vessels lose their elasticity, become progressively narrower and thus restrict the flow of blood to the heart, the walls of which are poorly nourished and begin to deteriorate.

Electrocardiagrams and X-rays tell the story of the change of activity and appearance of the heart under continued influence of chronic nicotine poisoning. The delicate, tensed muscles become relaxed and gradually change to a dirty brown color. If a person's heart muscles constantly suffer from lack of adequate nourishment, they will begin to look like those of a very old person. Pathological anatomy speaks of "brown atrophy" in describing such cases, because the worn out brownish pigments are deposited in individual cells of the heart muscles. In addition, a number of small, white streaks are noticeable. These indicate that minute particles of the muscle itself have been destroyed and are now replaced by connective and cicatrice tissues. Once the tissues of the heart muscles have been destroyed, they cannot be replaced, not even by the best possible natural remedies. All one can do is to strengthen whatever undamaged tissue is left so that it can now do the work that had previously been done by the scarred tissue.

If one values life, ought one not take great care of the heart muscle? It brings to mind words of ancient wisdom: "Treasure your heart above all things, for from it, comes life." If the heart fails, death rapidly follows. Anyone who has witnessed a heart failure is extraordinarily affected by this tragedy – the sudden change from life to death. The pathologist will say that the heart muscles were starved of blood for many years. The information that nicotine had been responsible for the fatal damage is then, unfortunately no longer of any use. It is too late.

The mere fact that the effects of nicotine poisoning become apparent long before its possible fatal consequences take place, should make the addicted one decide to give up smoking before it is too late.

The blood pressure and the pulse beat also react adversely to nicotine. In extensive tests it was found that the average rise in blood pressure after inhaling one cigarette was 15 m/m while the pulse beat increased by 15 per minute.

Tobacco can also damage plants, as a simple experiment will prove. Place cress seeds in two small dishes and when they begin to sprout, place a glass cover over them. When the plants are about an inch high, under one of the glass covers blow cigarette or cigar smoke; repeat next day. Within a few days the smoked plants will be dead, completely shrivelled up while the one in the uncontaminated dish will be perfectly healthy. Any gardener will tell you that tobacco extract kills insect life and this particular use of tobacco can be recommended, as long as it is not sprayed on fruit.

There is a general idea that tobacco is only dangerous because of its nicotine content. This is incorrect. There is yet another evil inherent in tobacco and that is the phenols and tarry substances that are released in the process of smoking. The latter is, to a great extent, responsible for the development of cancer. Smoker's cancer usually starts on the tongue or in the throat and results directly from tar contamination rather than the nicotine. Thus, there is no reason to draw a conclusion that low nicotine or nicotine-free tobacco is safe to smoke.

Despite the warning by the Surgeon General of the United States and governmental authorities in Great Britain that smoking is hazardous to one's health, and all advertisements for tobacco must be accompanied by this warning, it appears to have made very little progress in discouraging young people from taking up smoking. It appears that smoking is linked with personal freedom and when the medical profession sets such a poor example, as it has been observed that many doctors are habitual smokers, what can be expected from the lay person except to follow the example. The fact that lung cancer and pulmonary diseases can be directly connected to the use of tobacco is not a sufficient deterrent to disuade or discourage people from taking up the habit. It is not surprising that Dr. A. H. Roffo, university professor, should write: "I consider tobacco a narcotic such as cocaine, morphine and other drugs. In my opinion, tobacco is much more dangerous, for the number of people who indulge in hard drugs is small in comparison to the ever growing number of tobacco users. Besides, cocaine and morphine addicts, more often than not, are sick people, while tobacco, for the most part, attracts healthy young people." Though narcotic poisons are much more dangerous than tobacco, the latter is a far greater menace to humanity from a health standpoint because it has become so widespread.

BREATH IS LIFE

The peculiar connections between our psychic and physical life mirror themselves in the sentence "Breath is life". Again and again we find this subject discussed in journals and lecture halls from a scientific as well as a practical point of view. Research has definitely shown that mental depression can have a very potent effect on general health. It is safe to say that over 50% of present day illnesses have their origin in mental and emotional problems; and endemic and chronic diseases can be greatly aided by what our mind feeds on. Particularly, a negative outlook will greatly delay improvement of any kind.

Those who frequently are forced into a position contrary to the position taken by a majority often are faced with hostility. Those who are not emotionally equipped to face such problems are doomed from the beginning. But, if one stands up for morally correct convictions and has the proper thickness of skin, so to speak, of resisting the corrosive effect of wrong thinking, he will be able to sail triumphantly through such storms with calm imperturbability and the ability to overcome attacks. Nevertheless, it sometimes happens that adverse criticism, slander and calumny affect one's mental state to such an extent that it saps his physical resistance causing a breakdown in general health and nerves and even certain organs, as a result, fail to properly function.

Anger, worry, disgust, disappointment and frustration are bad companions for health as they nag at our nerves and eventually, the liver and pancreas are affected; and this is what happened to me. In the face of professional adversity, my stomach began to go awry in spite of maintaining the best possible diet. Flatulence followed. Breathing became difficult and heart problems appeared. Soon afterwards, an operation for appendicitis was necessary.

BREATHING EXERCISES

Thinking things over, I developed the idea of exercising the abdominal organs by rhythmic breathing. At first I practiced this by drawing the abdomen in when I inhaled, and pressing it out when I exhaled. On further consideration, however, I decided to reverse the order of things and draw in the abdomen when I exhaled and press it out when I inhaled. This resulted in considerable relief after a little while. The gases escaped and I felt better.

My first task in the morning was this breathing exercise, another session followed after lunch and finally one before going to sleep. I began to sleep better because after this intensive exercise, I felt pleasantly tired and relaxed. Now I began to enjoy long deep sleep, oblivious to the cares, worries and annoyances of the day.

From a physical point of view, my abdominal muscles seemed to be the first to benefit. They became stronger, my diaphragm developed and my digestion became better. I no longer felt any trace of pains and the inflammations had by now disappeared. A natural diet helped considerably and stood me in good stead, but without breathing exercises it would have been difficult to achieve success. A long time after this experiment, I saw a chiropractor, who was also a good friend of mine. The X-rays he took showed a normal spine, no arthritis, in fact, no signs of degeneration. He assured me that my diphragm muscles were exceptionally well developed which I attributed to breathing exercises. Apart from that these exercises enabled me to take a more cheerful outlook on life again.

NOSE BREATHING

An experience I had quite some years ago, quite by chance, was most helpful to me. My lungs were damaged in a motor accident and the resulting problem could have posed difficulties for me. However, I went to the mountains for the sake of pure air, adopted a natural diet and was making satisfactory progress. The "finishing touches", however, were provided by regular deep breathing exercises. I concentrated on thorough exhalation, followed by equally thorough inhalation. I began these exercises in front of an open window in fairly cold weather. In spite of the cold, this strenuous exercise made me perspire. I then took a short rest before starting on the exercise again. The air seemed to flow through my body like a warm stream and if I had been breathing through my mouth, undoubtedly I would have caught a chill with the possibility of pneumonia resulting. Thus I became aware of the importance of breathing through the nose and could appreciate why this is recommended in all health books. We possess a heating element in our nose which warms the air as we breathe it in; thus air below freezing will be warmed up to natural body temperature as it passes through the nostrils. That is why it is important in cold climates to breathe through the nose and when real cold to wrap a woolen scarf over the mouth and nose to protect the membranes. In the tropics, the nose acts as a thermostat and when hot air passes through it is cooled down to approximately blood heat.

Correct nose breathing will help avoid certain types of headaches. If in spite of having a good night's rest, you are still tired in the morning, or if you wake up with catarrh, then you must pay particular attention to breathing through the nose. You can tie a handkerchief around your mouth, or put a piece of adhesive tape over it at night, until such a time as breathing through the nose comes easily and naturally. Once you establish the habit of nose breathing you will wake up refreshed and ready for the day ahead. Also, if you snore, you will soon overcome it through nasal breathing.

There is no doubt that correct breathing has a salutary effect on the brain, since the air passes beneath the bony roof of the post-nasal cavity over which the important brain cells lie. Every anatomical detail of the human body serves a specific purpose. For example, why is the nasal space divided into three corridors through which air must pass before it can enter the nasopharyngal canal and the bronchial tubes? In flowing past the blood vessel-lined interior of the nose, the air is warmed and prepared for the lungs. In addition, the anterior nostrils are considerably smaller than the posterior nares and this causes a partial vacuum in the nasal interior, which sucks the warm air from accessory nasal cavities and mixes it with cold air coming in with each breath. With what extraordinary genius the construction of the nose has been planned! If the smallest detail in its structure was altered the normal airflow would be diverted and fail to accomplish its purpose. Everything is perfectly planned and in its right place to functionally serve the lungs, the heart, the body and keep one alive.

Favorable effects upon other diseases:

Correct breathing not only affects the head, heart, lungs and stomach, but the whole body. It influences and stimulates the activity of the sympathetic and para-sympathetic nervous systems. These interesting anatomical arrangements, which make, one might say, a brainless life possible, are responsible for the involuntary or subconscious functions of the body. Correct, deep breathing via these systems, will improve the functions of all internal organs. Even conditions such as *Angina pectoris, asthma, constipation* and *obesity* may be improved if other curative measures are employed at the same time. In the case of *constipation* at least fifteen minutes, mornings, afternoons and evenings should be devoted to deep breathing exercises. Within a week, if the exercise is kept up, the bowels will begin to function better and within at least a month regular bowel function will result.

A slim figure can be kept by correct breathing. The stomach with the "spare tire" look will disappear more quickly if, at the same time, attention is given to the diet. Even if one is careless with the diet, correct breathing alone will insure a 50% success in achieving a good figure.

Incorrect breathing can lead to the formation of polypi, whereas correct breathing will prevent and even cure them. If women would but breathe properly, most of their abdominal complaints could be prevented. Confinements would be much easier and nervous congestions would disappear. Tight clothing, belts, tight fitting elastic girdles should be avoided if abdominal breathing is to remain unrestricted. It is preferable to exercise the abdominal muscles to maintain their elasticity rather than to control their shape by girdles that restrict, which only serves to weaken the muscles. As soon as such an artificial contrivance is removed, the muscles which have been kept in place by pressure, will again bulge out, thus defeating the purpose of maintaining a pleasant appearance.

Breathing exercises in school:

If school children were taught correct breathing, their lungs, chests and diaphragms would develop properly and respiratory problems of the chest and lungs would largely remain unknown.

Professional singers never lose sight of the importance of correct breathing, for it is one of the main avenues that leads to a successful vocal career. Correct breathing is necessary for not only controlling the voice but in enhancing its quality.

How long should breathing exercises be practiced? To begin with, one minute may be sufficient. Gradually the time should be extended until the exercises become habitual and we no longer have to repeat them as conscious activities. Regularity of the exercises is of the utmost importance because this helps to promote new rhythm into the body better than anything else.

Physical exercises should not be ignored because they are important to the well-being of the whole body, but the results achieved cannot compare with those attained by breathing exercises done in the correct manner.

This is a form of "Medicine" that is within the reach of everyone and its regular application will bring truly amazing results. It can make the difference between good health and misery. It is always at hand and needs no written prescription; only a little energy, concentration and patience and it costs absolutely nothing.

We recognize with gratitude the help obtained from natural remedies and foods; from rest and proper exercise, but are we aware that it is only through correct breathing that we will crown the other successes and will add the finishing touches to their results?

NATURAL SLEEP

The question of how much sleep a person really needs has occupied the thoughts of many clever people who, try as they might, have never arrived at a satisfactory answer.

Some say that seven or eight hours sleep are necessary if one really wants to be rested and ready for work, while others seem to think that one can manage well with four or five hours. Regarding those who sleep fewer hours, it is question-able whether the nerve cells have had sufficient time to

478

become regenerated and whether, in time, some deficiency will become apparent. Failing strength, short attention spans and easy tiring are definite indications that one is getting insufficient sleep, no matter what kind of theories anyone has on the subject. Failure to remedy these symptoms can eventually produce a host of physical and mental problems.

The initial question can best be answered by nature herself. She sets before us a splendid example of the lively, ever active world of the birds. They begin their songs at the break of dawn when the average person is wasting the sunny hours of an early spring morning lying asleep in bed. They are already about their business and do not return to rest until the last traces of twilight have died out. For the birds this seems to be a natural and proper way of life and indeed, primitive people have adopted it. Ideally, our eyes were given to us by our Creator to enjoy and explore the light and what each day unfolds. In days of old, man rose early in the morning and took advantage of the daylight hours to accomplish his work and when night came he was ready to close his eyes in rest. Why otherwise was man given alternate light and darkness? Modern man, however, came along and invented artificial light for himself that enables him to prolong the day indefinitely. Today, our work can be prolonged indefinitely too, as a result. No longer can we say, as once was said: "Come, let us make an end to the day, for we have endured its cares for long enough." Now we can think of other ways, besides sleep, for banishing the cares of the day by dissipating our night hours in pleasures to help us forget our troubles. Thus, artificial light seems useful and practical to us, and we have forgotten that we have changed the natural rhythm of life to suit our own transient mood, personal need, or perhaps just to comply with a set of circumstances. Instead of waking with the first ray of sunshine so as to use every moment of natural light, we sleep through the most beautiful hours of the day and, of course, it is impossible to get our work done before the departing light invites us to sleep once more. In summer, we would have longer working hours. Could we but follow the natural rhythm of life, we would then have a wonderful opportunity of resting and becoming regenerated in the winter. We don't have to hibernate but by having a really good sleep before midnight, we should be well enough rested to rise with the dawn and work during the daylight hours. Nature's sleep lasts from sunset to sunrise and this was the correct rhythm of life planned for mankind from the beginning of his creation.

What would our civilization say to such a way of living? Obviously a resounding and uncompromising "NO!" How could habits and customs be changed so drastically? From a social and practical viewpoint it would, at this time, seem impossible to adapt to this once natural way of life, although it would be healthier for us. Try this form of life as an experiment either during your holidays or when you are convalescing from an illness. Instead of going out in the evenings on some social occasion that may last far into the night, take the opportunity to enjoy sleep several hours before midnight. If, during our holidays, we accustom ourselves to this way of life, perhaps, when we return from vacation, we will find our body and mind completely regenerated and strengthened with natural sleep. Our business and social life will actually benefit from this, for with our strength renewed, we will find ourselves in a position to work and play better. If, on the other hand, we behave like most people during their holiday and stay up all hours of the night enjoying social life to the full, then we should not be surprised if our body and mind demands a vacation once our holiday is over. So often I have said, sleeping far into the day does not compensate for those hours lost before midnight. An old proverb says: "One hour of sleep before midnight equals two hours after." This is no illusion, but a fact, that anyone can prove to himself over a two week period or even less, by going to bed when the sun goes down and getting up when it rises. He will find his nerves have become regenerated and his general health and vitality greatly improved. A clinical experiment carried out for one week showed interesting results: one person went to bed every night at midnight and slept for twelve hours until midday, while another slept from seven or eight o'clock in the evening until four or five o'clock in the morning. Even though the second person slept three or four hours less than the first person, it was found that he was more refreshed, more rested and in better physical condition. Without doubt, this was obvious proof that hours spent in rest before midnight are far more beneficial than the hours after midnight. Natural sleep is a simple easy way to help the body stay strong and healthy. The adage that "early to bed and early to rise, makes a man healthy, wealthy and wise" may seem trite for having been repeated so often but, nevertheless, no truer words were ever spoken. Give the experiment a try when your vacation time arrives and you will be surprised at the benefits derived from natural sleep before midnight.

THE HEALING POWER OF MUSIC

If harsh, clashing sounds such as that made by a factory gets on our nerves and could damage our health, it is easy to believe that harmony would do just the opposite for us. Science has studied the effects on humans produced by sounds of various kinds, and the consensus is that the right sort of music has definitely beneficial effects on our health.

Isn't the lullaby a mother sings at a child's bedside a good example of how a soft melody can have a calming effect? On the other hand, doesn't the loud blare of rock-and-roll music coming from a neighbor's open window, when one is trying to relax and rest, have just the opposite effect? How often have Mozart's delightful melodies raised our morale? How many troubled and wrinkled brows have been smoothed by listening to the works of great masters? The power of a Beethoven symphony has quieted many an agitated heart. Even the twittering of a bird song on a spring morning is often able to disperse worry and anxiety to such an extent, that those who see no solution to their troubles, return home from a walk in the woods, comforted and strengthened, hardly realizing from what source the power came. A child falls and immediately begins to scream to attract attention and assuage his pain. If, just then, a robin or a blackbird in the garden hedge sings, the child stops wailing. At first he is interested in where the voice is coming from, then comforted by the cheerful little minstrel; soon the pain is forgotten and the little face is all smiles again.

It is not surprising that intelligent doctors assert that music has a soothing influence on their patients when under stress and pain. It relaxes cramped muscles, improves the function of the glands and influences good digestion, which is directly dependent on glandular secretions. The dentist also is aware of the calming and soothing influence of soft music to such an extent that it is part of his office equipment. Not only is music available for the patient, but in some dental offices the patient may request the type of music he especially enjoys. Thus, while the drill is whirling around at high speed in the patient's mouth, his mind is distracted from the work as his attention is drawn to the music.

The choice of music:

It is quite understandable that every sort of music does not have the same effect. Some lovers of light music might think it strange that classical music has the best effect on some sick people. It must also seem strange that musicians very often do not react to music in the same way as those who do not make music a part of their daily lives. Perhaps this is the same sort of professional diffidence as that of the gardener who is never overjoyed at the sight of a beautiful garden as is the city dweller who knows little about gardens.

Music for the invalid must be chosen just as carefully as medicine, even in regards to "dosage", so that its healing power can work properly. We should bear in mind the homeopathic principle, that strong stimulants are destructive and weak stimulants vitalizing. It is interesting to note that there is a resemblance between all biological laws and principles. Just as a stimulating and invigorating medicine is given in the morning and a sedative at night, in the same way, lively music will be found suitable for mornings and soothing, soft music for evenings, which helps to produce relaxation and sleep. It is also important to understand the administering of music for the most therapeutic benefit and the part that volume, tone and tempo play in helping the patient.

As with all biological healing methods, it is necessary to apply intuition, understanding and feeling. Those who lack this sensitivity and do not have the ability to develop this method of healing with music should, nevertheless, protect the patient at home or in the hospital from constantly blaring noises that go under the name of "music" today. In recent years television has become available to distract attention from personal problems, but so few programs of therapeutic value are available, that, by and large, the violence and bloodshed that is projected from the TV screen has very little to recommend it as a health restorative.

HAPPINESS AND HEALTH

The encouragement of health through happiness is an interesting pursuit. The poet, Conrad Ferdinand Meyer, thought much about it, and concluded that a heavy heart is not cured by wild gaiety, but responds very quickly to even a little happiness.

Imagine a beautiful peach tree espaliered against the wall of your house as is the custom in European countries. Each spring it blossoms anew and a few months later it brings forth delicious fruit. How should we think it could be otherwise? Yet suddenly, the unexpected happens. The peach tree flowers as usual, but just as the flowers open, they fall to the ground. The bark of the tree dries up and the tree dies. What has happened? The tree was the pride of the household; its healthy growth, its beautiful blossoms and delicious fruit were the talk of the village. How could this tree die so quickly and unexpectedly? What malicious enemy could have attacked it?

483

You ask yourself all this but you can only get the answer by digging up the tree. It is then that you see that field rats have gnawed the roots and so killed the beautiful tree. Negligence, ignorance, inexperience, ineptitude, often force of circumstances as well as a lack of knowledge on how to sustain health and prolong life are all, metaphorically speaking, rodents, which are gnawing away at our life and bringing us eventually to ruin. Knowledge is the antidote and the only thing that can save our lives from an untimely end and assure us of a measure of health. Sometimes the damage is so great it is too late to do anything about it by the time discovery takes place. What a joy it would be to see the tree recover and again send forth its blossoms. Sometimes it is by losing things, either material or spiritual, that we become aware of their value. Young people would not be so casual about their health if they could but know that they might soon lose it. How bewildered we are by the loss of health and until we know the cause there is not much we can do about it. Good health should be treasured and never be abused, for good health leads to happiness.

Life is like good garden soil, which brings forth nothing if we do not sow, till, water and care for it. If we do not put anything into life, we cannot hope to get anything out of it. Again the poet's words come to mind: "Know that the noble mind puts goodness into life, but does not seek it there"! All that raises our spirit and gives us strength are like valuable and beautiful plants in our lives. The useless things that hang about us, imperfect men that we are, are as weeds, which should be pulled out and destroyed. Undoubtedly one of the best and most useful plants or attributes that we possess, is happiness. This not only brings peace to our spirit but also cures to our body. If we possess this wonderful thing, let us pass it on to others for does not an old proverb say: "Happiness which we give to others, returns to rejoice our own hearts."

HAPPINESS AS A REMEDY

Happiness can be spoken of as a remedy. Mysterious functions take place in our bodies which are responsible for equally mysterious and inexplicable effects. No less puzzling is the interaction between mind and nervous system. What a wonderful way the central nervous system executes the orders of the mind! Millions of muscle fibers work like obedient little horses, harnessed and driven by millions of reins and guided by our will – the driver. To this wonder-system of divine technique we owe the movement and rhythm of life.

How differently the sympathetic nervous system works! Unguided by the cerebrum and uninfluenced by the will, it performs those functions which could not possibly be maintained and attended to by our conscious minds. The circulation, digestion, etc. as well as all the other organs involved in these processes are all regulated by the autonomous nerves, on which our physical and mental well-being depends. Although the will has no power over them, they can nevertheless be influenced by our imaginative faculties, by our feelings and emotions. Joy will get hold of the hidden gear-levers of the sympathicus, release cramps and flood away the congestions in the liver, the kidneys and the pancreas. Even the heart cannot escape the positive influence of joy and happiness. By helping those around us to achieve happiness, we are administering to them the best biological medicine possible. If you know a diabetic patient, teach him to enjoy the good and beautiful life. Point out the beauty of the spring blossoms to him, encourage him to rejoice in the golden splendor of the ripe corn fields of the summer, to take pleasure in the autumnal symphony of colors and to admire the ornate beauty of wintry ice and snow crystals. To experience this happiness will touch his heart, improve his breathing and instill him with vitality that will carry him through the woods and over the hills with opened eyes and a thankful heart. The pancreas will begin to function better, the secretion of digestive ferments and consequently the digestion, will improve. Less food intake will be of advantage to him in his condition. The inner secretions will be stimulated, the islets of Langerhans will increase production of insulin and the sugar in the blood will be oxydized. Aided by physical measures such as hot abdominal packs, and plenty of raw vegetables in the diet, his health will visibly improve and he will be able to eat less and before long he may be fortunate enough to have regained it altogether.

You can help people who suffer from liver disorders, too, by telling them of this happiness cure. If your own liver, the most important gland in your body, is not working as it should, let happiness set about casting out trouble and anxiety. It can wage a successful war against these saboteurs and will effectively counteract the damage done by them. Take and use this help which, though sometimes buried deep within you, is always ready to come to your assistance. Let your life be filled with the rhythm of the pulsating life of happiness; be glad, even if the gladness at first is somewhat artificial and forced. Breathe deeply and at the same time concentrate upon something of beauty and value. Eventually you will find that happiness will pervade your whole being and so master your body and all its functions.

Happiness is like warmth. Even the thickest ice of a cold heart must melt, if this warmth is allowed to penetrate long enough. If whatever you do can somehow help your neighbor, the resulting happiness you receive will permeate your entire being. Whether you are a farmer, salesman, housewife, office worker, doctor, lawyer, butcher, candlestick maker, or whatever, your fellow man needs your skill and by rendering a service to him it should bring happiness to you. Do not go about your work sullenly, thereby spoiling the blessing of it. If you are a teacher or a doctor and perhaps you feel that your work does not get its proper recognition, at least take comfort and happiness from the fact that you are in a position to help those who need and want to be helped. Those who work just for the sake of making money or because they are forced to work because of circumstances gain very little, if anything, from their work. If there is no pleasure to be found in what you are doing or in your achievements, then you are betrayed in the truest sense of the word. If your eight or nine hour workday is pervaded by ill-will and discontentment, and you sleep for another eight hours, it is fairly certain that you will not have many happy, cheerful and thankful feelings during whatever time remains. Such a life is one of slavery and drudgery. Your work would be so much easier and enjoyable and it would make fewer demands on you, if only it could be permeated with happiness. In the evening you would be much less tired, your dinner would taste better and your morale would be higher. The hours of leisure spent with your family and friends would be filled with pleasure and peace of mind. Even though others contaminate the atmosphere with hate and discontent, your happiness would be strong enough to triumph over such discord. Even envy and jealousy are powerful enemies – luxuries you cannot afford to indulge in – that contaminate the mind. They can destroy and gnaw away the plant of happiness in the garden of your heart and lay hold of your innermost being.

There once was an Indian prince who marvelled at one of his fellow believers, a poor man, who in spite of his poverty, could rejoice without envy at the prince's wealth. The prince, puzzled, questioned him and the poor man explained: "Why should I not rejoice in beauty, especially if it does not occasion me any worry or responsibility. You have the burden of overseeing all your wealth and of providing for your family while I, on the other hand, can rejoice in your treasures by just looking at them."

Those who can enjoy the wealth of others without feeling envious, have passed their first big test, which will ensure them happiness and peace throughout their lives. Possessions always mean responsibility but there are many things we can enjoy without care. Our walks can be taken not only for the healthy exercise they bring but also for the joy of seeing the beauty of the flowers, of the distant mountains, of the fine woods and fields. We need not consider the fact that the cool blue lake and the rushing stream do not belong to us. We can rejoice in the graceful gambols of someone elses young animals without feeling that, by some mischance, we might lose them. We can enjoy all these things so much better than their owner, because ownership is a heavy burden that demands work and care. Many who strive for it with envy or jealousy in their hearts perhaps could not enjoy such a burden successfully. So if you wish to enjoy beauty to the full, do not let envy and jealousy encroach upon your joy in appreciating the possessions of others.

If one day you find yourself robbed of happiness, just exert yourself by doing something to please others and you will find that it will come back again. A kind, friendly word, an understanding smile, a comforting remark are the things that can do much good in giving pleasure to others. If you have the capacity to comfort someone in his sorrows, you will undoubtedly find comfort for yourself, for it is well known that one receives more pleasure in giving than in receiving.

Is not every day a gift from heaven? Why spoil it then with grumbling and discontent? How much more sensible it would be to fill the day with useful thoughts and deeds, for each day comes but once and by nightfall it is gone forever. Even though troubles arise, happiness and thankfulness can offset them and thus the day never needs to be lost and wasted.

If you are alone, you can rejoice in the quiet and collect your thoughts. If you are among friends, then rejoice in their company and make good use of the occasion to profit by such companionship. Avoid empty chatter. Instead, build one another up by conversation that gives moral improvement and thus benefit one another in a profitable way.

When you go to bed, the last thing you should do before going to sleep is to thank your Maker for the day he has given you. Rejoice in the good you have been able to do and if you have received a kindness, then remember it with quiet happiness and breathe deeply, for joy comes from the depths of the spirit and is borne on the breath of life. When borne aloft to higher spheres by this feeling of joy, you will realize how small and insignificant everyday troubles are. The higher we get in the spiritual realm of joy and peace, the more peaceful our inner lives will be.

To change our way of life so that we can find this deep, satisfying joy in the midst of our everyday life, must, of course, take a little time and practice. Our nature is not used to controlling our mind and spirit as it is used to ordering our muscles and sinews.

When the new day dawns, do not hurry agitatedly into the unknown, wondering what new worries it will bring. Try to remember that it has been given to you completely new, to do with it what you will. Thank your Maker for this gift, as thankfulness always fills the heart with appreciation and happiness. Those who begin their day in a happy frame of mind have better than an even chance of ending it in the same way.

Take pleasure in your food and be careful to see that your diet is both tasty and natural. Do not be a slave to time with an eye on the clock. Eat peacefully and slowly, chewing your food well. In this way you will get all the nourishment possible from your food. Your internal organs will benefit from the work your teeth and salivary glands have done for them. Those who enjoy and value what nature's garden so generously gives should remember to be grateful and not take the well-laden table for granted. There are so many things in which we can rejoice that almost no time remains for discontentment.

If, however, some sorrow strikes you down, face things bravely with determination to overcome it. Eventually you will reach the heights and the warm sun of peace and happiness again will soothe or even heal your pain completely.

Should the enemy of all living things rob you of one of your loved ones, try not to be overwhelmed by inconsolate grief. There have been prophetic words written which are no illusion, and which promise us a time when there will be no more sorrow, when pain and death will no longer exist. The God of life will put a stop to evil and destruction and the resurrection of the dead will become a reality for all. This faith in a happier future brings a warm glow of comfort and hope to our hearts. Nothing can strengthen our morale as much as the thought of the restoration of all things to a state of perfection. What a comfort it is to know that our pain and fear ridden world will one day be freed from all destructive forces! No one who willfully wielded evil power will be allowed to return from death to spread sorrow and anguish once more. Those who mourn their dead show a lack of understanding of the natural channels wrought by death. They must no longer let themselves be deprived of the joyful hope and faith in the resurrection. The superficiality of our lives and the cares of day to day living are apt to obscure our understanding of these things. We think that things have been and always will be the same. We cannot envisage a time when blood will no longer flow, when swords will be turned into plowshares, spears into pruning knives and man will no longer learn the art of war. This must now seem a quite unbelievable blessing for our war weary and warmongering times. However, the God of Life, the God of Peace will make good on his promises. Each one will have his own vineyard and sit beneath his own fig tree, at peace with the world and without fear for the future. These are sacred words of hope and comfort spoken under inspiration by the prophets of old and can be considered as good as fulfilled. The kingdom for which we learned to pray for as children will be an Edenic Paradise, no matter how much the worldly wise may scoff at the idea. Those who believe these words must eventually be filled with hope, even though they may have many trials and tribulations to overcome.

"Yes" some sigh, "if only we could understand and believe." Because many love the dissipations which have become common and seemingly necessary to their superficial lives, they cannot achieve real happiness in life and the joy of worth-while things. For them the future is gloomy and will remain so, to the extent that they seek pleasure in drugs, alcohol and immorality. While they get a certain amount of pleasure from these things, they are neither healthy nor lasting nor do they contribute to their well-being or real happiness.

Our pleasures should be healthy so that they can impart a sense of well-being. Some people become slaves to an enthusiasm and regard it as their real and only pleasure in life and it is quite possible that indulging this passion is doing them great harm. This applies very much to the passion for sports. From a healthy pleasure in movement and rhythm, sports have now become so exaggerated that they can damage and sometimes destroy one's health. An enthusiasm for violent sports cannot really be a pleasure and, if it is not kept under restraint, may well dig an early grave for the participant.

If you take pleasure in the beauties of nature you will find that other passions cannot make too many demands on you, especially passions that blind you to all true happiness. Concentrate on and enjoy the bounteous riches of creation which are limitless and offered to you for your pleasure. Only the normal biological rhythm of a healthy way of life can insure for you the happiness which strengthens and regenerates. For example, you will not be able to enjoy the fresh, clean mountain air, nor the perfume of the meadows and the larch or fir trees, if you have ruined your sense of smell by smoking unrestrainedly.

Happiness is a soothing balm for a sick heart and the best remedy for a wounded spirit. Even when you lose all that you thought was worth living for, or when the friends you thought you could depend upon, desert you, you will still find that happiness is inexhaustible, once you know where and how to find it. A ray of sunshine coming through your bedroom, your cell or your barrack room transforming, as it can, the unnoticed spider's web into a silver diadem, ought to fill one with joy. Light, air and sun are possessions which we value too little, for they enrich our lives by scattering many joys in our lives. Even when the sun's light is withdrawn, the inner light which we should have stored in our hearts should continue to illuminate our lives. Unfortunately, it does not seem to be a characteristic of our times to seek out and enjoy the little things in life. So much unhappiness has embittered people's hearts, too many hopes have been raised to no purpose; and peace, that great giver of happiness, has too often been destroyed. It is very difficult for an over-tired nervous system to be relaxed and at ease so that strength and peace-bringing happiness can enter and do its good work. It is never easy to rid oneself of unhappy memories and impressions, but if you wish to regain your health through happiness, then you must do your utmost to forget. Happiness then can take root and a healthy, happy spirit will provide the best conditions for making and keeping your body healthy.

Much advice has been given and I hope that it will help many of you. There is so much that we can do for ourselves by natural means. With the proper intelligent attitude perhaps we can live with the things that cannot be remedied, by leading as healthy a life as possible and permitting our spirit to rise above our physical suffering.

More could certainly be said about our mental attitude toward life and health but this would take us into another book. The important thing to remember is that we should regulate our lives according to nature's rules. The more we feel and think in a healthy way, the less will those damaging influences, which are so difficult to disperse, make their way into our bodies.

If we admit the value of the good, which is always at hand for ourselves and those around us, we will achieve something for our health and spiritual balance in these insecure and restless times. How we react to life depends upon our inner-most selves. The hurrying stream of time tries to blot out the healthy habits established in our youth and thus lead us along strange paths that make it so easy to go astray.

Open this book when you need advice on matters of health. It will save you many disappointments and you will avoid useless and perhaps harmful treatments. In any event, most of the advice given here can never do any harm, even if you use the treatments incorrectly. I am convinced that the advice in the book can relieve many a sorrow-laden moment. Indeed, it may even be a cure for the seemingly accursed times in which we live.

GLOSSARY

ALKALOID – Organic mixture containing nitrogen and forming water soluble salts with acids; bitter tasting.

ANTIPERSPIRANT – Reduces perspiration.

ANTIPHLOGISTIC – Prevent or arrest inflammation.

ANTISEPTIC/ANTISEPSIS – Prevent infection.

ANTISPASMODIC – Calming nerves and muscular spasms.

ANTIURIC – Conteracting acid in the urine.

APERIENT – Mild laxative.

APERITIVE – Stimulating appetite.

ASTRINGENT – Shrinks tissues and checks the flow of blood by contracting blood vessels, as Alum

BACTERIA – Microscopic organisms usually single-celled, multiplying by fission and spore formation.

BACTERICIDE – Substance that destroys bacteria.

BACTERIOPHAGE – Bactericide produced within the body and normally present in the intestines, urine, blood, etc.

CARMINATIVE – A medication that expels gas from the stomach and intestines.

CARTHARTIC – A strong laxative, i.e. Epsom Salts, Castor Oil.

COMPRESS – Cloth soaked in a decoction or infusion, usually cold, with excess squeezed out of cloth, and applied to affected body area until warmed to body temperature.

DECOCTION – An extraction of desired substances from plants or herbs by boiling in water and filtering the resulting solution when cooled.

DECONGESTANT – Disperse excess local blood supply.

DEMULCENT – A soothing medication or ointment.

DEPURATIVE – Causing excess perspiration and urine to cleanse impurities from the body.

DIURETIC – To increase the flow of urine.

EMETIC – Taken to induce vomiting.

EMOLLIENT – Skin softener.

ESSENTIAL OIL – Oil extracted from a plant by means of low heat.

EXCIPIENT – Binder into which a substance is mixed to form a pill under pressure.

EXTRACT – Concentrated preparation of a substance, i.e. vanilla extract to which alcohol or water is usually added.

FLATULENCE – Having gas in the stomach or intestines.

GRANULOMA – Dental abscess.
GLUCOSIDE – Glycoside containing sugar.
GLYCOSIDE – Compound containing sugar and non-sugar units.

HAEMOSTATIC – Arresting flow of blood.
HEARTBURN – Hyperacidity of the stomach.
HEPATIC – Anything beneficial to the liver.
HOMEOPATHIC DOSE – Herbal or mineral preparation triturated and diluted, i.e. 2x, 6x, 12x, etc.

INFUSION – A liquid preparation made by pouring boiling water over a herb or plant part; usually strained when cooled.
IRRITANT – Excessively irritating resulting in inflammation.

LACTATION – suckling a baby; time during which a mother produces milk, i.e. lactate, produce milk.
LACHRYMATION – Free flowing of tears usually from irritation of tear ducts.
LACTIC ACID – Colorless, odorless acid formed in sour milk.
LACTIFUGE – Arresting or diminishing the secretion of milk.

MACERATE – Seeds or other substance soaked in liquid to soften or dissolve, i.e. flax seed.
MASTICATION – Substance chewed thoroughly to increase the flow of saliva.
MUCILAGE – Gelatinous substance, i.e. psyllium seed or flax seed that softens and swells but does not dissolve in water.

NARCOTIC – Any drug that induces drowsiness or sleep.

PACKS (COLD OR HOT) – A paste, made up of herbs and alcohol, applied as cosmetic, i.e. mud pack; wrapping body area with several wet cloths, previously soaked, for medicinal purposes.
PECTORAL – Preparation for the relief of coughs and to induce expectoration. Some preparations are taken internally, others rubbed on throat or chest.

PHLEBITIS – Inflammation of a vein.

PHLEBOTOMY – Opening a vein to let blood; bleeding.

PLASTER – A soft, semi-solid preparation spread on a gauze and placed on skin over affected area.

POTENCY – Result of blending a remedy with a neutral substance such as alcohol. Potentising is accomplished by discarding nine parts of the original and keeping one part. By repeating the process, each time adds one degree of potency. After repeating performance six times, one part in a million remains which is called Potency Six.

POULTICE – A soft paste made from herbs, plants, etc., hot or cold, folded into a cloth and applied to the skin area affected.

PRURITIS – Itching of the skin.

REFLEX – involuntary; direct response to a stimulation of a sensory nerve. Sneezing, vomiting, shivering are reflexes.

REFRACTORY – Not yielding readily to treatment, i.e. a refractory cough.

RESOLVENT – Arresting inflammation and reducing swelling.

RETENTION – Holding back; retaining fluid, i.e. urine.

RUBEFACIENT – Drawing blood into the capillaries of the skin.

SEDATIVE – Substance that produces a calming and soothing effect on the nerves.

SOMNIFEROUS – Causing drowsiness and sleepiness.

SOPORIFIC – Causing or tending to cause sleep.

STIMULANT – Activating or exciting the functions of an organ of the body.

STYPTIC – Astringent, checks bleeding.

SUDORIFIC – Promotes and stimulates sweating.

SUPPURATION – Discharging pus or festering.

TINCTURE – Extraction of properties from plants or drugs which is dissolved in alcohol.

TRITURATE – Crush or grind into a very fine powder.

VERMIFUGE – Medication for expelling worms from the intestines.

WHITLOWS – Painful swelling of fingers.

ALPHABETICAL LIST OF HERBS, PLANTS AND MINERALS USED IN THIS BOOK

LATIN NAME	COMMON NAME
Achillea millefolium	Yarrow
Aconitum napellus	Monkshood, Wolfbane
Aesculus hippocastannum	Horse chestnut
Agrimonia eupatoria	Agrimony
Alchemilla vulgaris	Lady's mantle
Allium cepa	Onion
Allium sativum	Garlic
Allium ursinum	Wild leek
Aloe vera	Aloe
Anemone ranunculoides	Yellow wood anemone
Angelica archangelica	Angelica
Anthemis nobilis	Camomile
Apium petroselinum	Parsley
Apocynum androsaemifolium	Bitterroot
Arctium lappa	Burdock
Arnica montana	Arnica
Artemisia absinthum	Wormwood, Absinthe
Artemisia vulgaris	Mugwort
Atropa belladonna	Belladonna, Deadly Nightshade
Avena sativa	Oats
Berberis vulgaris	Barberry
Betula alba	White birch
Betula lenta	Black birch
Brassica alba	White mustard
Brassica nigra	Black mustard
Bryonia dioica	Bryony, red
Calendula officinalis	Marigold
Capsella bursa-pastoris	Shepherd's purse
Capsicum	Red pepper
Carica Papaya	Papaya
Castanea	Chestnut
Ceratonia siliqua	Carob
Cetraria islandica	Icelandic moss
Chelidonium majus	Celandine

LATIN NAME	COMMON NAME
Chichorium intybus	Chicory
Cochlearia armoracia	Horseradish
Convallaria majalis	Lily of the Valley
Crataegus oxyacantha	Hawthorne
Cynara scolymus	Artichoke
Digitalis purpurea	Foxglove
Echinacea augustifolia	Coneflower
Echinacea purpurea	Purple Coneflower
Elettaria cardamonum	Cardamon
Equisetum arvense	Horsetail
Erythraea centaurium	Centaury
Euphrasia officinalis	Eyebright
Foeniculum vulgare	Fennel
Fructus juniperus	Juniper berry
Fructus sorbi	Rowanberry
Galeopsis ochroleuca	Hemp nettle
Geranium pratense	Cranesbill
Glycyrrhiza glabra	Licorice
Grindelia robusta	Grindelia
Guaiacum officinale	Lignum vitae, resin of
Hamamelis virginiana	Witch hazel
Hippophae rhamnoides	Sea buckthorn
Hydrastis canadensis	Goldenseal
Hypericum perforatum	St. John's wort
Ilex aquifolium	Holly
Illicum verum	Anise
Imperatoria ostruth	Masterwort
Laurus nobilis	Bay laurel
Lepidium sativum	Gardencress
Linum usitatissimum	Linseed, Flax
Lycopus europaeus	Wolfstrap

LATIN NAME	COMMON NAME
Medicago sativa	Alfalfa
Melissa officinalis	Balm
Mezereum daphne	Daphne
Nasturtium officinalis	Watercress
Natrium chloratum	Table salt, sodium chloride
Natrium muriaticum	Cooking salt
Natrium sulphuricum	Glauber's salt
Petasites officinalis	Butterbur
Peumus boldus	Boldo
Pimpinella saxifraga	Pimpernel Burnet saxifrage
Pinus cembra	Swiss stone pine
Plantago major	Plantain
Plantago psyllium	Psyllium
Potentilla anserine	Silverweed
Potentilla tormentilla	Tormentil
Prunus amygdalus	Bitter almond
Quercus ilex	Acorn
Rauwolfia serpentina	Rauwolfia
Rhamnus carthartica	Common buckthorn
Rhamnus frangula	Alder buckthorn
Rheum undulatum	Rhubarb
Rhus toxicodendron	Poison Ivy
Ribes nigrum	Black currant
Ricinus communis	Castor oil plant
Rosmarinus officinalis	Rosemary
Rubus idaeus	Raspberry
Salvia officinalis	Sage
Sanguinaria canadensis	Bloodroot
Scilla maritima	Squill
Solanum dulcamara	Woody nightshade
Solidago virgaurea	European goldenrod
Stellaria media	Chickweed
Symphytum officinalis	Comfrey
Symphytum peregrinum	Siberian comfrey

LATIN NAME	COMMON NAME
Tamus communis	Black bryony
Taraxacum officinalis	Dandelion
Thymus serpyllum	Wild thyme
Thymus vulgaris	Thyme
Trigonella foenum graecum	Nasturtium
Tropaeolum majus	Fenugreek seeds
Urtica dioica	Stinging nettle
Vaccinium myrtillus	Bilbery (Whortleberry)
Valeriana officinalis	Valerian
Vinca major	Periwinkle
Viola tricolor	Wild Pansy, Heartsease
Viscum album	Mistletoe

COMMON NAME	LATIN NAME
Acorn	Quercus ilex
Agrimony	Agrimonia eupatoria
Alder buckthorn	Rhamnus frangula
Alfalfa	Medicago sativa
Almond, bitter	Prunus amygdalus
Aloe	Aloe vera
Angelica	Angelica archangelica
Anise	Illicum verum
Arnica	Arnica montana
Artichoke	Cynara scolymus
Balm, lemon balm, melissa	Melissa officinalis
Barberry	Berberis vulgaris
Bay laurel	Laurus nobilis
Belladonna, Deadly nightshade	Atropa belladonna
Bilberry (Whortleberry)	Vaccinium myrtillus
Birch, black	Betula lenta
Birch, white	Betula alba
Bitterroot	Apocynum androsaemifolium
Black bryony	Tamus communis
Black currant	Ribes nigrum
Bloodroot	Sanguinaria canadensis

COMMON NAME	LATIN NAME
Bloodwort	Potentilla tormentilla
Boldo	Peumus boldus
Bryony, red	Bryonia dioica
Buckthorn (Alder)	Rhamnus frangula
Buckthorn (Common)	Rhamnus carthartica
Buckthorn (Sea)	Hippophae rhamnoides
Burdock	Arctium lappa
Burnet saxifrage	Pimpinella saxifraga
Butterbur	Petasites officinalis
Camomile	Anthemis nobilis
Cardamon	Ceratonia siliqua
Carob	Elettaria cardamonum
Castor oil plant	Ricinus communis
Celandine	Chelidonium majus
Centaury	Erythrae centaurium
Chestnut	Castanea
Chickweed	Stellaria media
Chicory	Cichorium intybus
Comfrey	Symphytum officinalis
Coneflower	Echinacea augustafolia
Cranesbill	Geranium pratense
Dandelion	Taraxacum officinale
Daphne	Mezereum daphne
Deadly nightshade	Atropa belladonna
Eyebright	Euphrasia officinalis
Fennel	Foeniculum vulgare
Fenugreek	Trigonella foenum graecum
Flax, Linseed	Linum usitatissimum
Foxglove	Digitalis purpurea
Gardencress	Lepidium sativum
Garlic	Allium sativum
Glauber's salt	Natrium sulphuricum
Goldenrod, European	Solidago virgaurea
Goldenseal	Hydrastis canadensis
Grindelia	Grindelia robusta

COMMON NAME	LATIN NAME
Hawthorne	Crataegus oxyacantha
Heartsease, Wild Pansy	Viola tricolor
Hemp nettle	Galeopsis ochroleuca
Holly	Ilex aquifolium
Horse chestnut	Aesculus hippocastannum
Horse radish	Cochlearia armoracia
Horsetail	Equisetum arvense
Icelandic moss	Cetraria islandica
Juniper berry	Fructus juniperus
Lady's mantle	Alchemilla vulgaris
Leek (wild)	Allium ursinum
Licorice	Glycyrrhiza glabra
Lignum vitae, resin of	Guaiacum officinale
Lily of the Valley	Convallaria majalis
Linseed (Flax)	Linum usitatissimum
Marigold	Calendula officinalis
Masterwort	Imperatoria osthruth
Mistletoe	Viscum album
Monkshood	Aconitum napellus
Mugwort	Artemisia vulgaris
Mustard (black)	Brassica nigra
Mustard (white)	Brassica alba
Nasturtium	Tropaeolum majus
Nettle	Urtica
Nightshade, deadly	Atropa belladonna
Oats	Avena sativa
Onion	Allium cepa
Pansy (wild)	Viola tricolor
Papaya	Carica papaya
Parsley	Apium petroselinum
Periwinkle	Vinca major
Pimpernel	Pimpinella saxifraga
Plantain	Plantago major

COMMON NAME	LATIN NAME
Poison ivy	Rhus toxicodendron
Psyllium	Plantago psyllium
Purple coneflower	Echinacea purpurea
Raspberry	Rubus idaeus
Red pepper	Capsicum
Rhubarb	Rheum undulatum
Rosemary	Rosemarinus officinalis
Rowanberry	Fructus sorbi
Sage	Salvia officinalis
Salt, cooking	Natrium muriaticum
Salt, Glauber's	Natrium sulphuricum
Salt, sodium chloride	Natrium chloratum
St. John's wort	Hypericum perforatum
Sea buckthorn	Hippophae rhamnoides
Shepherd's purse	Capsella bursa-pastoris
Silverweed	Potentilla anserine
Squill	Scilla maritima
Stinging nettle	Urtica dioica
Stone pine (Swiss)	Pinus cembra
Thyme	Thymus vulgaris
Thyme (wild)	Thymus serpyllum
Tormentil	Potentilla tormentilla
Valerian	Valeriana officinalis
Watercress	Nasturtium officinalis
Whortleberry, Biberry	Vaccinium myrtillus
Wild Pansy, Heartsease	Viola tricolor
Witch hazel	Hamamelis virginiana
Wolfbane	Aconitum napellus
Wolfstrap	Lycopus europaeus
Woody nightshade	Solanum dulcamara
Wormwood	Artemisia ansinthium
Yarrow	Achillea millefolium
Yellow wood anemone	Anemone ranunculoides

ALPHABETICAL SUBJECT INDEX